I0065979

Essentials of Pediatrics

Essentials of Pediatrics

Edited by **Alice Kunek**

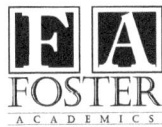

FOSTER
ACADEMICS

New Jersey

Published by Foster Academics,
61 Van Reypen Street,
Jersey City, NJ 07306, USA
www.fosteracademics.com

Essentials of Pediatrics
Edited by Alice Kunek

© 2016 Foster Academics

International Standard Book Number: 978-1-63242-466-2 (Hardback)

This book contains information obtained from authentic and highly regarded sources. Copyright for all individual chapters remain with the respective authors as indicated. All chapters are published with permission under the Creative Commons Attribution License or equivalent. A wide variety of references are listed. Permission and sources are indicated; for detailed attributions, please refer to the permissions page and list of contributors. Reasonable efforts have been made to publish reliable data and information, but the authors, editors and publisher cannot assume any responsibility for the validity of all materials or the consequences of their use.

The publisher's policy is to use permanent paper from mills that operate a sustainable forestry policy. Furthermore, the publisher ensures that the text paper and cover boards used have met acceptable environmental accreditation standards.

Trademark Notice: Registered trademark of products or corporate names are used only for explanation and identification without intent to infringe.

Printed in the United States of America.

Contents

Preface

The world is advancing at a fast pace like never before. Therefore, the need is to keep up with the latest developments. This book was an idea that came to fruition when the specialists in the area realized the need to coordinate together and document essential themes in the subject. That's when I was requested to be the editor. Editing this book has been an honour as it brings together diverse authors researching on different streams of the field. The book collates essential materials contributed by veterans in the area which can be utilized by students and researchers alike.

This book discusses the fundamentals as well as modern approaches of pediatrics. As a field of medical science, pediatrics refers to the study of disorders related to infants, children, pre-teens and teens. It has many sub-specialities like neonatology, social paediatrics, adolescent medicine, pediatric nephrology, etc. This book includes a detailed explanation of various concepts and essential theories related to this field. It elucidates the new techniques and applications emerging in this subject. It is a valuable compilation of topics, ranging from the basic to most complex advancements in the field of pediatrics. It includes contributions of experts and practitioners from across the globe to provide readers with in-depth knowledge about this area. Students, experts, researchers and paediatricians will find this book full of crucial and beneficial content.

Each chapter is a sole-standing publication that reflects each author's interpretation. Thus, the book displays a multi-facetted picture of our current understanding of applications and diverse aspects of the field. I would like to thank the contributors of this book and my family for their endless support.

Editor

Empyema Necessitans Complicating Pleural Effusion Associated with *Proteus* Species Infection: A Diagnostic Dilemma

M. S. Yauba,[1] **H. Ahmed,**[2] **I. A. Imoudu,**[2] **M. O. Yusuf,**[2] **and H. U. Makarfi**[2]

[1]*Department of Paediatrics, University of Maiduguri College of Medical Sciences, Maiduguri 752106, Nigeria*
[2]*Department of Paediatrics, Federal Medical Centre, Azare 751101, Nigeria*

Correspondence should be addressed to M. S. Yauba; saadyko@yahoo.co.uk

Academic Editor: Mohammad M. A. Faridi

Background. Empyema necessitans, a rare complication of pleural effusion, could result in significant morbidity and mortality in children. It is characterized by the dissection of pus through the soft tissues and the skin of the chest wall. *Mycobacterium tuberculosis* and *Actinomyces israelii* are common causes but Gram negative bacilli could be a rare cause. However, there were challenges in differentiating between *Mycobacterium tuberculosis* and nontuberculous empyema in a resource poor setting like ours. We report a child with pleural effusion and empyema necessitans secondary to *Proteus* spp. infection. *Methods*. We describe a 12-year-old child with empyema necessitans complicating pleural effusion and highlight management challenges. *Results*. This case was treated with quinolones, antituberculous drugs, chest tube drainage, and nutritional rehabilitation. *Conclusion*. Empyema necessitatis is a rare condition that can be caused by Gram negative bacterial pathogens like *Proteus* species.

1. Introduction

Empyema necessitans is a rare long-term complication of poorly or uncontrolled empyema thoracis characterized by the dissection of pus through the soft tissues and skin of the chest wall [1]. The pus collection bursts and communicates with the exterior, forming a fistula between the pleural cavity and the skin [1]. Pleural effusion with empyema necessitans is usually caused by *Mycobacterium tuberculosis* and *Actinomyces israelii* [2]. The most common nontubercular etiological agent is *Staphylococcus* [3]. Other microbial causes include Pneumococci, *Escherichia coli*, *Pseudomonas*, *Klebsiella*, and anaerobes [3]. Pleural fluids are usually diagnostic and help in the choice of appropriate antibiotics. However, it is very difficult to differentiate tuberculous from a nontuberculous empyema, especially in malnourished children and resource poor countries, because of the difficulty in diagnosing tuberculosis in children and lack of modern facilities for diagnosis of tuberculosis. Further investigations and management depend on the stage of the disease. Treatment of this condition would include antibiotics, tube drainage, and decortication for obliterating the cavity and regenerating pulmonary function.

2. Case Presentation

This is a 12-year-old boy who presented with low grade fever and cough for 3-month duration and chest pain for 7-week duration. Cough was insidious in onset and productive of purulent and nonbloody sputum. No history of contact with tuberculosis or chronically coughing adult. Seven weeks prior to presentation, he developed right sided dull aching chest pain that was nonradiating. There was associated difficulty in breathing but no discoloration of the mucous membrane. Fifteen days before presentation, he developed a swelling on the right side of the chest wall which became fluctuant and later ruptured and started discharging foul smelling pus. Appetite had been good but there was associated weight loss. There were no other systemic symptoms and he was not a known sickle cell anaemia subject. Developmental and nutritional history was uneventful. He was only given oral and topical traditional concoction at home with no relief of

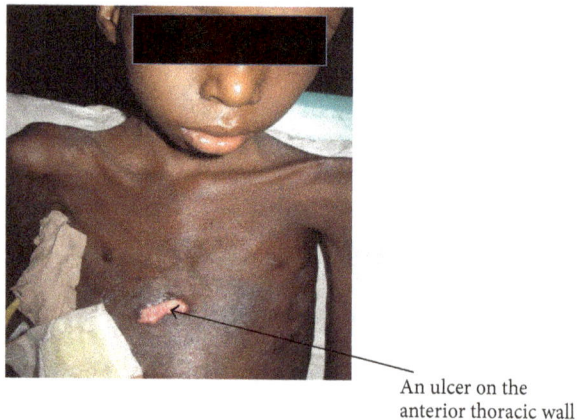

FIGURE 1: A picture of the child showing empyema necessitans.

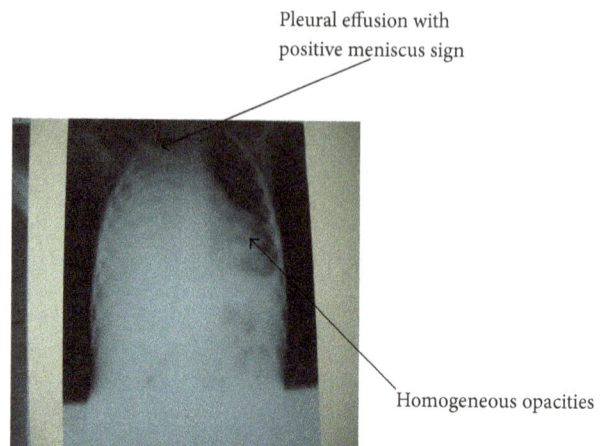

FIGURE 2: Chest X-ray showing pleural effusion with consolidation.

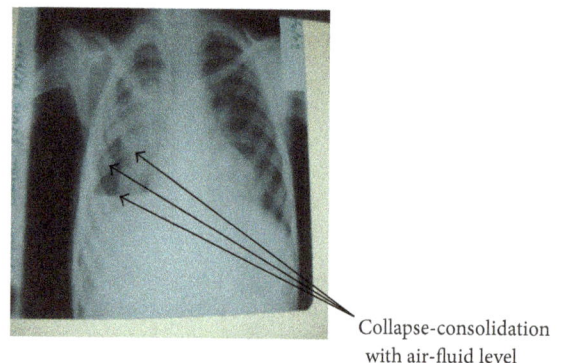

FIGURE 3: A chest X-ray after two-week course of antibiotics.

symptoms and the past medical history was not significant. He has not had any vaccination due to sociocultural factors.

On examination he was found to be chronically ill-looking, wasted, and stunted, with a Z-score of <-3 standard deviation according to the World Health Organization classification of malnutrition. He was febrile (37.8°C), severely pale, and in obvious respiratory distress and had significant axillary lymphadenopathy. Respiratory system examination revealed flattening of the right chest wall with a purulent discharging tender ulcer with necrotic base on the right side of the chest wall. He was tachypneic with respiratory rate of 44 cycles/min. He was also dyspnoeic with reduced chest expansion on the right hemithorax. There was a stony dull percussion note on the right hemithorax but dull percussion notes on the left hemithorax. There was markedly reduced breath sounds intensity on the right hemithorax with widespread crepitation. He had tachycardia of 140 beats/min with displaced apex beat and grade two haemic murmurs. There was soft tender hepatomegaly of 4 cm below the right costal margin. Another systemic examination was normal. An initial diagnosis of pleural effusion with empyema necessitans secondary to pulmonary tuberculosis in anaemic heart failure was made (Figure 1). Chest X-ray showed right sided pleural effusion with homogeneous opacity and left sided opacities (Figure 2). Full Blood Count revealed haemoglobin of 5.8 g/L, white blood cell count of $10.1 \times 10^3/\mu L$, lymphocytes of 46.4%, neutrophils of 47.7%, and erythrocyte sedimentation rate of 105 mm/hour. Both pus from the pleural aspirate and wound swab culture grew *Proteus* spp. sensitive to quinolones and ceftriaxone. Pus Ziehl-Neelsen stains revealed no acid fast bacilli and Mantoux test was nonreactive. He initially had intravenous crystalline penicillin and intramuscular gentamycin which was later changed to quinolones based on the antimicrobial sensitivity for 6 weeks. He was also commenced on frusemide, antituberculous drugs, and nasogastric tube feeding and transfused with packed red blood cells. Patient was comanaged with surgeons who inserted chest tube for drainage and the child had clinical and radiological improvement after 2 weeks of treatment (Figure 3). Patient was discharged after 3 weeks of admission and followed up by the managing paediatric

doctors. Patient was finally referred to the cardiothoracic surgeons for further management.

Management of this case was challenging in terms of diagnosis and treatment. Diagnosis of tuberculosis in this case was based on history only since investigation did not support the diagnosis. Low diagnostic yield of gastric aspirate for acid fast bacilli and negative Mantoux test due to anergy associated with malnourished children make it difficult to diagnose tuberculosis in this case. Contrast enhanced computed tomographic (CECT) scan which is the diagnostic study of choice that will show lung and mediastinal windows and reveal the extent and nature of the disease was not available. The isolation of *Proteus* species from the pleural fluid aspirate and wound swab suggests *Proteus* as the etiologic agent of the parapneumonic effusion. The dramatic resolution of symptoms in this case with anti-*Proteus* antibiotics could also suggest empyema necessitans complicating pleural effusion secondary to *Proteus* species.

3. Discussion

Pleural effusion with empyema necessitans is a cause of morbidity and mortality in children. It is characterised by pus collection in the thorax which bursts and communicates with the exterior, forming a fistula between the pleural cavity and the skin [1]. Empyema necessitans complicating pleural effusion is rare in our environment. This was the first case seen in our hospital for the past 12 years confirming the rarity of the condition. It is also reported to be rare by other workers elsewhere [2, 4]. Akgül et al. [2] reported only nine cases of empyema necessitans over a 4-year period in Turkey. Hoffman [5], in United Kingdom, also reported its rarity where he reported a prevalence of 3.2% (4/125). This patient's empyema and chest wall swelling were present for three months before presenting to our hospital for intervention. If pleural effusion is left for several months without intervention, this can lead to developing this complication, empyema necessitans [6, 7]. This might have contributed to the development of empyema necessitans in our patient.

The isolation of *Proteus* species from the pleural fluid in our patient indicates that this condition is probably due to the isolated organisms. This is in conformity with the reports by some workers [7, 8] who documented the etiologic agents to be Gram negative bacilli, *Streptococcus pneumoniae*, *Staphylococcus aureus*, and Blastomycosis. This finding contrasted with the reports by others where they documented more indolent pathogens, *Mycobacterium tuberculosis* and *Actinomyces israelii*, as a common cause of empyema necessitans [6]. Our finding also contrasted with the report [4] that most cases occur in immunocompromised patients because our case was seronegative for HIV. Our patient might be immunocompromised since he was severely malnourished.

Management of this case was challenging as this case was malnourished and features of TB may not be prominent. It was only the chest X-ray that suggested TB. Other investigations like Mantoux test, sputum, and pleural pus AFB were not diagnostic of tuberculosis. Differentiating tuberculous from nontuberculous empyema was very difficult because of low diagnostic yield of gastric aspirate for acid fast bacilli. Furthermore, malnutrition in children may suppress the tuberculin sensitivity leading to a negative Mantoux test which explains the difficulty in diagnosing tuberculosis in this case.

This patient's diagnosis was based on clinical, chest X-rays, and pleural fluid and wound swab microscopy culture and sensitivity. Contrast enhanced CT (CECT) scan was not done due unavailability of the facilities. Studies [8, 9] also revealed that the majority of empyema thoracis studied was based on a chest radiograph and not on a CT scan as was the case in our report. This may lead to incorrect judgment of the stage of the disease as well as delay in surgical intervention posing a challenge in managing the patient. However, a chest radiograph will only show opacity occupying a certain area of the hemithorax, which may be secondary to consolidated parenchyma, pleural peel, or a lung abscess. The CECT scan is the diagnostic study of choice with lung and mediastinal windows and reveals the extent and nature of the disease like demonstrating a communication of empyema into subcutaneous tissue [3, 8–10]. However, chest CECT could not be done in many centres, including ours, due to lack of facilities in most developing countries.

Early diagnosis and management of pleural effusion would prevent the development of empyema necessitans but our patient was not diagnosed and managed early

necessitating the development of this complication [11]. The management consists of antimicrobials, tube drainage, and decortication for obliterating the cavity to prevent fibrosis and facilitate lung expansion [11]. Our case had antimicrobials therapy, tube drainage, and nutritional rehabilitation and was referred to the cardiothoracic surgeons for other management.

4. Conclusion

Empyema necessitans is a rare complication of pleural space infection. It is commonly associated with pulmonary tuberculosis, *Actinomyces*, and nontuberculous organisms like *Staphylococcus aureus*. Pulmonary infections with Gram negative organisms like *Proteus* spp. should also be considered as a cause of pleural effusion with empyema necessitans. The management of this case was challenging since it was difficult to differentiate between tuberculous and nontuberculous effusion in this case.

Conflict of Interests

The authors declare that they have no competing interests.

References

[1] A. U. Francis, E. M. Donald, and S. B. Eric, "Pleural effusion and empyema," in *Paediatric Surgery: A Comprehensive Text for Africa*, E. A. Ameh, S. W. Bickler, B. C. Nwomeh, and D. Poenaru, Eds., pp. 299–303, Global Health Organization, Seattle, Wash, USA, 2011, http://www.global-help.org/.

[2] A. G. Akgül, A. Örki, T. Örki, M. Yüksel, and B. Arman, "Approach to empyema necessitatis," *World Journal of Surgery*, vol. 35, no. 5, pp. 981–984, 2011.

[3] D. K. Gupta and S. Sharma, "Management of empyema—role of a surgeon," *Journal of Indian Association of Pediatric Surgeons*, vol. 10, no. 3, pp. 142–146, 2005.

[4] S. A. Kono and T. D. Nauser, "Contemporary empyema necessitatis," *The American Journal of Medicine*, vol. 120, no. 4, pp. 303–305, 2007.

[5] E. Hoffman, "Empyema in childhood," *Thorax*, vol. 16, pp. 128–137, 1961.

[6] S. P. Kellie, F. Shaib, D. Forster, and J. P. Mehta, "Empyema necessitatis," *Chest*, vol. 138, article 39A, 2010.

[7] S. Ayik, A. Qakan, N. Aslankara, and A. Ozsöz, "Empyema necessitates," *Monaldi Archives for Chest Disease*, vol. 71, pp. 39–42, 2009.

[8] W. Chan, E. Keyser-Gauvin, G. M. Davis, L. T. Nguyen, and J.-M. Laberge, "Empyema thoracis in children: a 26-year review of the Montreal children's hospital experience," *Journal of Pediatric Surgery*, vol. 32, no. 6, pp. 870–872, 1997.

[9] B. Satish, M. Bunker, and P. Seddon, "Management of thoracic empyema in childhood: does the pleural thickening matter?" *Archives of Disease in Childhood*, vol. 88, no. 10, pp. 918–921, 2003.

[10] F. Gun, T. Salman, L. Abbasoglu, N. Salman, and A. Celik, "Early decortication in childhood empyema thoracis," *Acta Chirurgica Belgica*, vol. 107, no. 2, pp. 225–227, 2007.

[11] S. A. Edaigbini, N. Anumenechi, V. I. Odigie, L. Khalid, and A. D. Ibrahim, "Open drainage for chronic empyema thoracis; clarifying misconceptions by report of two cases and review of literature," *Archives of International Surgery*, vol. 3, no. 2, pp. 161–165, 2013.

The Combination of Gastroschisis, Jejunal Atresia, and Colonic Atresia in a Newborn

Zachary Bauman[1] and Victor Nanagas Jr.[2]

[1]Henry Ford Macomb Hospital, Clinton Township, MI 48038, USA
[2]Dayton Children's Hospital, Dayton, OH 45404, USA

Correspondence should be addressed to Zachary Bauman; zbauman1@hfhs.org

Academic Editor: Ursula Kiechl-Kohlendorfer

We encountered a rare case of gastroschisis associated with jejunal atresia and colonic atresia. In our case, the jejunal atresia was not discovered for 27 days after the initial abdominal wall closure. The colonic atresia was not discovered for 48 days after initial repair of the gastroschisis secondary to the rarity of the disorder. Both types of atresia were repaired with primary hand-sewn anastomoses. Other than the prolonged parenteral nutrition and hyperbilirubinemia, our patient did very well throughout his hospital course. Based on our case presentation, small bowel atresia and colonic atresia must be considered in patients who undergo abdominal wall closure for gastroschisis with prolonged symptoms suggestive of bowel obstruction. Our case report also demonstrates primary enteric anastomosis as a safe, well-tolerated surgical option for patients with types of intestinal atresia.

1. Introduction

Atresia of the colon is an uncommon cause of intestinal obstruction in the newborn patient, with classic etiologic factors resulting from intrauterine mesenteric vascular obstruction associated with internal hernia, volvulus, intussusception, or strangulation in tight gastroschisis [1]. It occurs between 1.8 and 15 percent of all patients affected by atresia of the bowel, with most studies quoting less than 10 percent of patients reviewed [2]. Reported incidences range from 1 in 1500 to 1 in 66,000 live births [3, 4]. Furthermore, approximately 5 to 15 percent of all infants born with gastroschisis will have intestinal stenosis or atresia resulting in increased time to full enteral feeds, prolonged parenteral nutrition, increased hospital stay, and increased mortality [5, 6]. Isolated colonic atresia is an extremely rare condition with limited information published about management and outcomes. Here, we report an even greater rarity in which a patient born with a known gastroschisis was later found to have both jejunal atresia and colonic atresia.

2. Case Report

A 35-week-old gestational age male weighing 2,495 grams was admitted to our neonatal intensive care unit (NICU) shortly after he was born secondary to previously diagnosed gastroschisis. The child was born to a 17-year-old gravida 1 para 1 female. The pregnancy was uncomplicated other than a traumatic event that occurred at 17 weeks resulting in placental abruption but no loss of the pregnancy. The mother did receive appropriate prenatal care. The child was born via an uncomplicated vaginal delivery with APGAR scores of 9 and 9 at one and five minutes, respectively. There is no family history of gastroschisis or intestinal atresia. The mother's only medical history included celiac disease.

Upon presentation to the NICU, the child was examined by the surgical service and deemed to be an appropriate candidate for reduction of the gastroschisis and primary closure of the abdominal wall defect. Only a small amount of bowel was protruding from the abdominal wall defect without signs of compromised bowel viability. The patient was subsequently taken to the operating room where a nasogastric tube was placed for decompression. Furthermore, the rectum of the patient was emptied of meconium by gentle anal dilatation and irrigation, providing standard of care prior to reduction and closure of the abdomen for the gastroschisis. The patient's gastroschisis was reduced and the abdominal wall was primarily closed without any complications. The extracorporeal bowel was found to be mildly edematous with minimal inflammatory peel and no signs of atresia. The patient was transferred back to the NICU where he was extubated within the first 24 hours postoperatively. A peripherally inserted central catheter was placed on postoperative day one and the patient was started on total peripheral nutrition (TPN), awaiting return of bowel function before starting enteral feeds. Postoperatively, the patient never developed any signs or symptoms of abdominal compartment syndrome or necrotizing enterocolitis. The patient was continued on IV antibiotics for a total of 72 hours from the date of surgery.

The patient remained hemodynamically stable with nasogastric decompression and parenteral nutrition. He continued to demonstrate high output from the nasogastric tube, which, over the course of his first three weeks of life, became more mucus-like and nonbilious. His abdomen remained mildly distended but, as Snyder et al. pointed out, patients can often suffer from severe ileus for up to 3 to 4 weeks after closure of the gastroschisis [7]. Further studies have also demonstrated prolonged ileus from closure of a gastroschisis. A study from 2000 by Driver et al. showed the median time to full oral feedings and resolution of ileus was 30 days (range: 5 to 160 days) [8] and a 2011 study by Bradnock et al. showed a median duration of 21 days (range: 9 to 39 days) [9] to reach full oral intake [9]. For this reason, we never became alarmed as we felt our patient was just suffering a prolonged ileus. However, as the patient approached four weeks since the initial gastroschisis closure, the concern for a possible bowel obstruction became evident as the patient never developed any further bowel function since the original passage of meconium at the initial surgery. Therefore, an upper gastrointestinal study with small bowel follow-through was obtained (Figure 1). The study demonstrated multiple dilated loops of proximal small bowel, consistent with a small bowel obstruction. Therefore, on day of life 27, the decision was made to take the patient back to the operating room for exploratory laparotomy.

After an extensive enterolysis, it was found that the patient had type III proximal jejunal atresia, which is when the blind ends of bowel are separated by a V-shaped defect of the mesentery [1]. Eight centimeters of the distal atretic jejunum was resected secondary to questionable viability; however, the remaining bowel appeared healthy and without inflammatory peel. A catheter was inserted into the distal atretic enterotomy and sterile normal saline was injected, demonstrating patency of the bowel through to the ascending colon. At this point, a primary end-to-end hand-sewn enteroenterostomy was created followed by a proximal jejunal plication secondary to the size difference of the two ends of bowel. The abdomen was primarily closed and the patient was transferred to the NICU in a stable condition.

Once again, the patient did well postoperatively. His TPN was continued and the nasogastric tube remained in place for decompression secondary to the anticipated postoperative ileus. Three weeks following the second surgery, there was again concern for an obstructive process, as the patient was still demonstrating high, nonbilious output from the nasogastric tube with chronic abdominal distension and no progression of bowel function. Furthermore, the patient also

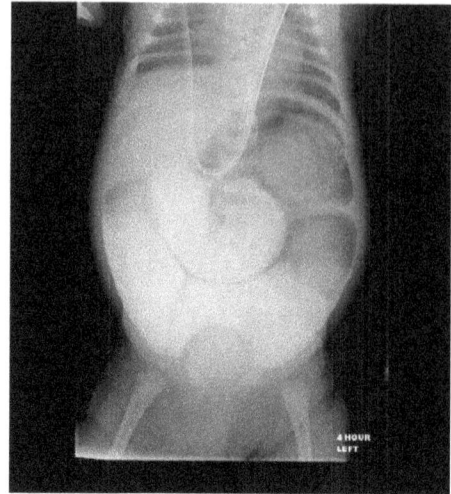

FIGURE 1: Upper gastrointestinal small bowel follow-through at 4 hours showing dilated loops of proximal small bowel and no progression of contrast through to the colon, suggestive of small bowel obstruction.

developed elevated bilirubin levels due to the extended period of time receiving TPN. At this point, we attributed the prolonged ileus to the previous two extensive surgeries experienced by the patient; however, in retrospect, we probably observed the patient too long this second time. The average postoperative ileus for jejunal atresia is approximately 5 days with a range of 3 to 10 days [10]. Additional imaging, such as an abdominal ultrasound, may have been beneficial during this time to help determine why the patient was not having bowel function. Nonetheless, a barium enema was obtained (Figure 2) after our allotted observation time demonstrating no progression of contrast beyond the midtransverse colon as well as significant microcolon, highly suggestive of colonic obstruction. Furthermore, an upper gastrointestinal study with small bowel follow-through was again performed (Figure 3). It demonstrated patency of the previously created jejunojejunostomy and propagation of contrast into the distal small bowel and proximal colon but was also suggestive of a distal colonic obstruction. Due to a work-up and clinical presentation highly suggestive of a colonic obstruction, the patient was taken back to the operating room on day of life 48 for a second exploratory laparotomy.

Again, extensive enterolysis was performed after entrance into the abdominal cavity. The previous jejunojejunostomy with the proximal plication was found to be patent. The bowel was followed to the colon where we discovered type II transverse colonic atresia, which is when the blind ends of bowel are separated by a fibrous cord [1]. An enterotomy was made in the distal atretic segment and 60cc of normal saline was injected into the distal colon with conformation of patency demonstrated by fluid excreted by the anus. The decision was made to perform a hand-sewn end-to-end anastomosis by spatulating the distal atretic segment. Once this was completed, the abdomen was closed and the patient was transferred to the NICU in a stable condition. The patient tolerated the procedure well.

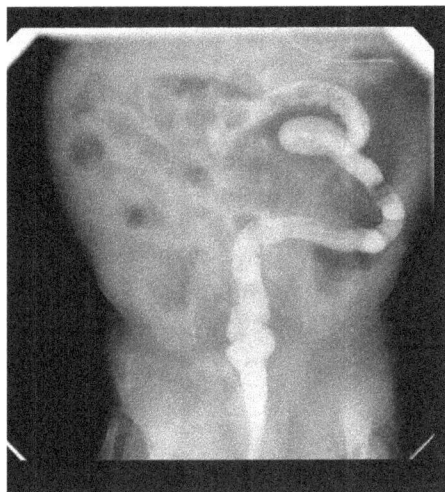

FIGURE 2: Barium enema showing microcolon and no progression of contrast proximal to the midtransverse colon suggestive of colonic obstruction.

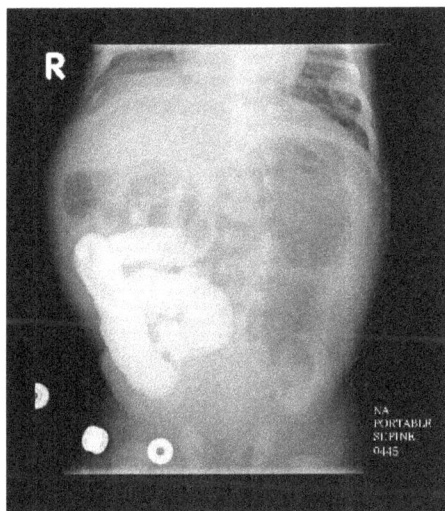

FIGURE 3: Upper gastrointestinal small bowel follow-through showing no progression of contrast beyond the right side of the abdomen after 4 days suggestive of obstruction. Previous enteroenterostomy appears patent.

The patient was continued on TPN and his nasogastric tube remained in place. A few days after the final surgery, the patient finally had his first bowel movement. Enteric tubes feeds were introduced slowly as his TPN was weaned. With the introduction of enteric feeds and weaning of TPN, the patient's hyperbilirubinemia gradually resolved.

3. Discussion

Although the incidence of gastroschisis, jejunal atresia, and colonic atresia found concomitantly in the same patient is not well defined in the current literature, only a signal case report has been described where one of a pair of dichorionic, diamniotic twins was found to have all three anomalies [6].

Diagnosis of intestinal atresia at the initial presentation of gastroschisis can be difficult secondary to a thick inflammatory peel covering the bowel [7], as well as poor visualization of bowel within the peritoneal cavity. Similar to the review by Kronfli et al., our missed intestinal atresia patient continued to demonstrate abdominal distension with prolonged feeding intolerance and high nasogastric tube output [5]. We were, however, able to recognize this obstructive jejunal atresia within 27 days of life, as opposed to the 41–57-day range cited in this review [5].

Our management of this patient was certainly not ideal as the patient required three operations in total. We believe this to be related to the rarity of having all three anomalies simultaneously. The classic surgical approach to managing patients with both gastroschisis and small bowel atresia has been to create a stoma in the acute setting with delayed primary anastomosis after a period of nasogastric decompression [5]. A similar surgical approach has been described for colonic atresia in which a primary anastomosis is performed for colonic atresia found proximal to the splenic flexure, and a colostomy with delayed anastomosis is performed for colonic atresia distal to the splenic flexure [1]. More recently, bowel resection with primary anastomosis has been demonstrated as a reasonable treatment for patients with gastroschisis and intestinal atresia [1, 5]. Of course, this is only possible when the bowel is healthy enough to undergo primary anastomosis, which is left to the judgment of the pediatric surgeon [7].

In our case presentation, the types of intestinal atresia were not initially diagnosed at abdominal wall closure secondary to a lack of bowel protruding through the abdominal wall defect and a low suspicion. Unfortunately, during our patient's second operation, transverse colon atresia was missed resulting in a third operation at day of life 48. Etensel et al. demonstrated in their meta-analysis of 224 cases of colonic atresia a statistically significant increase in mortality if time from birth to colonic atresia repair is greater than 72 hours [1]. Although our case does not support this increase in mortality from delayed repair, our patient was not without multiple comorbidities including hyperbilirubinemia, chronic TPN requirements, extended period of nasogastric tube insertion with high volume output, constant electrolyte abnormalities, inappropriate weight gain, and intestinal motility dysfunction.

Isolated colonic atresia is very uncommon, meaning its association with gastroschisis and jejunal atresia is even more so. Although the management of gastroschisis and intestinal atresia still remains contentious among various pediatric surgeons, the ultimate goal of restoring normal bowel function remains the focus of care for these patients. Healthcare providers must have a high suspicion of intestinal atresia associated with gastroschisis, something we lacked throughout this case, if neonates demonstrate intractable bilious vomiting, abdominal distension, and feeding intolerance on physical examination. We delayed the second operation because what we felt was a prolonged ileus from the gastroschisis itself, but that was obviously an incorrect assumption. Once the jejunal atresia was discovered, diagnostic dilemmas such as the false positive intraoperative saline injection test, not completely imaging the rectum and colon prior to surgery, and the initial passage of meconium during the initial gastroschisis closure plagued us causing the patient to require a third operation. Additionally, once the jejunal atresia was discovered, we should have had a higher suspicion for colonic atresia as jejunal atresia is associated with a greater number of simultaneous congenital malformations than ileal atresia [10].

The diagnosis of gastroschisis is fairly obvious and often diagnosed prior to birth. Intestinal atresia, however, can be more challenging, especially in the presence of other pathologic abnormalities. Although the use of both upper and lower contrast gastrointestinal studies should be included in the work-up of intestinal atresia, simply monitoring of bowel movements is extremely sensitive in assessing bowel obstruction. As clinicians, we were misled by the passage of a small amount of meconium at the initial surgery followed by the already known extended ileus that can result from these various pathologies. Utilizing bowel movement frequency with appropriate imaging modalities will allow for early and more accurate diagnosis of obstructive pathology in neonates, which would have been very beneficial for the patient described in our case report. Once intestinal atresia is diagnosed, time should not be wasted in repairing the obstructive pathology in order to decrease morbidity and mortality. When patients with such anomalies are managed appropriately, outcomes are generally favorable.

Disclosure

Drs. Zachary Bauman, D.O., and Victor Nanagas, M.D., had full access to all the information in the case report and take responsibility for the integrity of the information and the accuracy of the information analysis.

Conflict of Interests

There is no conflict of interests or financial interests to disclose for any of the contributing authors.

Authors' Contribution

All authors contributed substantially to this project. All authors involved in this project collectively reviewed and agreed upon the information as presented. Furthermore, all authors reviewed and approved the decision to submit this paper for publication.

References

[1] B. Etensel, G. Temir, A. Karkiner et al., "Atresia of the colon," *Journal of Pediatric Surgery*, vol. 40, no. 8, pp. 1258–1268, 2005.

[2] M. Baglaj, R. Carachi, and B. MacCormack, "Colonic atresia: a clinicopathological insight into its etiology," *European Journal of Pediatric Surgery*, vol. 20, no. 2, pp. 102–105, 2010.

[3] C.-T. Hsu, S.-S. Wang, J.-F. Houng, P.-J. Chiang, and C.-B. Huang, "Congenital colonic atresia: report of one case," *Pediatrics and Neonatology*, vol. 51, no. 3, pp. 186–189, 2010.

[4] S. Kim, S. Yedlin, and O. Idowu, "Colonic atresia in monozygotic twins," *The American Journal of Medical Genetics*, vol. 91, no. 3, pp. 204–206, 2000.

[5] R. Kronfli, T. J. Bradnock, and A. Sabharwal, "Intestinal atresia in association with gastroschisis: a 26-year review," *Pediatric Surgery International*, vol. 26, no. 9, pp. 891–894, 2010.

[6] M. A. Saxonhouse, D. W. Kays, D. J. Burchfield, R. Hoover, and S. Islam, "Gastroschisis with jejunal and colonic atresia, and isolated colonic atresia in dichorionic, diamniotic twins," *Pediatric Surgery International*, vol. 25, no. 5, pp. 437–439, 2009.

[7] C. L. Snyder, K. A. Miller, R. J. Sharp et al., "Management of intestinal atresia in patients with gastroschisis," *Journal of Pediatric Surgery*, vol. 36, no. 10, pp. 1542–1545, 2001.

[8] C. P. Driver, J. Bruce, A. Bianchi, C. M. Doig, A. P. Dickson, and J. Bowen, "The contemporary outcome of gastroschisis," *Journal of Pediatric Surgery*, vol. 35, no. 12, pp. 1719–1723, 2000.

[9] T. J. Bradnock, S. Marven, A. Owen et al., "Gastroschisis: one year outcomes from national cohort study," *British Medical Journal*, vol. 343, no. 7832, Article ID d6749, p. 1036, 2011.

[10] V. C. Shakya, C. S. Agrawal, P. Shrestha, P. Poudel, S. Khaniya, and S. Adhikary, "Management of jejunoileal atresias: an experience at eastern Nepal," *BMC Surgery*, vol. 10, article 35, 2010.

Abdominal Lymphonodular Cryptococcosis in an Immunocompetent Child

Mehjabeen Zaidi,[1] **Sonia Qureshi,**[1] **Sadia Shakoor,**[2] **Saira Fatima,**[3] **and Fatima Mir**[1]

[1]*Department of Pediatrics and Child Health, Aga Khan University, Stadium Road, Karachi 74800, Pakistan*
[2]*Microbiology, Department of Pathology, Aga Khan University, Stadium Road, Karachi 74800, Pakistan*
[3]*Histopathology, Department of Pathology, Aga Khan University, Stadium Road, Karachi 74800, Pakistan*

Correspondence should be addressed to Fatima Mir; fatima.mir@aku.edu

Academic Editor: Maria Moschovi

We describe our experience with an apparently immunocompetent child presenting with pyrexia of unknown origin without focal signs. Investigations revealed lymphadenopathy at lung hila, mesentery, and porta hepatis. The child had received at least two months of empiric antituberculous therapy (ATT) before she came to us. A CT-guided biopsy revealed granulomatous inflammation. PAS stain showed yeasts which stained blue with Alcian blue, suggesting *C. neoformans*.

1. Background

Lymphonodular cryptococcosis has been reported in the past in immunocompromised and immunocompetent children [1, 2]. The two species, *C. neoformans* and *C. gattii*, enter the respiratory system through inhalation and disseminate hematogenously to various sites in the body [3]. Disease manifestations range from localized disease such as meningitis, pulmonary infiltrates, and lymphadenopathy to disseminated cryptococcosis with multiorgan involvement [3]. Cryptococcosis has classically been associated with acquired and inherited T-cell deficiencies [4]. Though antiretroviral therapy has decreased the incidence of cryptococcosis in HIV patients, it is increasingly being reported in a non-HIV, nontransplant cohort [5]. The underlying pathophysiology is not clear. We report the case history of a 5-year-old female child with Fever of Unknown Origin (FUO) and abdominal lymphadenopathy. A CT-guided lymph node biopsy showed granulomatous inflammation and encapsulated yeasts resembling *Cryptococcus* species. Culture was negative for Acid Fast Bacillus (AFB) and bacterial and fungal cultures could not be sent due to inadequate tissue sample. The child responded clinically and serologically to 6 months of oral fluconazole and remains well to date.

2. Case History

A 5-year-old female child had remained well and thriving till 10 weeks before presentation when she developed high grade, continuous fever associated with nonradiating, central abdominal pain and anorexia. She had started taking three-drug antituberculous therapy (ATT) (isoniazid, rifampicin, and pyrazinamide) based on a general practitioner's prescription/physician discretion due to the clinical finding of nontender lymphadenopathy and unabated fever for 2 weeks. The modified Keith Edwards scoring had not been done and neither had the tissue culture been sought. By week 8 of empiric ATT for presumed TB adenitis, there was no clinical improvement and a weight loss of 2.5 kg was observed.

She was the second amongst 3 siblings and a student of kindergarten. She had a positive BCG scar with immunization complete for age as per Pakistan's Expanded Programme of Immunization (EPI) schedule. There was no contact history for tuberculosis (TB), no family pets, or travel beyond her hometown. She belonged to a middle-income family and was a resident of a neighbouring city (approximately 160 km away from Karachi). The father was a civil servant, and the mother was a housewife.

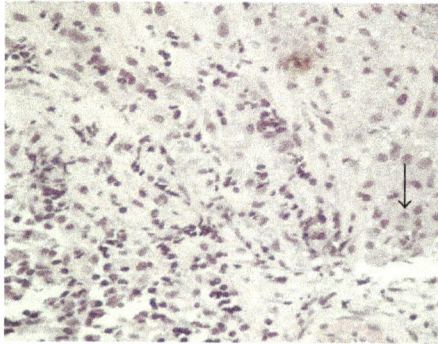

FIGURE 1: H&E stain of mesenteric lymph node biopsy showing granuloma formation, 400x.

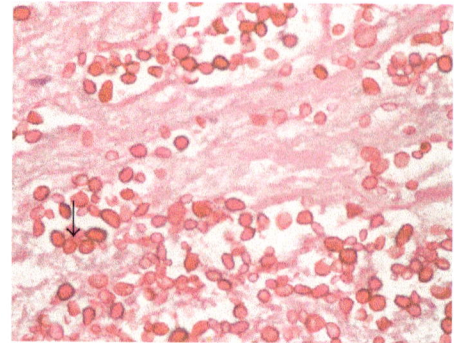

FIGURE 2: PAS stain of mesenteric lymph node biopsy showing yeasts, 1000x.

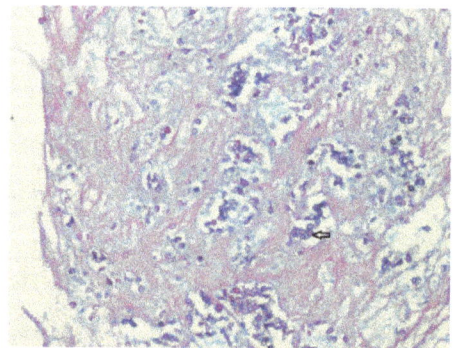

FIGURE 3: PAS stain with Alcian blue, 1000x.

On examination, the child was febrile, icteric, and pale with hepatomegaly. There was no peripheral adenopathy.

Investigations done prior to presentation in the Infectious Disease (ID) clinic revealed normochromic, normocytic anemia (Hb 7.4 mg/dL), a progressively rising white count over twelve weeks of fever (21×10^9/L at outset to 32×10^9/L at presentation in ID clinic), high inflammatory markers: Erythrocyte Sedimentation Rate (ESR 135 mm/hr) and C-reactive protein (CRP29), direct hyperbilirubinemia (total bilirubin 4.6 with 3.7 direct component), and an episode of *E. coli* Urinary Tract Infection (UTI), along with lymphadenopathy seen at the lung hila (chest X-Ray), mesentery, and porta hepatis 3.9×7 cm in AP and transverse dimension in the mesentery and 4×5 cm AP and transverse dimension at the porta hepatis (CT abdomen).

Tests conducted in the ID clinic as workup for "pyrexia of unknown origin" were negative for malaria, typhoid (blood and bone marrow culture), malignancy (bone marrow smear and trephine results showing normal erythropoiesis, myelopoiesis, and megakaryocytes), and autoimmune disease (negative dsDNA, rheumatoid factor, and Coombs test).

A chest X-ray and abdominal ultrasound were repeated to monitor size of lymph nodes after 2 months of ATT. They remained as before. Tissue diagnosis was stressed on and a CT-guided mesenteric lymph node biopsy was carried out and sent for histopathology and an AFB culture, keeping our top differentials of malignancy and multidrug resistant tuberculosis (MDR-TB) in mind. Fungal and bacterial cultures could not be sent due to inadequate tissue.

Histopathology sections revealed extensive necrosis with aggregates of epithelioid histiocytes forming granulomas in the core tissue (see arrow in Figure 1). Few Langhans-type giant cells were also seen. Periodic acid-Schiff (PAS) stain showed yeasts (see Figure 2) and capsules stained blue with Alcian blue (arrow Figure 3) suggesting *C. neoformans*.

Additional tests done after the biopsy result revealed a very high cryptococcal antigen titre (>1 : 1024) and a negative HIV antibody. Though the underlying T-cell deficiency was considered, quantitative evaluation (flow cytometry) was deferred because of the absence of a clinical history suggesting immune compromise and also because cryptococcosis is not exclusively an immunocompromised-host disease.

The parents refused lumbar puncture because of scepticism of occult CNS disease in the absence of signs and symptoms. The child was assumed to have high antigenemia with lymph node involvement and unknown CNS status. Amphotericin was started at a dose of 0.5 mg/kg/day and increased over 2-3 days to 1.5 mg/kg/day. Flucytosine, recommended by the IDSA in conjunction with amphotericin for cryptococcosis, was not available in Karachi. The child was ultimately discharged home on oral fluconazole monotherapy (6 mg/kg/day) as the parents were reluctant to administer prolonged parenteral amphotericin at home.

At one-month follow-up, the patient had gained 2 kg, had defervesced, and resumed normal home and school activities. At 3 months, she was clinically well with improvement in lymph node size on abdominal ultrasound and chest X-ray. Therapy was monitored by repeat cryptococcal antigen titres which progressively decreased over 6 months of therapy (more than 1 : 1024 during admission, 1 : 1024 one month, 1 : 256 three months, and 1 : 32 five months of therapy). The family did not return to our center for a follow-up or immune workup beyond 6 months. The patient is doing well after cessation of therapy and continues to thrive as per telephonic contact with parents.

3. Discussion

Pathogenesis of cryptococcosis in "phenotypically normal" hosts like our patient, without predisposing factors such as

HIV, transplant, clinical history suggesting T-cell immunodeficiency, or chronic conditions such as end-stage liver disease and renal insufficiency, has been studied [4]. It involves innate (macrophages, complement and Natural Killer) (NK) defense mechanisms, and cell-mediated (CD4 cells) and humoral immunity (facilitation of phagocytosis) [6]. Pathogen factors such as the capsule and host factors such as surfactant at the alveolar level have been implicated in helping the organism evade detection by macrophages. Although precisely how the human host controls cryptococci remains unclear, clinical practice suggests that immunosuppressive agents like corticosteroids allow cryptococci to reactivate, CD4 cell numbers are critically important to host immunity, and cryptococcal proliferation in humans is clearly contained by a vigorous granulomatous response [7, 8]. Cryptococcosis should therefore be considered as a differential in the workup for PUO, especially in the presence of granulomatous inflammation.

Our patient had an uneventful first 5 years of life till the onset of this illness. Changing trends in epidemiology of cryptococcosis in China shows that the majority of cases occurred in a non-HIV, nontransplant "phenotypically normal" cohort [5]. Kiertiburanakul et al. in a retrospective review (1987–2003) of HIV-negative patients with positive cryptococcal cultures showed that 35% patients had no underlying conditions [9]. Idiopathic CD4 lymphocytopenia (ICL) was found in 11 patients with cryptococcosis reviewed over a 12-month period with features similar to those of cryptococcal infections in normal hosts [10]. Our threshold for suspecting immunodeficiency was very high. Ideally quantitative deficiencies, especially in the absence of the availability of qualitative immune tests in Karachi, would have been useful in deciding on the drug of choice, duration of treatment, and prognostication. The family was retrospectively counseled to get an immune workup in case of prolonged or unusual fever.

CNS is the commonest system affected in cryptococcosis [3]. Occult disease can occur without overt signs and symptoms. Though the parents refused a lumbar puncture, they were extensively counseled that this would mean a longer course of therapy and difficulty in prognostication. Pulmonary involvement has been reported in 10–36% of non-HIV patients [11]. Symptoms can be absent in up to one-third of the patients with abnormal X-rays. Our child had no pulmonary symptoms: her chest X-ray showed normal lung fields and hilar lymphadenopathy.

Tissue-based PCR is the gold standard for diagnosis on histopathology [12]. This was not done as it was unavailable in our institution. Liaw et al. report direct determination of cryptococcal antigen through latex agglutination system in transthoracic needle lung aspirate with a positive predictive value of 89% and a negative predictive value of 100% [13]. Fridlington et al. have also reported using Tzanck smear on skin biopsy which revealed narrow-based budding encapsulated yeasts, suggesting cryptococcosis, and was confirmed by fungal culture [14]. These may have additive value in the absence of tissue-PCR and fungal culture.

Cryptococcal lymphadenopathy has been reported in HIV and immunocompetent patients with some and apparently no immune deficiency [1, 15–17]. Karagüzel reported a child with mesenteric cryptococcal lymphadenitis who presented with acute abdomen [18].

Wu et al. reported on a 10-year-old boy with disseminated cryptococcosis resembling lymphoreticular malignancy [19]. Differentials of granulomatous inflammation on biopsy in countries like Pakistan should include cryptococcosis.

IDSA guidelines recommend that cryptococcemia or dissemination (involvement of at least 2 noncontiguous sites or evidence of high fungal burden based on cryptococcal antigen titer 1 : 512), as in our case, should be treated as CNS disease (2 weeks of induction therapy with IV amphotericin with flucytosine, followed by 8 weeks of maintenance therapy with oral fluconazole) [20]. Our patient received IV amphotericin while in hospital (approximately 3 days between histopathology reporting and discharge). The family refused parenteral therapy even though they were counseled about the drug of choice in the absence of ruling out CNS involvement. The patient was sent home on oral fluconazole therapy for 6–12 months with instructions to have cryptococcal antigen titre repeated every 2 months. She remained lost to follow-up for almost two years after 6-month therapy until the parents contacted the primary physician. The child remains well and asymptomatic to date. Induction with fluconazole has been recommended only for patients with no antigenemia and no CNS disease and only single site involvement. Our patient had very high antigenemia and lymphadenopathy (mesenteric and porta hepatis, the latter causing secondary cholestasis).

Heteroresistance and emerging resistance have been implicated as possible causes in reactivation of cryptococcosis in patients treated with fluconazole in induction phase [21].

We were relatively successful in monitoring therapy success with the help of progressively falling antigen titres over 6 months of therapy. However, patients like these should be ideally followed posttreatment and investigated for immune deficiency.

We should also send tissue for fungal and AFB cultures in addition to bacterial cultures when faced with lymphadenopathy and Fever of Unknown Origin, or empiric ATT failures.

4. Conclusion

Cryptococcosis should be considered as a differential of Fever of Unknown Origin and granulomatous lymphadenopathy in Pakistan. Patients should be investigated for immunodeficiency, and extent of disease should be established. Clinical suspicion must be communicated at the time of sending specimens to the laboratory so that optimal diagnostic tools can be resourced.

Consent

Written informed consent was obtained from the patient for publication of this case report and any accompanying images.

Conflict of Interests

The authors declare that there is no conflict of interests.

Authors' Contribution

Mehjabeen Zaidi wrote the first draft of the paper. Sadia Shakoor provided the photographs, interpreted laboratory findings, and contributed to the final paper. Saira Fatima helped in interpretation of histopathology slides. Fatima Mir modified and finalized the paper. All authors read and approved the final paper.

Acknowledgment

Dr. Fatima Mir received research training support from the National Institute of Health's Fogarty International Center (1 D43 TW007585-01).

References

[1] F. Bao, H. Tan, W. Liu, Y. Li, and H. Li, "Pediatric cryptococcal lymphadenitis in the absence of AIDS: case report and literature review," *Case Reports in Pediatrics*, vol. 2013, Article ID 563081, 4 pages, 2013.

[2] P. Dogbey, M. Golden, and N. Ngo, "Cryptococcal lymphadenitis: an unusual initial presentation of HIV infection," *BMJ Case Reports*, vol. 2013, 2013.

[3] C. B. Severo, M. O. Xavier, A. F. Gazzoni, and L. C. Severo, "Cryptococcosis in children," *Paediatric Respiratory Reviews*, vol. 10, no. 4, pp. 166–171, 2009.

[4] R. M. La Hoz and P. G. Pappas, "Cryptococcal infections: changing epidemiology and implications for therapy," *Drugs*, vol. 73, no. 6, pp. 495–504, 2013.

[5] C. Yuchong, C. Fubin, C. Jianghan et al., "Cryptococcosis in China (1985–2010): review of cases from Chinese database," *Mycopathologia*, vol. 173, no. 5-6, pp. 329–335, 2012.

[6] M. S. Price and J. R. Perfect, "Host defenses against cryptococcosis," *Immunological Investigations*, vol. 40, no. 7-8, pp. 786–808, 2011.

[7] C. A. Hage, K. L. Wood, H. T. Winer-Muram, S. J. Wilson, G. Sarosi, and K. S. Knox, "Pulmonary cryptococcosis after initiation of anti-tumor necrosis factor-α therapy," *Chest*, vol. 124, no. 6, pp. 2395–2397, 2003.

[8] D. Salmon-Ceron, F. Tubach, O. Lortholary et al., "Drug-specific risk of non-tuberculosis opportunistic infections in patients receiving anti-TNF therapy reported to the 3-year prospective French RATIO registry," *Annals of the Rheumatic Diseases*, vol. 70, no. 4, pp. 616–623, 2011.

[9] S. Kiertiburanakul, S. Wirojtananugoon, R. Pracharktam, and S. Sungkanuparph, "Cryptococcosis in human immunodeficiency virus-negative patients," *International Journal of Infectious Diseases*, vol. 10, no. 1, pp. 72–78, 2006.

[10] D. I. Zonios, J. Falloon, C.-Y. Huang, D. Chaitt, and J. E. Bennett, "Cryptococcosis and idiopathic CD4 lymphocytopenia," *Medicine*, vol. 86, no. 2, pp. 78–92, 2007.

[11] W.-C. Chang, C. Tzao, H.-H. Hsu et al., "Pulmonary cryptococcosis: comparison of clinical and radiographic characteristics in immunocompetent and immunocompromised patients," *Chest*, vol. 129, no. 2, pp. 333–340, 2006.

[12] P. J. Simner, S. P. Buckwalter, J. R. Uhl, N. L. Wengenack, and B. S. Pritt, "Detection and identification of yeasts from formalin-fixed, paraffin-embedded tissue by use of Pcr-electrospray ionization mass spectrometry," *Journal of Clinical Microbiology*, vol. 51, no. 11, pp. 3731–3734, 2013.

[13] Y.-S. Liaw, P.-C. Yang, C.-J. Yu et al., "Direct determination of cryptococcal antigen in transthoracic needle aspirate for diagnosis of pulmonary cryptococcosis," *Journal of Clinical Microbiology*, vol. 33, no. 6, pp. 1588–1591, 1995.

[14] E. Fridlington, M. Colome-Grimmer, E. Kelly, and B. C. Kelly, "Tzanck smear as a rapid diagnostic tool for disseminated cryptococcal infection," *Archives of Dermatology*, vol. 142, no. 1, pp. 25–27, 2006.

[15] B. S. Araújo, M. Bay, R. Reichert, and L. Z. Goldani, "Intra-abdominal cryptococcosis by *Cryptococcus gattii*: case report and review," *Mycopathologia*, vol. 174, no. 1, pp. 81–85, 2012.

[16] N. Jain, B. L. Wickes, S. M. Keller et al., "Molecular epidemiology of clinical *Cryptococcus neoformans* strains from India," *Journal of Clinical Microbiology*, vol. 43, no. 11, pp. 5733–5742, 2005.

[17] S. B. Memon, A. M. Memon, S. Faisal, N. Kapadia, and I. N. Soomro, "Cryptococcus—diversity of clinical presentation," *Journal of the Pakistan Medical Association*, vol. 51, no. 9, pp. 337–339, 2001.

[18] G. Karagüzel, B. Kiliçarslan-Akkaya, M. Melikoglu, and G. Karpuzoglu, "Cryptococcal mesenteric lymphadenitis: an unusual cause of acute abdomen," *Pediatric Surgery International*, vol. 20, no. 8, pp. 633–635, 2004.

[19] J. M. Wu, C. Y. Lee, L. M. Huang, K. H. Lin, K. H. Hsieh, and M. Z. Wu, "Disseminated cryptococcosis mimicking lymphoreticular malignancy: report of one case," *Zhonghua Min Guo Xiao Er Ke Yi Xue Hui Za Zhi*, vol. 31, no. 3, pp. 196–201, 1990.

[20] J. R. Perfect, W. E. Dismukes, F. Dromer et al., "Clinical practice guidelines for the management of cryptococcal disease: 2010 update by the infectious diseases society of America," *Clinical Infectious Diseases*, vol. 50, no. 3, pp. 291–322, 2010.

[21] E. Sionov, Y. C. Chang, H. M. Garraffo, and K. J. Kwon-Chung, "Heteroresistance to fluconazole in *Cryptococcus neoformans* is intrinsic and associated with virulence," *Antimicrobial Agents and Chemotherapy*, vol. 53, no. 7, pp. 2804–2815, 2009.

Nephrotic Syndrome in a Child Suffering from Tetralogy of Fallot: A Rare Association

Pépé Mfutu Ekulu,[1] **Orly Kazadi-wa-Kazadi,**[1]
Paul Kabuyi Lumbala,[2] **and Michel Ntetani Aloni**[1]

[1]*Division of Paediatric Haemato-Oncology and Nephrology, Department of Paediatrics, University Hospital of Kinshasa, Faculty of Medicine, University of Kinshasa, Kinshasa, Congo*
[2]*Division of Cardiology, Department of Paediatrics, University Hospital of Kinshasa, Faculty of Medicine, University of Kinshasa, Kinshasa, Congo*

Correspondence should be addressed to Michel Ntetani Aloni; michelaloni2003@yahoo.fr

Academic Editor: Larry A. Rhodes

Nephrotic syndrome is an uncommon complication of tetralogy of Fallot and has been rarely reported in pediatric population. We describe a 4-year-old female Congolese child who was referred for investigation for persistent dyspnea, edema, and cyanosis and nephrotic range proteinuria. Our patient presented with a tetralogy of Fallot and nephrotic syndrome. *Conclusion.* This case reminds us that children with tetralogy of Fallot may develop nephrotic proteinuria.

1. Introduction

Glomerular dysfunction can be found in cyanotic congenital heart disease (CHD) especially in older children and adults, being associated occasionally with proteinuria and microalbuminuria [1, 2]. The risk of developing renal impairment is particularly high in cyanotic patients particularly in patients with long-standing cyanotic CHD [1, 2]. However, nephrotic syndrome (NS) is an uncommon complication of cyanotic congenital heart disease and is rarely reported. This complication has not been documented in Congolese children.

2. Case Report

A 4-year-old girl with edema, dyspnea, and cyanosis was referred from Butembo at the East of the Democratic Republic of Congo (DRC) to a facility renal and cardiology investigations in Department of Pediatrics of University Hospital of Kinshasa, Kinshasa, DRC. The history of present illness dates back to about 13 months characterized by progressive cough, dyspnea, and orthopnea. Physical examination revealed respiratory distress with edema and episodes of squatting. She was cyanosed with finger and toes clubbing. Apex beat was at the fifth intercostal space anterior axillary line. Both heart sounds were noted with a systolic thrill and loud systolic ejection murmur grade 3. The blood pressure was 150/110 mmHg, and oximetry was 63%.

A complete blood count showed hemoglobin 23.2 g/dL, total proteins 45 g/L, and albumin 22 g/L. Dipstick urinalysis was 3 + while the 24-hour urinary protein was 154 mg/kg. Creatinine was 37 μmol/L, urea was 3.8 mmol/L, cholesterol was 4.3 mmol/L, and HDL was 1.3 mmol/L. HIV and hepatitis serology were negative. Anti-streptolysin O (ASLO) was <200 IU.

X-ray revealed "boot shaped" heart with an upturned cardiac apex (Figure 1). Echocardiography revealed tetralogy of Fallot with hypoplastic pulmonary artery and biventricular dysfunction. Cardiac catheterization was not performed due to technical reasons. A diagnosis of Fallot's tetralogy and NS was established. Renal biopsy was contraindicated because of the deteriorating renal condition and cardiac status.

During her hospitalization, the child received specific treatment for her blood hypertension, associated furosemide (1 mg/kg/dose, every six hours), Propranolol (2 mg/kg, every

TABLE 1: Results of the literature review of cyanotic CHD associated with nephrotic syndrome in African children.

Source	Our case	Adedoyin and Afolabi [2]	Ogunkunle et al. [1]	Ogunkunle et al. [1]
Country	Kinshasa, DRC	Ilorin, Nigeria	Ibadan, Nigeria	Ibadan, Nigeria
Year of description	2015	2006	2008	2008
Age (years)	4	9	12	7
Gender	Female	Male	Female	Male
Cyanotic CHD*	Tetralogy of Fallot	Truncus arteriosus	Tetralogy of Fallot	Tricuspid atresia

*CHD: congenital heart disease; DRC: Democratic Republic of Congo.

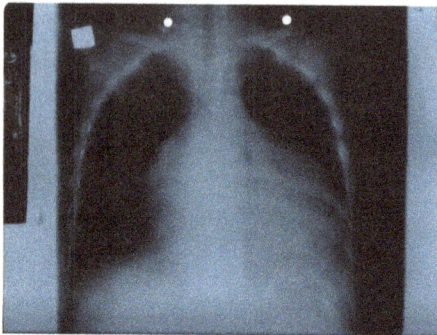

FIGURE 1: Plain film shows a "boot shaped" heart with an upturned cardiac apex due to right ventricular hypertrophy and concave pulmonary arterial segment.

six hours), and Enalapril (0.4 mg/Kg, every twelve hours). For her NS, the child received prednisone (60 mg/m^2/day during 30 days) for the first phase and diet.

Initial biologic and clinical improvement was observed with steroid and Enalapril therapies. Edema regressed with treatment. The 24-hour urinary protein decreased from 154 mg/kg to 6.7 mg/kg and creatinine remained stable. Death occurred 41 days after admission to an array of sudden hypoxic tet spells. She was stable enough to be discharged after six weeks on admission.

3. Discussion

Nephropathy among patients is an important complication of tetralogy of Fallot [1, 2]. The incidence and prevalence are unknown and epidemiological data are rare in Africa. In Central Africa, this affection was not previously noted. Our observation is the first description in our population. Only three cases in pediatric population could be found in Nigeria with the use of available computer-assisted medical literature search programs [1, 2]. The situation is probably due to the lack of the evaluation of renal function in highly resource-scarce settings and nephrologist pediatrician [3]. At the same time, it is probable that many children with cyanotic CHD die before the development of NS in our midst.

We have reviewed the literature on cyanotic CHD and NS (Table 1). The development of NS associated with cyanotic CHD remains unclear. However, some aetiopathogenetic

mechanisms have been suggested for the development of nephropathy. The patients with cyanotic CHD are exposed to chronic hypoxia. The risk of developing glomerular lesions rose sharply during the second decade of life if the cyanosis remains unchanged for more than ten years [4, 5]. Hyperviscosity due to polycythemia may induce an angiogenic increase in the glomerular capillary beds, in turn leading to glomerulomegaly. Glomerulomegaly is a consequence of the hyperperfusion of glomeruli associated with the chronic hypoxia and the increased hydrostatic pressure in the capillary wall. This situation is a causative factor of the deterioration and the decline of renal function, in the condition of polycythemia. Furthermore, the failure of a compensatory mechanism to respond to reduced RPF by hyperfiltration may be accompanied by the development and progression of microalbuminuria and proteinuria [4–6]. The pathogenesis and development of nephrotic proteinuria range are the result of these combined mechanisms. Although we could not perform the renal biopsy, the nephrotic range proteinuria is probably a consequence of focal and segmental glomerulosclerosis.

Our patient presented late. This case revealed the problem of early diagnosis, regular follow-up, and early detection of complications in African cyanotic CHD patients especially in case of Fallot's tetralogy during antenatal or neonatal period. It is known that untreated cardiac malformations in patient with Fallot's tetralogy have high likelihood of progression to glomerular damage [4–6]. In our context, diagnosis and management were generally delayed.

It is worth considering the use of ACE-I when nephropathy accompanies cyanotic CHD. In a previous study, Enalapril apparently reduced the urinary protein excretion in 80% of patients [7]. In our case, proteinuria decreased from 154 mg/kg/24 h to 6.7 mg/kg/24 h.

This case reminds us that children with tetralogy of Fallot may develop NS. This case report is pointing out the problem encountered in the early diagnosis and management of cyanotic CHD in resource-limited settings as in DRC. Considering the paucity of facilities available for medical and surgical management of Fallot's tetralogy in our midst, we recommend early detection of this congenital heart disease and regular renal screening of patients and thus allow, at least at this stage, the initiation of ACE-I. However, it has to be stated that, in countries such as the DRC, early corrective cardiac surgery should be the first choice particularly in patients who otherwise present severe complications of their cyanotic CHD and reduce the risk of the development of chronic renal failure.

Ethical Approval

This study was determined to be Non-Human/Non-Research by the Ethical Committee of the Public Health School of the University of Kinshasa, Kinshasa, DRC.

Conflict of Interests

The authors declare that there is no conflict of interests regarding the publication of this paper.

References

[1] O. O. Ogunkunle, A. O. Asinobi, S. I. Omokhodion, and A. D. Ademola, "Nephrotic syndrome complicating cyanotic congenital heart disease: a report of two cases," *West African Journal of Medicine*, vol. 27, no. 4, pp. 263–266, 2008.

[2] O. T. Adedoyin and J. K. Afolabi, "Sudden deterioration in the renal function of an African child with cyanotic congenital heart disease," *Journal of the National Medical Association*, vol. 98, no. 2, pp. 287–289, 2006.

[3] P. Cochat, C. Mourani, J. Exantus et al., "Pediatric nephrology in developing countries," *Medecine Tropicale*, vol. 69, no. 6, pp. 543–547, 2009.

[4] S. Dittrich, N. A. Haas, C. Bührer, C. Müller, I. Dähnert, and P. E. Lange, "Renal impairment in patients with long-standing cyanotic congenital heart disease," *Acta Paediatrica*, vol. 87, no. 9, pp. 949–954, 1998.

[5] F. Krull, J. H. H. Ehrich, U. Wurster, U. Toel, S. Rothgänger, and I. Luhmer, "Renal involvement in patients with congenital cyanotic heart disease," *Acta Paediatrica Scandinavica*, vol. 80, no. 12, pp. 1214–1219, 1991.

[6] J. Inatomi, K. Matsuoka, R. Fujimaru, A. Nakagawa, and K. Iijima, "Mechanisms of development and progression of cyanotic nephropathy," *Pediatric Nephrology*, vol. 21, no. 10, pp. 1440–1445, 2006.

[7] Y. Fujimoto, M. Matsushima, K. Tsuzuki et al., "Nephropathy of cyanotic congenital heart disease: clinical characteristics and effectiveness of an angiotensin-converting enzyme inhibitor," *Clinical Nephrology*, vol. 58, no. 2, pp. 95–102, 2002.

Pulmonary Epithelioid Hemangioendothelioma in a Patient with Crohn's Disease

Nanda Ramchandar and Henry A. Wojtczak

Naval Medical Center San Diego, Department of Pediatrics, 34800 Bob Wilson Drive, San Diego, CA 92134, USA

Correspondence should be addressed to Nanda Ramchandar; nandaramchandar@gmail.com

Academic Editor: Amalia Schiavetti

Pulmonary epithelioid hemangioendothelioma (PEH) is a rare neoplasm, largely unresponsive to chemotherapeutic medications, and with varied prognosis. Imaging on computerized tomography may demonstrate perivascular nodules, but diagnosis is ultimately made on biopsy with immunohistochemical analysis. Here we describe a case of PEH in a 14-year-old male with Crohn's disease, which, to our knowledge, has not previously been described in the literature.

1. Introduction

Originally described as an intravascular bronchoalveolar tumor by Dail and Liebow in 1975, pulmonary epithelioid hemangioendothelioma (PEH) is a rare vascular neoplasm that may arise as a primary tumor either in the lung or in the pleura [1–4]. The natural history and clinical course of PEH are poorly understood, and malignant potential ranges from benign hemangioma to malignant angiosarcoma. Diagnosis is made on histology, requiring immunohistochemical staining for markers specific to vascular endothelium. Response to chemotherapy is minimal at best with prognosis varying from complete spontaneous regression to rapid onset of end stage disease. To our knowledge, there is only one case in the literature of a hepatic epithelioid hemangioendothelioma and there are no cases of PEH described in the setting of inflammatory bowel disease [5]. We report a 14-year-old male with Crohn's disease (CD) and pulmonary epithelioid hemangioendothelioma.

2. Case Report

A 14-year-old male diagnosed with Crohn's disease in August of 2012 is referred to a pulmonologist for multiple pulmonary nodules found incidentally on abdominal computerized tomography during evaluation of his Crohn's disease. Initially, there was no complaint of respiratory symptoms, but over time, he developed a dry cough and back pain. Patient was well-developed and well-nourished on physical exam with symmetric chest. Lung exam was without crackles or wheeze, but with mildly prolonged expiratory phase. There was no hepatosplenomegaly, tenderness, or distension on the abdominal exam. Chest radiograph findings included multiple pulmonary nodules, and chest CT showed irregular ground glass nodules 2-3 cm in diameter, mild thickening of airway walls, no effusion, and reactive lymphadenopathy in the perihilar regions bilaterally (Figure 1).

Spirometry showed forced vital capacity (FVC) of 2.78 (78%), forced expiratory volume in 1 second (FEV1) of 2.10 (68%), FEV1/FVC of 76%, and forced expiratory flow 25–75% (FEF 25–75%) of 46%. Extensive pulmonary workup for pulmonary nodules including bronchoscopy, bronchoalveolar lavage (BAL), and thoracoscopic lung biopsy was completed. Results were negative for infectious, rheumatologic, or malignant processes. Of note, there was grossly bloody BAL fluid and numerous red blood cells. Lung biopsy revealed multifocal intra-alveolar collections of hemosiderin-laden macrophages with focal hemorrhage, scattered pulmonary artery branches showing collapse with luminal loss and mural calcification, and no vasculitis. Surrounding the degenerated arteries were areas of fibrosis with peripheral aerated alveolar spaces present. Final pathology reported arteriopathy with hemosiderosis, hemorrhage, and fibrosis. Despite regular infliximab infusions for his CD, pulmonary symptoms did

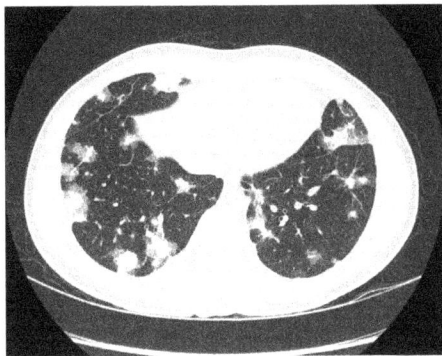

FIGURE 1: Chest computerized tomography scan. Multiple irregular ground glass nodules 2-3 cm in diameter, mild thickening of airway walls, no effusion, and reactive lymphadenopathy in the perihilar regions bilaterally.

not resolve. Patient was started on 3-week course of prednisone, but again to no avail. Patient underwent a second bronchoscopy and repeat thoracoscopic lung biopsy. Analysis of biopsies showed nodular cellular infiltrate intermixed with hemosiderin laden macrophages and plugs of fibrin. Atypical cells were epithelioid in appearance, consistent with PEH. Immunohistochemical staining confirmed endothelial lineage.

3. Discussion

PEH was originally described in 1975 as an aggressive form of bronchoalveolar cell carcinoma with invasion into surrounding vasculature [1, 2, 6]. Subsequent immunochemical analysis and electron microscopy revealed the endothelial nature of this neoplasm, and the current name of PEH was coined by Weiss et al. in 1982 [3, 4, 6]. Epithelioid hemangioendothelioma is not specific to the lung, arising as a primary lesion more commonly in the liver as well as bone and other soft tissues. It is more often diagnosed in women and in younger patients, with a median age of 35 years [6–8]. Imaging is not sufficient for diagnosis, but lesions often appear as either unilateral or bilateral perivascular nodules generally <2 cm in diameter [6, 9]. Histological characteristics include nodules with hypocellular sclerotic or necrotic center. Immunochemical staining for vimentin, erythroblast transformation-specific related gene (ERG), cluster of differentiation 31, cluster of differentiation 34, and factor VIII or friend leukemia integration 1 (FLI-1) transcription factor confirms diagnosis [4, 6, 10, 11]. Additionally, use of fluorescence in situ hybridization (FISH) or polymerase chain reaction (PCR) to detect CAMTA1-WWTR1 and YAP1-TFE3 rearrangements can be used as an adjunct to immunohistochemical analysis, tools that are useful in distinguishing epithelioid hemangioendothelioma from other epithelioid vascular neoplasms [10–13].

Prognosis is difficult to forecast, ranging from complete resolution without intervention to rapid progression and death. Poor prognostic indicators include low weight, anemia, pulmonary symptoms, pleural hemorrhagic effusions,

and hemoptysis [14, 15]. In patients with pleural effusion or hemoptysis, the median survival is less than 1 year [4, 10, 14]. Conversely, in patient with asymptomatic pulmonary nodules, average survival time is 15 years [8]. There is currently no gold standard for therapy given the relative rarity of this condition. Chemotherapeutic measures have been attempted with varying degrees of success, but PEH is often unresponsive to treatment [16]. Such agents used in the treatment of PEH include vincristine, cisplatin, 5-fluorouracil, mitomycin, cyclophosphamide, ifosfamide, and etoposide [16]. Radiation therapy has been attempted as well. In asymptomatic patients, careful observation can result in spontaneous regression [14, 15]. With regard to our patient, he developed hemoptysis 3 months after his repeat lung biopsy. Imaging did not demonstrate progression of nodules, and spirometry remained stable, so close observation was chosen as a reasonable treatment modality.

CD, an inflammatory bowel disease (IBD) characterized by chronic, granulomatous inflammation of the intestines, is associated with many concomitant respiratory ailments, including pulmonary nodules and bronchiectasis. The pulmonary nodules associated with CD are sterile necrobiotic lesions that are generally responsive to corticosteroid therapy [17–20]. However, this is hitherto the first case we know of describing PEH in a patient with IBD. Both MEDLINE and OVID searches for epithelioid hemangioendothelioma, Crohn's disease, ulcerative colitis, and inflammatory bowel disease yielded only one reference. No cases of PEH in the setting of IBD were identified. At least one previous case study has described hepatic epithelioid hemangioendothelioma in association with IBD [5]. Increased levels of vascular endothelial growth factor have been shown to be upregulated in patients with IBD, suggesting increased angiogenesis in the setting of IBD [5]. It may be that chronic increase in inflammatory cytokines prompting increased angiogenesis in the endothelium primes this site as a potential nidus for primary disease [5]. While there is currently insufficient data to fully explore this, further study may shed light on a possible association between chronic inflammatory conditions and this rare endothelial neoplasm.

Disclaimer

The views expressed herein are those of the authors and do not necessarily reflect the official policy or position of the Department of the Navy, Department of Defense, or the U.S. Government.

Conflict of Interests

The authors declare that there is no conflict of interests regarding the publication of this paper.

References

[1] D. Dail and A. Liebow, "Intravascular bronchioalveolar tumor," *The American Journal of Pathology*, vol. 78, no. 1, pp. A6–A7, 1975.

[2] D. H. Dail, A. A. Liebow, J. T. Gmelich et al., "Intravascular, bronchiolar, and alveolar tumor of the lung (IVBAT): an analysis of twenty cases of a peculiar sclerosing endothelial tumor," *Cancer*, vol. 51, no. 3, pp. 452–464, 1983.

[3] S. W. Weiss and F. M. Enzinger, "Epithelioid hemangioendothelioma a vascular tumor often mistaken for a carcinoma," *Cancer*, vol. 50, no. 5, pp. 970–981, 1982.

[4] D. Rosengarten, M. R. Kramer, G. Amir, L. Fuks, and N. Berkman, "Pulmonary epithelioid hemangioendothelioma," *The Israel Medical Association Journal*, vol. 13, no. 11, pp. 676–679, 2011.

[5] J. Y. Chang, R. S. Marks, D. M. Nagorney, S. O. Sanderson, and S. Kane, "Ulcerative colitis, infliximab, and hepatic epithelioid hemangioendothelioma: who is to blame? Case report," *Therapeutic Advances in Gastroenterology*, vol. 3, no. 3, pp. 203–206, 2010.

[6] P. Cronin and D. Arenberg, "Pulmonary epithelioid hemangioendothelioma: an unusual case and a review of the literature," *Chest*, vol. 125, no. 2, pp. 789–792, 2004.

[7] M. J. Rock, R. A. Kaufman, T. E. Lobe, S. D. Hensley, and M. L. Moss, "Epithelioid hemangioendothelioma of the lung (intravascular bronchioloalveolar tumor) in a young girl," *Pediatric Pulmonology*, vol. 11, no. 2, pp. 181–186, 1991.

[8] J. Shao and J. Zhang, "Clinicopathological characteristics of pulmonary epithelioid hemangioendothelioma: a report of four cases and review of the literature," *Oncology Letters*, vol. 8, no. 6, pp. 2517–2522, 2014.

[9] Y. Mizuno, H. Iwata, K. Shirahashi, Y. Hirose, and H. Takemura, "Pulmonary epithelioid hemangioendothelioma," *General Thoracic and Cardiovascular Surgery*, vol. 59, no. 4, pp. 297–300, 2011.

[10] T. Anderson, L. Zhang, M. Hameed, V. Rusch, W. D. Travis, and C. R. Antonescu, "Thoracic epithelioid malignant vascular tumors: a clinicopathologic study of 52 cases with emphasis on pathologic grading and molecular studies of WWTR1-CAMTA1 fusions," *The American Journal of Surgical Pathology*, vol. 39, no. 1, pp. 132–139, 2015.

[11] U. Flucke, R. J. C. Vogels, N. de Saint Aubain Somerhausen et al., "Epithelioid Hemangioendothelioma: clinicopathologic, immunhistochemical, and molecular genetic analysis of 39 cases," *Diagnostic Pathology*, vol. 9, no. 1, p. 131, 2014.

[12] V. Wiwanitkit, "CAMTA1 immunostaining is not useful in differentiating epithelioid hemangioendothelioma from its potential mimickers," *Turkish Journal of Pathology*, vol. 31, no. 1, p. 80, 2014.

[13] S. Y. Ha, I. H. Choi, J. Han et al., "Pleural epithelioid hemangioendothelioma harboring CAMTA1 rearrangement," *Lung Cancer*, vol. 83, no. 3, pp. 411–415, 2014.

[14] P. Bagan, M. Hassan, F. L. P. Barthes et al., "Prognostic factors and surgical indications of pulmonary epithelioid hemangioendothelioma: a review of the literature," *The Annals of Thoracic Surgery*, vol. 82, no. 6, pp. 2010–2013, 2006.

[15] C. Celikel, P. F. Yumuk, G. Basaran, B. Yildizeli, N. Kodalli, and R. Ahiskali, "Epithelioid hemangioendothelioma with multiple organ involvement," *APMIS*, vol. 115, no. 7, pp. 881–888, 2007.

[16] D. Márquez-Medina, J. C. Samamé-Pérez-Vargas, N. Tuset-DerAbrain, A. Montero-Fernández, T. Taberner-Bonastre, and J. M. Porcel, "Pleural epithelioid hemangioendothelioma in an elderly patient. A case report and review of the literature," *Lung Cancer*, vol. 73, no. 1, pp. 116–119, 2011.

[17] R. Golpe, A. Mateos, J. Pérez-Valcárcel, J. A. Lapeña, R. García-Figueiras, and J. Blanco, "Multiple pulmonary nodules in a patient with Crohn's disease," *Respiration*, vol. 70, no. 3, pp. 306–309, 2003.

[18] B. A. Nelson, J. L. Kaplan, C. M. El Saleeby et al., "Case 39-2014: a 9-year-old girl with crohn's disease and pulmonary nodules," *The New England Journal of Medicine*, vol. 371, no. 25, pp. 2418–2427, 2014.

[19] G. Warwick, T. Leecy, E. Silverstone, S. Rainer, R. Feller, and D. H. Yates, "Pulmonary necrobiotic nodules: a rare extraintestinal manifestation of crohn's disease," *European Respiratory Review*, vol. 18, no. 111, pp. 47–50, 2009.

[20] B. Basseri, P. Enayati, A. Marchevsky, and K. A. Papadakis, "Pulmonary manifestations of inflammatory bowel disease: case presentations and review," *Journal of Crohn's and Colitis*, vol. 4, no. 4, pp. 390–397, 2010.

Cardiac Tamponade Associated with the Presentation of Anaplastic Large Cell Lymphoma in a 2-Year-Old Child

Gema Mira-Perceval Juan,[1] Pedro J. Alcalá Minagorre,[1] Ana M. Huertas Sánchez,[1] Sheila Segura Sánchez,[1] Silvia López Iniesta,[2] Francisco J. De León Marrero,[3] Estela Costa Navarro,[4] and María Niveiro de Jaime[4]

[1]Department of Pediatrics, University General Hospital of Alicante, C/Pintor Baeza 12, 03010 Alicante, Spain
[2]Department of Pediatric Hematology and Oncology, University General Hospital of Alicante, C/Pintor Baeza 12, 03010 Alicante, Spain
[3]Department of Dermatology, University General Hospital of Alicante, C/Pintor Baeza 12, 03010 Alicante, Spain
[4]Department of Pathological Anatomy, University General Hospital of Alicante, C/Pintor Baeza 12, 03010 Alicante, Spain

Correspondence should be addressed to Gema Mira-Perceval Juan; gema.mpj@gmail.com

Academic Editor: Denis A. Cozzi

The anaplastic large cell lymphoma is a rare entity in pediatric patients. We present an unusual case of pericardial involvement, quite uncommon as extranodal presentation of this type of disorder, that provoked a life-risk situation requiring an urgent pericardiocentesis. To our knowledge, this is the first report on a child with pericardial involvement without an associated cardiac mass secondary to anaplastic large cell lymphoma in pediatric age. We report the case of a 21-month-old Caucasian male infant with cardiac tamponade associated with the presentation of anaplastic large cell lymphoma. Initially, the child presented with 24-day prolonged fever syndrome, cutaneous lesions associated with hepatomegaly, inguinal adenopathies, and pneumonia. After a 21-day asymptomatic period, polypnea and tachycardia were detected in a clinical check-up. Chest X-ray revealed a remarkable increase of the cardiothoracic index. The anaplastic large cell lymphoma has a high incidence of extranodal involvement but myocardial or pericardial involvements are rare. For this reason, we recommend a close monitoring of patients with a differential diagnosis of anaplastic large cell lymphoma.

1. Introduction

The anaplastic large cell lymphoma (ALCL) is a rare entity in pediatric patients. It represents approximately 10% of lymphomas in children [1] and it is included in the non-Hodgkin lymphomas group according to the 2008 WHO classification [2]. Two entities are identified according to clinical and molecular criteria, the primary cutaneous anaplastic large cell lymphoma (c-ALCL) and the primary systemic anaplastic large cell lymphoma (s-ALCL), which is divided into 2 subtypes according to the expression of the anaplastic lymphoma kinase (ALK) [2].

Up to 70% of the pediatric patients with s-ALCL present with a disseminated stage of the disease at diagnosis [3]. Constitutional symptoms and signs appear quite often: fever,

asthenia, anorexia, and weight loss. This lymphoma has a high incidence of extranodal involvement and it is the pediatric lymphoma with the highest skin affinity. The central nervous system (CNS), lungs, bone marrow, spleen, and liver may also be involved. Cases of ALCL with myocardial [4] or pericardial [5] involvement are rare. To the best of our knowledge, this is the first report on a child with pericardial involvement without an associated cardiac mass secondary to ALCL in pediatric age.

2. Case Presentation

A 21-month-old baby with a 24-day prolonged fever syndrome, cutaneous lesions associated with hepatomegaly, inguinal adenopathies, and pneumonia located in the middle

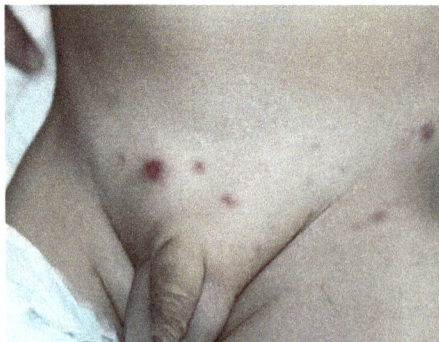

FIGURE 1: Papulosquamous lesions located in the inguinal region.

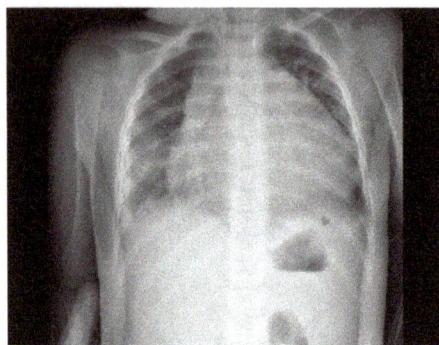

FIGURE 2: Chest X-ray. Increase of the cardiothoracic index at the time of diagnosis of cardiac tamponade. The patient had a normal chest X-ray 10 days before.

lobe with a small pleural effusion was admitted to our centre. Cutaneous lesions were papulosquamous and located in the inguinal region and trunk (Figure 1).

Initially, amoxicillin-clavulanate therapy was administered. An expectant attitude was adopted before the pleural effusion due to its small size. The patient progressed favorably in the short run; he was afebrile within 24 hours; respiratory involvement was less severe; in the following days, cutaneous lesions progressively disappeared and adenopathies were reduced.

Complete blood count, blood culture, and the tuberculin skin test did not show pathologic results. Peripheral blood studies did not report atypical cells. The serum test showed a weak positive IgM for *Chlamydia pneumoniae*. However, due to the cutaneous lesions and the history of prolonged febrile syndrome, a lymphoproliferative disorder was considered as possible diagnosis. A biopsy of the cutaneous lesions was performed for anatomopathological and immunohistochemical analysis. Chest X-ray showed disappearance of the lobe consolidation and the pleural effusion 2 weeks after admission. Before the clinical stability, the patient was discharged and followed ambulatory care.

After a 21-day asymptomatic period, polypnea and tachycardia were detected in a clinical check-up. Chest X-ray revealed a remarkable increase of the cardiothoracic index (Figure 2). The echocardiographic study showed a massive

pericardial effusion causing cardiac tamponade. A pericardiocentesis was performed to drain 180 mL of serohematic fluid.

The pericardial fluid analysis showed infiltration due to anaplastic lymphoma CD30+. Cutaneous biopsy revealed a CD30+, ALK+ lymphoproliferative process (Figure 3). Cutaneous and pericardial involvement in addition to the prolonged fever history and the likely respiratory involvement led to the diagnosis of anaplastic lymphoma s-ALCL, ALK+ stage IV-B. Assessment of tumor extension (CT scan, bone marrow aspiration, abdominal ultrasound, pulmonary CT angiography, head MRI, and CSF analysis) did not show other affected organs.

Chemotherapy treatment was administered according to ALCL international protocol (2003) high risk subgroup. It consisted of an initial cytoreductive phase followed by 6 cycles (AM/BM) administered alternately every 21 days.

Twelve months after completion of therapy, the patient has progressed favorably without evidence of residual disease.

3. Discussion

Diagnosis of systemic ALCL is based on morphological (large cells with a kidney-shaped eccentric nucleus), immunohistochemical, and genetic criteria [6]. ALK protein is overexpressed when translocation occurs (2;5) (p23;q35) and has been described in more than 80% of ALCL cases in children. Positive ALK lymphomas have a better prognosis than negative ALK lymphomas [7]. Protein expression is normally found by immunohistochemical techniques in the tumor cells of the CD30 antigen, the epithelial membrane antigen (EMA), and the interleukin-2 receptor (CD25).

Neoplastic cells in c-ALCL rarely express ALK and a spontaneous resolution is produced in up to 40% of cases. Thus, primary c-ALCL may be difficult to distinguish from lymphomatoid papulosis (LyP) clinically and histologically. Both entities are rare in children. Isolated or multiple lesions concentrated on an anatomic region suggest a c-ALCL, whereas the disseminated lesions are more common in the LyP [8]. The difference between c-ALCL and LyP may be difficult in clinical practice, because they are clinically, histologically, and immunohistologically similar and even some authors consider them as spectrum within the same disorder [9]. Moreover, distinguishing between systemic and primary cutaneous ALCL may be complicated [10], especially at an initial stage.

In our case, diagnosis was difficult at an early stage due to the self-limited character of the pulmonary process and the initial clinical improvement. Due to the lack of biological sample, it could not be established whether the lobe consolidation and the effusion were related to the extranodal involvement that occurs in 10% of cases or it was a recurrent infectious process (weak positive IgM for *Chlamydia pneumoniae*). Diagnosis was precipitated by the appearance of cardiac tamponade and the cytologic and immunohistochemical findings of the pericardial fluid together with the final results of the cutaneous biopsy.

Pericardial involvement is quite uncommon as extranodal presentation of s-ALCL, but it may provoke a life-risk

(a) H&E, 40x: dermis with dense cellular infiltrate

(b) H&E, 400x: at high magnification, the infiltrate shows histiocytes, lymphocytes, and atypical large cells with a kidney-shaped eccentric nucleus

(c) Immunohistochemistry: large cells show cytoplasmic CD30 staining

(d) Immunohistochemistry: nuclear and cytoplasmic ALK staining

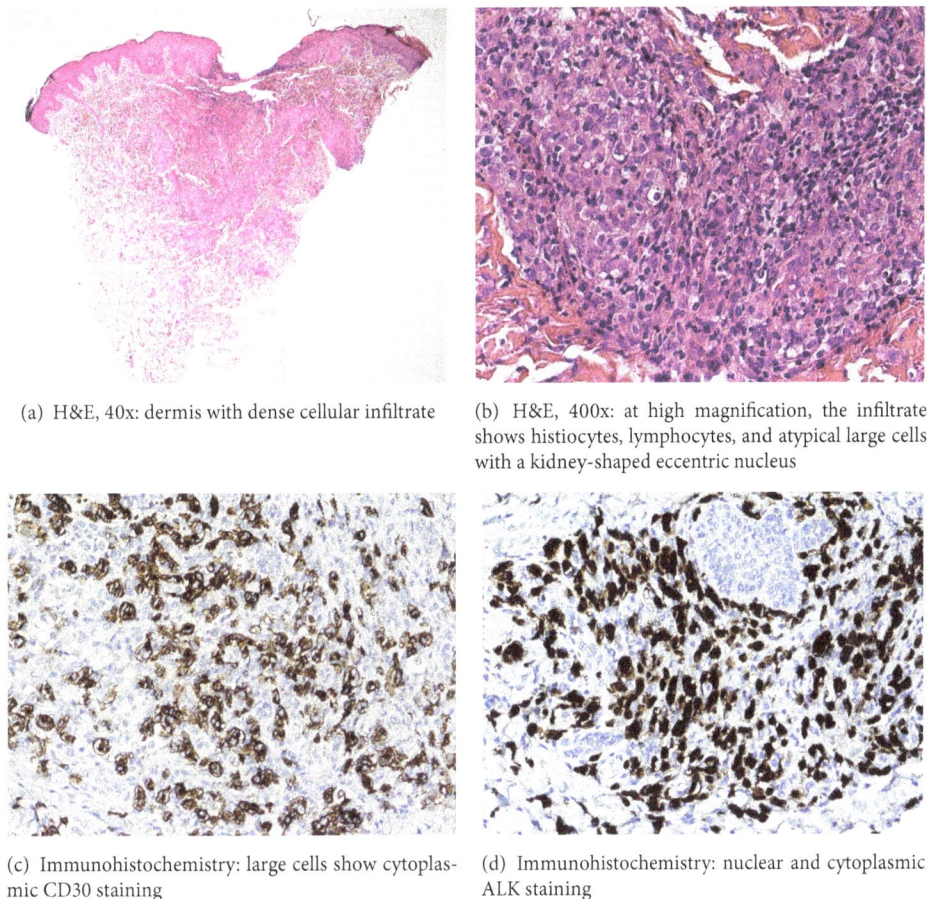

FIGURE 3: Skin biopsy.

situation requiring an urgent pericardiocentesis, as was the case in our patient. For this reason, we recommend a close monitoring of patients with a differential diagnosis of CD30+ lymphoproliferative disorder.

Abbreviations

ALCL: Anaplastic large cell lymphoma
ALK: Anaplastic lymphoma kinase
CNS: Central nervous system
c-ALCL: Primary cutaneous anaplastic large cell lymphoma
EMA: Epithelial membrane antigen
LyP: Lymphomatoid papulosis
s-ALCL: Systemic anaplastic large cell lymphoma.

Consent

Additional informed consent was obtained from their patient and any accompanying images.

Disclosure

The authors would of course be ready to provide further information about their clinical data.

Conflict of Interests

The authors declare that there is no conflict of interests regarding the publication of this paper.

Authors' Contribution

All the authors have contributed sufficiently to the scientific work and therefore share collective responsibility.

References

[1] O. M. E. Sánchez, A. H. Hernández, and T. A. García, "Linfoma anaplásico de células grandes endobronquial en la infancia," *Anales de Pediatría*, vol. 70, no. 5, pp. 449–452, 2009.

[2] S. Swerdlow, E. Campo, N. Harris et al., *IARC WHO Classification of Tumours of Haematopoietic and Lymphoid Tissues*, IARC Press, Lyon, France, 4th edition, 2008.

[3] E. J. Lowe and T. G. Gross, "Anaplastic large cell lymphoma in children and adolescents," *Pediatric Hematology and Oncology*, vol. 30, no. 6, pp. 509–519, 2013.

[4] M. Lauten, S. Vieth, C. Hart et al., "Cardiac anaplastic large cell lymphoma in an 8-year old boy," *Leukemia Research Reports*, vol. 3, no. 2, pp. 36–37, 2014.

[5] P. Muthusamy, S. Ebrom, S. D. Cohle, and N. Khan, "Pericardial involvement as an initial presentation of anaplastic large cell

lymphoma," *Canadian Family Physician*, vol. 60, no. 7, pp. 638–641, 2014.

[6] L. J. Medeiros and K. S. J. Elenitoba-Johnson, "Anaplastic large cell lymphoma," *American Journal of Clinical Pathology*, vol. 127, no. 5, pp. 707–722, 2007.

[7] W. Kempf, K. Pfaltz, M. H. Vermeer et al., "EORTC, ISCL, and USCLC consensus recommendations for the treatment of primary cutaneous CD30-positive lymphoproliferative disorders: lymphomatoid papulosis and primary cutaneous anaplastic large-cell lymphoma," *Blood*, vol. 118, no. 15, pp. 4024–4035, 2011.

[8] R. Willemze, E. S. Jaffe, G. Burg et al., "WHO-EORTC classification for cutaneous lymphomas," *Blood*, vol. 105, no. 10, pp. 3768–3785, 2005.

[9] L. Calzado-Villarreal, I. Polo-Rodríguez, and P. L. Ortiz-Romero, "Primary cutaneous CD30$^+$ lymphoproliferative disorders," *Actas Dermo-Sifiliograficas*, vol. 101, no. 2, pp. 119–128, 2010.

[10] H. Stein, H.-D. Foss, H. Durkop et al., "CD30$^+$ anaplastic large cell lymphoma: a review of its histopathologic, genetic, and clinical features," *Blood*, vol. 96, no. 12, pp. 3681–3695, 2000.

Cystic Fibrosis in a Female Infant with Cardiac, Ocular, and Musculoskeletal Anomalies

Azhar Farooqui,[1] **Susan Gamal Eldin,**[2] **Muna Dawood Ali,**[2]
Ali AlTalhi,[2] **and Ahmad AlDigheari**[2]

[1]*College of Medicine, Alfaisal University, Riyadh 11533, Saudi Arabia*
[2]*Department of Pediatrics, Security Forces Hospital, Riyadh 12625, Saudi Arabia*

Correspondence should be addressed to Azhar Farooqui; afarooqui@alfaisal.edu

Academic Editor: John B. Amodio

Cystic fibrosis (CF) remains the most common hereditary disease in the western population. Its concomitant presence with other congenital abnormalities is a rare phenomenon with very little documentation. In this case report we describe a case of cystic fibrosis in a female infant with cardiac, ocular, and musculoskeletal abnormalities. A brief literature review is also provided.

1. Introduction

Cystic fibrosis remains as the commonest hereditary disorder in the western population. The incidence of this autosomal recessive disorder has been estimated to be around 1 in 4100 live births in the United States [1]. Pulmonary symptoms are often the mode of presentation at the time of diagnosis with up to 95% of the affected patients observed to have recurrent pulmonary infections [2]. Gastrointestinal complications are a common finding; pancreatic insufficiency remains the commonest reported complication. Diagnosis of cystic fibrosis before the age of 14 years has been associated with a greater risk of pancreatic exocrine insufficiency [3].

Association of cystic fibrosis with other diseases or congenital anomalies is rare. In Saudi Arabia, only a few of these associations including sickle cell anemia, Ehler-Danlos syndrome (EDS), insulin dependent diabetes mellitus, and congenital adrenal hyperplasia have been documented from a single center experience [4]. In this case report, the authors describe a case of cystic fibrosis with multiple cardiac, ocular, and musculoskeletal abnormalities. A brief literature review is also presented.

2. Case

A 3-month-old baby girl presented to our emergency department (ER) with cough, shortness of breath, and difficulty in breathing as noticed by the mother. The baby is a product of spontaneous pregnancy, delivered at full-term via cesarean section at her local hospital due to breech presentation. The baby was admitted in the neonatal intensive care unit (NICU) of her local hospital immediately after delivery due to possibility of perinatal asphyxia; however, she was discharged in stable condition without complications. Further history revealed that the patient was admitted to her local hospital at the age of one month as a case of bronchiolitis, received supportive therapy, and was discharged in stable condition.

Upon presentation to our ER, patient was vitally stable with 98% oxygen saturation on room air; weight was 2.56 kg (<5th percentile), head circumference 32 cm (<5th percentile), and height 52 cm (<5th percentile). Cardiac examination demonstrated preserved 1st and 2nd heart sounds with a pan-systolic murmur at the left sternal border. Chest examination revealed decreased air entry bilaterally, with bilateral crepitation. Central nervous system examination demonstrated generalized hypotonia (upper limbs greater than lower limbs) with presence of head lag. The patient had blue sclera with left eye esotropia (Figure 1), thin ears, arched palate, and depressed nasal bridge. There was a significant pectus excavatum (Figure 2). Also appreciated was a transparent appearing skin with extremely prominent scalp veins. There was increased elasticity in the skin over the chest (2-3 cm) and increased mobility in the thumb with

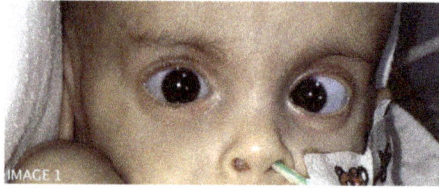

FIGURE 1: An image of the patient to demonstrate the blue sclera and left eye esotropia.

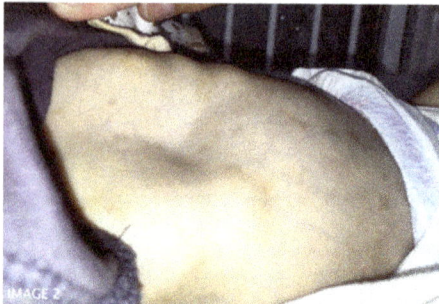

FIGURE 2: An image of the patient demonstrating pectus excavatum.

a positive thumbs sign. However, there was no other joint laxity or hypermobility in axial or other peripheral joints. Patient was admitted as a case of community acquired pneumonia and failure to thrive. Appropriate antibiotics and supportive managements were initiated.

Blood work-up demonstrated a positive nasopharyngeal culture for *Pseudomonas aeruginosa*. Sweat chloride test was carried out which was positive in two different sets with results 90 and 137 mmol/L, respectively (range 3–60 mmol/L). Stool test for pancreatic elastase demonstrated exocrine pancreas insufficiency. Chromosomal study was unremarkable. Blood samples were sent for mutations in cystic fibrosis genes to the United States, which were negative. However, the diagnosis of cystic fibrosis could not be ruled out due to lack of data on the sensitivity of the genetic study in the Saudi population, with the laboratory suggesting a clinical correlation. A diagnosis of cystic fibrosis was made after careful review of the patient's history and clinical presentation, positive sweat chloride tests, signs of pancreatic insufficiency, and multiple bouts of upper respiratory infections growing *Pseudomonas aeruginosa* on blood cultures.

Echocardiogram demonstrated bicuspid aortic valve with mild to moderate aortic stenosis, dilated ascending aorta, dilated superior vena cava, mild left ventricular hypertrophy, and a moderate restrictive patent ductus arteriosus with left to right shunt (PDA). Ultrasound of the brain, ultrasound of the abdomen, and CT scan of the brain were all unremarkable.

The patient was discharged home in a stable condition with pancreatic amylase supplementation, vitamin supplementation, fluticasone and Ventolin inhalers, and prophylactic antibiotics with close outpatient follow-up.

3. Discussion

Acute cardiac failure in pathologic myocardial fibrosis often characterizes cardiac involvement of cystic fibrosis in infants. Cor pulmonale as a result of chronic hypoxemia with resultant effect on the pulmonary vasculature is the dominant and a more serious presentation of cardiac involvement in older affected individuals [5, 6]. However, there is very little documentation regarding congenital cardiac anomalies in patients with cystic fibrosis and their effect in the prognosis of these patients [4]. From the Arab population, only Banjar and Mogarri [7] have reported a single case of twins affected by cystic fibrosis with concomitant cardiac anomalies; one sibling was affected by an atrial septal defect, which was treated surgically, while the other sibling was affected by a ventricular septal defect which closed spontaneously. In our case, there is a bicuspid aortic valve with mild to moderate stenosis of the aortic valve. Also associated is a PDA with left to right shunt, which may accelerate cardiac dysfunction in such cases. Ascending aortic dilatation may be explained by an underlying collagen defect as described below.

Although extremely rare, collagen fiber disorders such as EDS have also been reported to occur in patients with cystic fibrosis. To date, there are only two published studies describing cases of cystic fibrosis with classical concomitant presentation of EDS. One was an association of type 6 (kyphoscoliosis type) where two siblings from consanguineous Turkish parents were observed to have marfanoid habitus, generalized hypotonia, progressive kyphoscoliosis, and joint dislocations [8]. The other case had type 3 (hypermobility type) EDS with hypermobility of all joints and elastic skin [4]. In our case there is an element of possible collagen defect disorder though it does not fit the typical clinical criteria for the 10 different types described in the literature. The patient had blue sclera, which is a feature of the rare spondylocheirodysplasia EDS [9]. The patient also had pectus excavatum, generalized hypotonia, prominent scalp veins, and thin, stretchable skin. However, apart from hypermobility in the thumb joints, with a positive thumbs sign, there was no joint laxity in other axial or other distal joints.

The incidence of cystic fibrosis in the Saudi population has been estimated to be around 1 : 4200 live births [10]. It has been associated with various other anomalies in the Saudi population. Banjar [4] described an association of cystic fibrosis with sickle cell disease, insulin dependent diabetes mellitus, and congenital adrenal hyperplasia. No other publications can be found in the literature to demonstrate association of congenital anomalies with cystic fibrosis in the Arab population.

Conflict of Interests

The authors declare that there is no conflict of interests regarding the publication of this paper.

References

[1] S. C. FitzSimmons, "The changing epidemiology of cystic fibrosis," *The Journal of Pediatrics*, vol. 122, no. 1, pp. 1–9, 1993.

[2] I. Durieu, G. Bellon, D. Vital Durand, L. Calemard, Y. Morel, and R. Gilly, "Cystic fibrosis in adults," *Presse Médicale*, vol. 24, no. 39, pp. 1882–1887, 1995.

[3] I. Modolell, A. Alvarez, L. Guarner, J. De Gracia, and J.-R. Malagelada, "Gastrointestinal, liver, and pancreatic involvement in adult patients with cystic fibrosis," *Pancreas*, vol. 22, no. 4, pp. 395–399, 2001.

[4] H. H. Banjar, "Cystic fibrosis: presentation with other diseases, the experience in Saudi Arabia," *Journal of Cystic Fibrosis*, vol. 2, no. 3, pp. 155–159, 2003.

[5] G. Chéron, K. Paradis, D. Stéru, G. Demay, and G. Lenoir, "Cardiac involvement in cystic fibrosis revealed by a ventricular arrhythmia," *Acta Paediatrica Scandinavica*, vol. 73, no. 5, pp. 697–700, 1984.

[6] A. J. Moss, "The cardiovascular system in cystic fibrosis," *Pediatrics*, vol. 70, no. 5, pp. 728–741, 1982.

[7] H. Banjar and I. Mogarri, "Twins and cystic fibrosis: a case report and review of the literature," *Current Pediatric Research*, vol. 5, no. 1-2, pp. 11–17, 2001.

[8] A. Jarisch, C. Giunta, S. Zielen, R. König, and B. Steinmann, "Sibs affected with both Ehlers-Danlos syndrome type VI and cystic fibrosis," *American Journal of Medical Genetics*, vol. 78, no. 5, pp. 455–460, 1998.

[9] F. Malfait, D. Syx, P. Vlummens et al., "Musculocontractural Ehlers-Danlos Syndrome (former EDS type VIB) and adducted thumb clubfoot syndrome (ATCS) represent a single clinical entity caused by mutations in the dermatan-4-sulfotransferase 1 encoding CHST14 gene," *Human Mutation*, vol. 31, no. 11, pp. 1233–1239, 2010.

[10] H. Nazer, E. Riff, N. Sakati, R. Mathew, M. A. Majeed-Saidan, and H. Harfi, "Cystic fibrosis in Saudi Arabia," *European Journal of Pediatrics*, vol. 148, no. 4, pp. 330–332, 1989.

Postdural Puncture Superior Sagittal Sinus Thrombosis in a Juvenile Case of Clinically Isolated Syndrome

Miriam Michel,[1] **Edda Haberlandt,**[1] **Matthias Baumann,**[1] **Andreas Entenmann,**[1] **Michaela Wagner,**[2] **and Kevin Rostasy**[3]

[1]*Department of Pediatrics, Medical University of Innsbruck, Anichstrasse 35, 6020 Innsbruck, Austria*
[2]*Department of Neuroradiology, Medical University of Innsbruck, Anichstrasse 35, 6020 Innsbruck, Austria*
[3]*Medical University of Witten/Herdecke, Department of Neuropediatrics, Dr.-Friedrich-Steiner Strasse 5, 45711 Datteln, Germany*

Correspondence should be addressed to Miriam Michel; miriam.michel@i-med.ac.at

Academic Editor: Albert M. Li

Background. The causes of cerebral venous thrombosis (CVT) are manifold as is its clinical presentation. *Case.* We report the case of a CVT following lumbar puncture and intravenous glucocorticosteroid therapy in a female adolescent with a clinically isolated syndrome and risk factors for thrombosis. *Conclusion.* In adolescent patients with acute inflammatory disease undergoing lumbar puncture followed by intravenous high-dose glucocorticosteroid therapy, one should be aware of the elevated risk for thrombosis. A persistent headache with change in the headache pattern and loss of a postural component might be a sign for CVT, requiring emergency imaging of the brain.

1. Introduction

The causes of cerebral venous thrombosis (CVT) in children and adults are manifold as is its clinical presentation. In children, CVT is observed at any age with a higher incidence in neonates [1]. We report the case of a CVT following lumbar puncture and intravenous glucocorticosteroid therapy in a female adolescent with a clinically isolated syndrome and risk factors for thrombosis.

2. Clinical Presentation

A 17-year-old female with a prior medical history of idiopathic focal epilepsy with EEG continuous spike-and-wave during slow sleep (CSWSS), treated with sultiame for the last five years, and mild cognitive developmental delay presented with an unprovoked seizure during which she sustained a mild head trauma. A few days later her right arm and right leg felt "strange," and she was unable to move her right body properly. Moreover, her parents noticed that she was slightly aggressive and that she was speaking less clearly. She was brought to the local hospital where an intracerebral haemorrhage was excluded by cranial computed tomography scan. She was referred to our clinic for further assessment and management. Neurological examination revealed a right-sided hemiplegia and a mild dysarthria. She further had a bilateral resting tremor worsening on finger-nose testing. Routine laboratory testing (complete blood cell count, electrolytes, protein, and liver and renal function parameters) was normal. There was no sign of systemic infection.

Cerebral magnetic resonance imaging (MRI) showed four supratentorial white matter lesions of high signal intensity in T2 and FLAIR enhancement in T1, the largest of them located in the posterior limb of the left-sided internal capsule and central region, and smaller lesions in the left temporal, right frontal, and right parietal region. Two lesions revealed contrast-medium enhancement (Figures 1(a), 1(b), and 1(d)). The venogram was completely normal without any evidence of poor flow, asymmetry, or stenoses of the sinuses.

A spinal MRI did not reveal any lesions. A lumbar puncture was conducted with a traumatic needle, revealing normal cerebral spinal fluid (CSF) pressure and normal total protein level. White cell count was elevated ($14/\mu L$), and numerous additional CSF oligoclonal IgG bands were

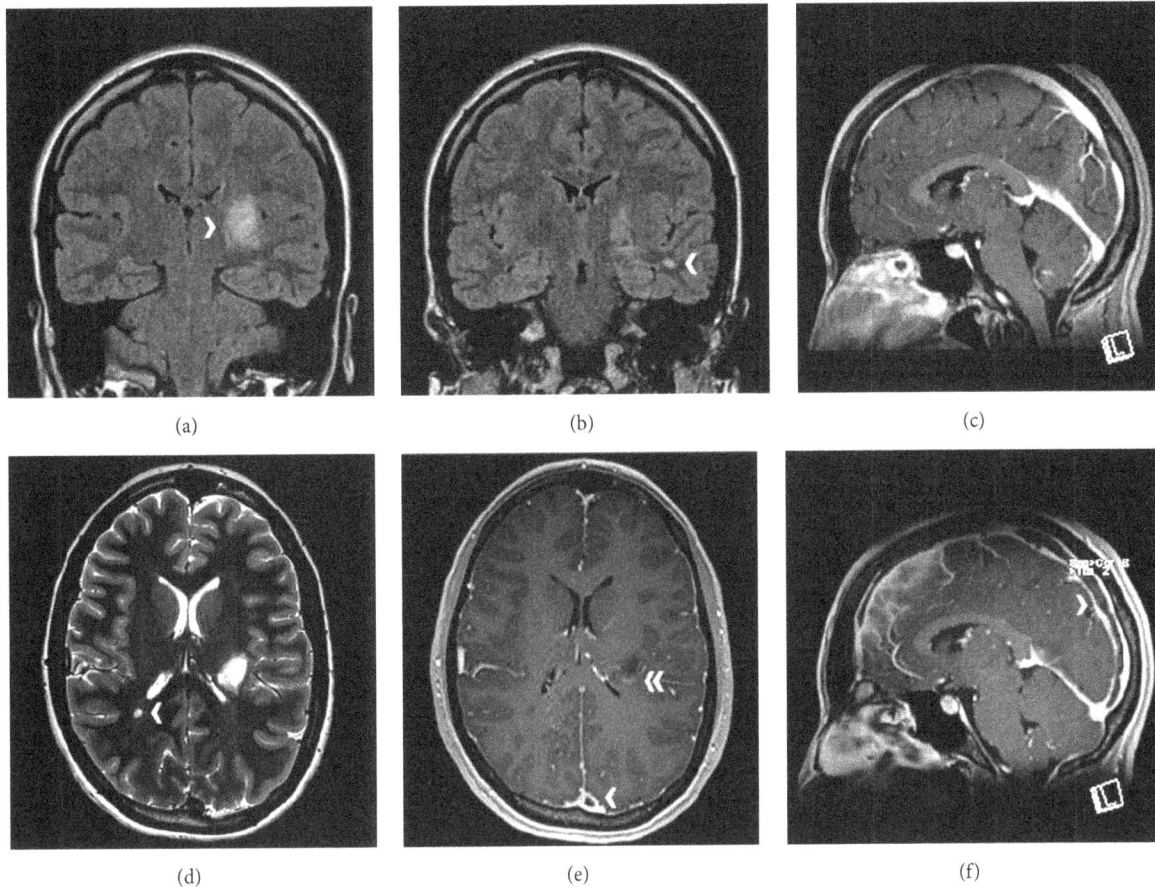

Figure 1: The magnetic resonance imaging of the patient reveals a large hyperintense lesion on FLAIR (a) and T2 (d) in the posterior limb of the left-sided internal capsule, probably extending to the thalamus. The other supratentorial lesions are much smaller (in the right occipital (d) and left temporal white matter ((b) FLAIR)). In the initial imaging the blood flow in the sagittal sinus was free ((c) gadolinium (Gd) enhanced T1w). 8 days later the white matter lesions were unchanged ((d) T2w, arrowhead pointing out a small lesion behind the occipital horn of the right ventricle) and some lesions were still Gd enhancing ((e) double arrowhead, Gd enhanced T1w). But now a thrombosis of the superior sagittal sinus can be seen ((e), (f) arrowheads, Gd enhanced T1w).

identified. Bacteriological findings were negative. Based on the aforementioned findings a diagnosis of a clinical isolated syndrome was made and the patient was treated with intravenous methylprednisolone pulse therapy (1 g daily) administered for five days [2, 3]. On the fourth day of steroid treatment, she developed severe and continuous frontotemporal headache, vertigo, and vomiting. The headache did not have any postural component and was unresponsive to intravenous analgesics. At first, these symptoms were assigned to the lumbar puncture and the steroid treatment. Because of persisting headache, a second cerebral MRI was performed showing a thrombosis of the superior sagittal sinus. There were no signs of venous congestion edema and no new white matter lesions (Figures 1(d)–1(f)). Anticoagulant treatment was started with low molecular weight heparin intravenously (2 mg/kgBW/d) and Phenprocoumon was introduced, shifting the international normalized ratio ((PT)-INR) to 2-3 [4]. In addition intravenous fluid therapy was administered. Under this therapy, headache and vomiting decreased and vanished within two days and the patient was discharged in good condition after ten days. Both the patient's and the family's thrombophilia history (deep vein thrombosis included)

were negative. The patient's thrombophilia screening revealed normal values for the platelet count, antithrombin III, C and S protein, plasmatic homocysteine, fibrinogen, antinuclear antibodies, lupus anticoagulant, and cardiolipin antibodies. However, our patient carried a heterozygous mutation for factor II G20210A and a rather high lipoprotein A serum level, two factors known to increase the risk for thrombosis. Phenprocoumon therapy was planned for six months. Six weeks later the patient reported that she has had few minor headache episodes but no other symptoms. Her neurological examination was normal apart from the resting tremor of her hands. Ten weeks later the superior sagittal sinus was completely recanalised. The white matter lesion in the posterior limb of the left-sided internal capsule appeared smaller. None of the remaining lesions showed contrast-medium enhancement. There were no new lesions.

3. Discussion

CVT in paediatric patients is seen in various clinical settings such as infection, dehydration, trauma, renal failure, cancer, and haematological disorders [5]. Many children show additional prothrombotic risk factors [6]. In adults with multiple sclerosis CVT has been reported occurring shortly after a diagnostic lumbar puncture followed by intravenous high-dose glucocorticosteroid therapy [7–11], and only recently Presicci et al. reported a paediatric patient [12]. In our case the patient had a history of normal pregnancy, birth, neonatal period, and early childhood without any severe cases of trauma or dehydration [1]. She was not dehydrated during her hospital stay before the incident, nor was she obese, nor did she smoke. She did not take any medication (oral hormonal contraceptives included) other than sultiame which is not known for prothrombotic effects. However, our juvenile female patient was diagnosed with an acute inflammatory disease of the central nervous system and she underwent lumbar puncture followed by high-dose intravenous glucocorticosteroid treatment. Both factors, puncture and glucocorticosteroid treatment, raise the risk for the development of a thrombosis. By using a traumatic needle CSF leakage might appear, which might even be increased under the anti-inflammatory effect of the corticosteroid treatment possibly also inhibiting the reduction of the loss of dural tissue after the puncture. Thus, intracranial hypotension and a "rostrocaudal sagging" effect might be exerted on the intracranial contents. By a negative spinal-cranial pressure gradient, this hypotension might at the same time lead to venous endothelial traumatic damage from stretching of the cerebral vessels or to a stasis of the blood flow via venous dilatation, again possibly provoking the development of a central nervous thrombosis [9, 13]. Another important aspect is the fact that our patient carried a heterozygous mutation for factor II G20210A and a rather high lipoprotein A serum level, two factors known to increase the risk for thrombosis [14, 15]. The importance of hereditary and acquired prothrombotic disorders has been emphasized in recent series of paediatric CVT [1, 6, 12]. In our patient the epilepsy syndrome and the cephalalgia our patient suffered from might be regarded as an additional risk factor in the cascade of CVT [16, 17]. Interestingly, CSWSS is reported to possibly be related to prior sinus venous thrombosis, for example, in the straight sinus leading to thalamic compromise. Even if there is no imaging footprint this might at least subclinically have been the case in our patient. Thus, the episode after the minor head injury might have even been a recurrence [18].

Patient outcome depends on extent and location of cerebral parenchymal damage, haemoglobin, patient age, and the time interval between onset of symptoms and diagnosis and start of treatment. Permanent occlusion of parts of the intracranial venous drainage system, with or without formation of collaterals, may have an unfavourable impact on the developing brain [5]. Moreover, knowledge about prothrombotic factors for recurrence is important. Kenet et al. reported that the heterozygous factor II G20210A mutation, which was present in our patient, is a significant risk factor for recurrence of CVT, while a heterozygous factor V G1691A mutation or a raised lipoprotein(a) is not associated with an increased risk for recurrence [15].

4. Conclusion

In adolescent patients with acute inflammatory disease undergoing lumbar puncture followed by intravenous high-dose glucocorticosteroid therapy one should be aware of the elevated risk for thrombosis. We recommend at least asking for any additional risk factor for thrombosis in patients undergoing this type of diagnostic and treatment and if a patient complains of a persistent headache with change in the headache pattern and loss of a postural component, emergency imaging of the brain is mandatory; otherwise the diagnosis is likely to be missed.

Conflict of Interests

The authors declare that there is no conflict of interests regarding the publication of this paper.

References

[1] G. deVeber, M. Andrew, C. Adams et al., "Cerebral sinovenous thrombosis in children," *The New England Journal of Medicine*, vol. 345, no. 6, pp. 417–423, 2001.

[2] M. Sailer, F. Fazekas, A. Gass et al., "Cerebral and spinal MRI examination in patients with clinically isolated syndrome and definite multiple sclerosis," *RöFo*, vol. 180, no. 11, pp. 994–1001, 2008.

[3] L. B. Krupp, M. Tardieu, M. P. Amato et al., "International Pediatric Multiple Sclerosis Study Group criteria for pediatric multiple sclerosis and immune-mediated central nervous system demyelinating disorders: revisions to the 2007 definitions," *Multiple Sclerosis*, vol. 19, no. 10, pp. 1261–1267, 2013.

[4] K. Einhäupl, J. Stam, M.-G. Bousser et al., "EFNS guideline on the treatment of cerebral venous and sinus thrombosis in adult patients," *European Journal of Neurology*, vol. 17, no. 10, pp. 1229–1235, 2010.

[5] G. Sébire, B. Tabarki, D. E. Saunders et al., "Cerebral venous sinus thrombosis in children: risk factors, presentation, diagnosis and outcome," *Brain*, vol. 128, no. 3, pp. 477–489, 2005.

[6] C. Heller, A. Heinecke, R. Junker et al., "Cerebral venous thrombosis in children: a multifactorial origin," *Circulation*, vol. 108, no. 11, pp. 1362–1367, 2003.

[7] S. Aidi, M.-P. Chaunu, V. Biousse, and M.-G. Bousser, "Changing pattern of headache pointing to cerebral venous thrombosis after lumbar puncture and intravenous high-dose corticosteroids," *Headache*, vol. 39, no. 8, pp. 559–564, 1999.

[8] J. F. Albucher, C. Vuillemin-Azaïs, C. Manelfe, M. Clanet, B. Guiraud-Chaumeil, and F. Chollet, "Cerebral thrombophlebitis in three patients with probable multiple sclerosis. Role of lumbar puncture or intravenous corticosteroid treatment," *Cerebrovascular Diseases*, vol. 9, no. 5, pp. 298–303, 1999.

[9] A. Mouraux, M. Gille, S. Dorban, and A. Peeters, "Cortical venous thrombosis after lumbar puncture," *Journal of Neurology*, vol. 249, no. 9, pp. 1313–1315, 2002.

[10] D. I. Gunal, N. Afsar, N. Tuncer, and S. Aktan, "A case of multiple sclerosis with cerebral venous thrombosis: the role of lumbar puncture and high-dose steroids," *European Neurology*, vol. 47, no. 1, pp. 57–58, 2002.

[11] N. Vandenberghe, M. Debouverie, R. Anxionnat, P. Clavelouc, S. Bouly, and M. Weber, "Cerebral venous thrombosis in four

patients with multiple sclerosis," *European Journal of Neurology*, vol. 10, no. 1, pp. 63–66, 2003.

[12] A. Presicci, V. Garofoli, M. Simone, M. G. Campa, A. L. Lamanna, and L. Margari, "Cerebral venous thrombosis after lumbar puncture and intravenous high dose corticosteroids: a case report of a childhood multiple sclerosis," *Brain and Development*, vol. 35, no. 6, pp. 602–605, 2013.

[13] D. Milhaud, C. Heroum, M. Charif, P. Saulnier, M. Pages, and J. M. Blard, "Dural puncture and corticotherapy as risks factors for cerebral venous sinus thrombosis," *European Journal of Neurology*, vol. 7, no. 1, pp. 123–124, 2000.

[14] G. Lippi, G. Targher, and M. Franchini, "Lipoprotein(a), thrombophilia and venous thrombosis," *Acta Haematologica*, vol. 117, no. 4, pp. 246–247, 2007.

[15] G. Kenet, F. Kirkham, T. Niederstadt et al., "Risk factors for recurrent venous thromboembolism in the European collaborative paediatric database on cerebral venous thrombosis: a multicentre cohort study," *The Lancet Neurology*, vol. 6, no. 7, pp. 595–603, 2007.

[16] E. Wilder-Smith, I. Kothbauer-Margreiter, B. Lämmle, M. Sturzenegger, C. Ozdoba, and S. P. Hauser, "Dural puncture and activated protein C resistance: risk factors for cerebral venous sinus thrombosis," *Journal of Neurology Neurosurgery and Psychiatry*, vol. 63, no. 3, pp. 351–356, 1997.

[17] M. Maurelli, R. Bergamaschi, E. Candeloro, A. Todeschini, and G. Micieli, "Cerebral venous thrombosis and demyelinating diseases: report of a case in a clinically isolated syndrome suggestive of multiple sclerosis onset and review of the literature," *Multiple Sclerosis*, vol. 11, no. 2, pp. 242–244, 2005.

[18] K. J. Kersbergen, L. S. de Vries, F. S. S. Leijten et al., "Neonatal thalamic hemorrhage is strongly associated with electrical status epilepticus in slow wave sleep," *Epilepsia*, vol. 54, no. 4, pp. 733–740, 2013.

9

Paravertebral and Retroperitoneal Vascular Tumour Presenting with Kasabach-Merritt Phenomenon in Childhood, Diagnosed with Magnetic Resonance Imaging

Gonca Keskindemirci,[1] Deniz Tuğcu,[1] Gönül Aydoğan,[1] Arzu Akçay,[2] Nuray Aktay Ayaz,[3] Ali Er,[4] Ensar Yekeler,[5] and Bilge Bilgiç[6]

[1]Department of Pediatric Hematology-Oncology, İstanbul Kanuni Sultan Süleyman Educational and Research Hospital, 34303 Istanbul, Turkey
[2]Department of Pediatric Hematology-Oncology, Faculty of Medicine, Acıbadem University, 34742 Istanbul, Turkey
[3]Department of Pediatric Rheumatology, İstanbul Kanuni Sultan Süleyman Educational and Research Hospital, 34303 Istanbul, Turkey
[4]Department of Radiology, İstanbul Kanuni Sultan Süleyman Educational and Research Hospital, 34303 Istanbul, Turkey
[5]Department of Radiology, İstanbul Faculty of Medicine, İstanbul University, 34093 Istanbul, Turkey
[6]Department of Pathology, İstanbul Faculty of Medicine, İstanbul University, 34093 Istanbul, Turkey

Correspondence should be addressed to Gonca Keskindemirci; keskindemirci@hotmail.com

Academic Editor: Jonathan Muraskas

Kasabach-Merritt phenomenon (KMP) is characterized by vascular tumour and consumptive coagulopathy with life-threatening thrombocytopenia, prolonged prothrombin time and partial thromboplastin time, hypofibrinogenemia, and the presence of high fibrin split products. We report a case of 3-year-old boy with local aggressive vascular lesions associated with KMP. Magnetic resonance imaging revealed an extensive lesion at paravertebral and retroperitoneal regions that was infiltrating vertebrae. Although we did not get any response to steroid or propranolol treatment, partial response was observed radiologically with interferon-alpha treatment. Unfortunately, the patient died because of the uncontrolled consumptive coagulopathy that led to intracranial hemorrhage which was caused by huge knee hematoma after minor trauma.

1. Introduction

Vascular anomalies include a spectrum of disorders from simple lesions to life-threatening entities [1]. Kasabach-Merritt phenomenon is characterized by vascular tumour and consumptive coagulopathy with life-threatening thrombocytopenia, prolonged prothrombin time (PT), and activated partial thromboplastin time (aPTT), hypofibrinogenemia, and the presence of D-dimer and fibrin split products [2]. Kaposiform hemangioendothelioma (KHE) is the responsible lesion most of the time. Mortality rate is around 10–37% [3]. Here, we describe a 3-year-old boy with unusual localization of extensive vascular lesions involving spinal vertebrae from T11 to L5 that caused fatal consumptive coagulopathy.

2. Case

A 3-year-old boy was referred to our hematology clinic because of ecchymosis on the legs and arms for 2 weeks in 2012, July. Medical history was unremarkable. Physical examination revealed ecchymosis on the legs, arms, and back. Muscle atrophy was evident on the upper legs and gluteal region, but there were no vascular lesions on the skin. It was also noted that the child had waddling gait. On the blood count, hemoglobin was 9 gr/dL, leukocyte count was 6100/μL, and platelet count was 7000/μL. On bone marrow examination, megakaryocytes were seen and exclusion of malignant diseases was made. On coagulation study, PT was 38.2 sec, aPTT was 52.4 sec, INR was 4, D-dimer was 2001 mg/dL, and

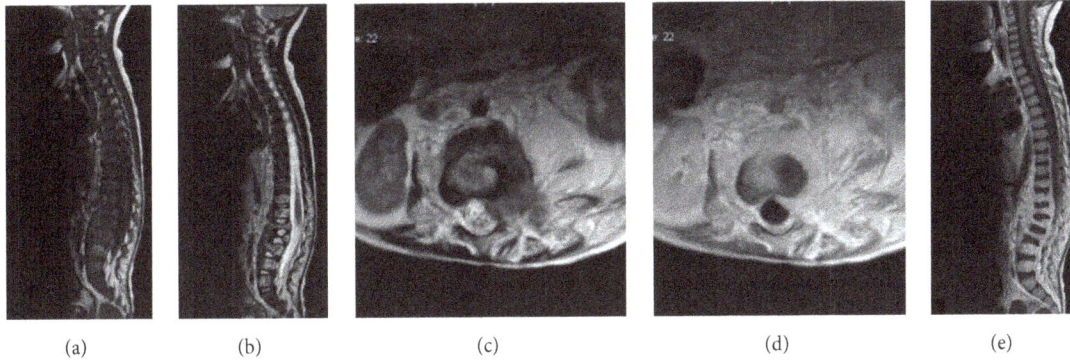

(a)   (b)   (c)   (d)   (e)

Figure 1: Lesion in the retroperitoneal and paravertebral area and infiltrating vertebrae from T11 to L5. Sagittal MR images show intermediate signal intensity on T1-weighted image (a) and high signal intensity on T2-weighted image (b). Transverse MR image shows high signal intensity on T2-weighted image (c). Transverse and sagittal contrast-enhanced T1-weighted images show homogeneous enhancement of the lesions (d-e).

fibrinogen level was 37.7 mg/dL. Abdominal ultrasonography and chest X-ray were normal. Because of the muscle atrophy in the legs and gait disturbance, spinal magnetic resonance imaging (MRI) was taken to exclude neurological problems. Diffusely infiltrating lesion in the paravertebral and retroperitoneal area from T11 to L5 vertebrae with extension into the left side of spinal canal was shown on the lumbar MRI examination. It was variable hypointermediate signal intensity on T1W images and predominantly hyperintense on the T2W images with heterogeneous areas. Postcontrast MRI showed diffuse contrast enhancement of all areas of lesions. The bony structure showed compression on especially central area of L1, L2, and L3 vertebrae corpus, and there was no signal change of the bone marrow of these vertebrae (Figure 1). There was no evidence of any other lesion in the brain or abdomen. With the thrombocytopenia, consumptive coagulopathy, ecchymosis in physical examination, and locally aggressive lesions in the radiologic evaluation, lesion was considered to be vascular lesions, KHE mostly. Prednisolone was started at a dose of 2 mg/kg/day. But, with this treatment, severe thrombocytopenia and abnormal coagulation profile persisted. On the third week, propranolol was added to the treatment at a dose of 2 mg/kg/day. After 2 months of these treatments, clinical, radiological, and laboratory improvements were not observed. To rule out hemangioblastoma, biopsy was taken after the replacement therapies with platelet and fibrinogen infusions. But, just after the surgery, bleeding from the surgical site could not be controlled, and massive amounts of thrombocyte, erythrocyte, fibrinogen, and fresh frozen plasma (FFP) transfusions were needed. Ten hours after the surgery, respiratory distress developed and the patient was transferred to intensive care unit. He was extubated on the sixth day and was taken back to the hematology clinic. Immunohistochemistry staining showed Glut-1 positive erythrocytes in pathological examination and any malign transformation was not detected (Figure 2). Propranolol and corticosteroid treatment did not improve thrombocytopenia and consumptive coagulopathy that was lasting for more than two months; interferon-α (IFN-α) treatment was started at a dose of 3 million U/m^2/day subcutaneously. Steroid and

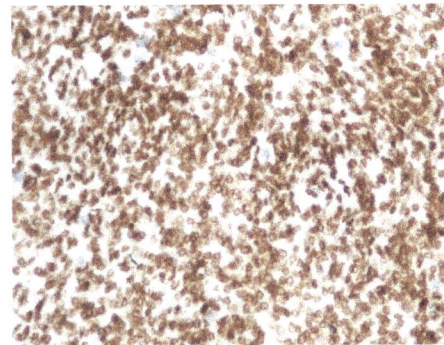

Figure 2: Extensive Glut-1 nuclear positivity in immunohistochemistry staining in biopsy (400x magnification in microscope).

propranolol treatments were stopped by tapering. On the third month of IFN-α treatment, the follow-up MRI showed moderate regression of lesion size, but there was no significant signal change before and after contrast images (Figure 3) and chronic disseminated intravascular coagulopathy symptoms persisted both clinically and in the laboratory tests. On the 4th month of IFN-α treatment, the patient had a minor knee trauma and the next day huge hematoma developed around the knee. Despite thrombocyte, fibrinogen, and FFP transfusions, bleeding in the knee and consumptive coagulopathy could not be kept under control. Two days after this incident, intracranial hemorrhage developed that caused the death of the patient, and while thrombocyte count was 5000/μL, fibrinogen level was 70 mg/dL and PT was 40 sec.

3. Discussion

Kasabach-Merritt phenomenon (KMP) is characterized by consumptive coagulopathy and vascular tumour that can be found in the skin, retroperitoneum, mediastinum, pelvis, visceral organs, and mesentery [2]. With the unexplained thrombocytopenia and consumptive coagulopathy, KMP should be considered. The diagnosis of visceral lesions can be

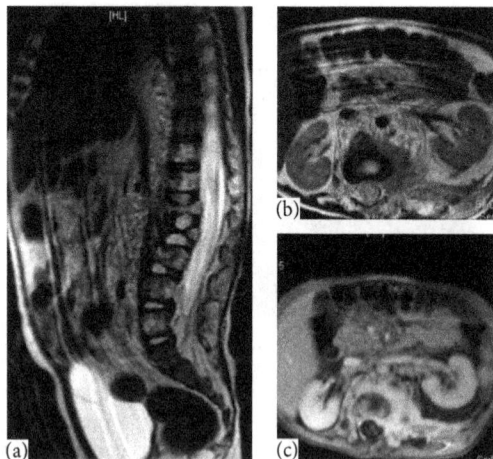

FIGURE 3: Partial response after interferon-α therapy. Sagittal and transverse MR images show high signal intensity on T2-weighted image (a-b). Transverse contrast-enhanced T1-weighted image shows homogeneous enhancement of the lesions (c).

difficult, especially when there are no vascular lesions on the skin. Retroperitoneal lesions are often large, easy to be missed clinically, and generally associated with a higher mortality [4, 5]. In the absence of the typical cutaneous findings, imaging techniques can be used to confirm the diagnosis and to determine the extent of the involvement. MRI is the gold standard technique according to the studies in this field [6, 7]. In our case, the diagnosis was made by radiological findings in MRI and we also used the diagnostic criteria for the consumptive coagulopathy developed by ISTH [8].

It has been recently shown that KMP is complicated with variety of vascular tumours not only with infantile hemangioma but also with KHE and tufted angioma [9]. According to the ISSVA classification, vascular lesions associated with thrombocytopenia and consumptive coagulopathy are KHE mostly [1]. On the light of this knowledge, locally aggressive vascular lesion is considered to be KHE in our case. Although Glut-1 is a unique immunohistochemical marker in endothelial cells in infantile hemangiomas, there is a literature of Glut-1 positive in KHE [1, 10]. In KMP treatment, there are two aims. One is the regression of the lesion and the other is controlling and preventing bleeding from thrombocytopenia and coagulopathy [2, 3]. Several treatment approaches are employed; however, it is unclear which is superior and there are no consensus guidelines for the treatment of KMP. Prednisolone is the first line therapy. Most patients respond to the therapy with a dose of 2-3 mg/kg/day within a few days [4]. Higher doses (5 mg/kg/day) or megadoses (30 mg/kg/day, for 3 days) can also be used [4, 11, 12]. The other option is propranolol treatment with a dose of 2 mg/kg/day. The most important advantages of propranolol over corticosteroids are efficacy, safety, fewer side effects, and low cost. In unresponsive cases, IFN-α is used to treat rapidly growing, life-threatening hemangiomas at a dose of 3 million U/m^2 subcutaneously per day. According to the literature, the success of the IFN-α treatment is 80% and 90% [13]. However, there are some side effects of IFN-α such, as influenza-like symptoms and fever,

somnolence, anorexia, diarrhea or constipation, neutropenia, high level of aminotransferases, and neurotoxicity [8, 13, 14]. Because of this, compared to the corticosteroids and propranolol, IFN-α should be used for proliferative hemangiomas as a second line therapy. There is currently no consensus on the second line management of KHE that was resistant to prednisone, propranolol, and IFN-α [15]. If there is no response to these therapies, cyclophosphamide, vincristine, pentoxifylline, ticlopidine, platelet derived growth factor, and imiquimod can be used [2, 4, 16]. Radiotherapy is an option for life-threatening hemangiomas, but, as it can cause secondary tumors, its use should be evaluated for its safety and efficacy [17, 18]. Surgical excision of hemangiomas is suggested only for cases involving eyelid or huge scalp hemangiomas [16]. Platelet transfusions should only be used when bleeding cannot be controlled or before surgical procedures. Everolimus or sirolimus, an inhibitor of the mammalian target of rapamycin (mTOR), was successfully used recently in the treatment of KHE [15]. Prognosis of KMP is related to lesion's location, size, and depth of invasion.

In our case, with corticosteroid and propranolol therapy, we did not get any response in clinical, radiological, and laboratory parameters. With IFN-α treatment, partial response was seen radiologically and the patient died under IFN-α treatment. Similar to our case, Hatley et al. were treated from a giant vascular tumour at the retroperitoneal lesion with IFN-α [19]. To the best of our knowledge, this is the first childhood vascular tumour with extensive involvement of paravertebral and retroperitoneal area and vertebral corpus diagnosed with MRI that responded partially to the IFN-α treatment radiologically. We also emphasize the importance of radiologic evaluation at the differential diagnosis of thrombocytopenia and consumptive coagulopathy without any visible etiological lesion in the skin.

Conflict of Interests

The authors declare that there is no conflict of interests regarding the publication of this paper.

References

[1] M. Wassef, F. Blei, D. Adams et al., "Vascular anomalies classification: recommendations from the International Society for the Study of Vascular Anomalies," *Pediatrics*, vol. 136, pp. 203–214, 2015.

[2] S. Wananukul, I. Nuchprayoon, and P. Seksarn, "Treatment of Kasabach-Merritt syndrome: a stepwise regimen of prednisolone, dipyridamole, and interferon," *International Journal of Dermatology*, vol. 42, no. 9, pp. 741–748, 2003.

[3] M. Kwok-Williams, Z. Perez, R. Squire, A. Glaser, S. Bew, and R. Taylor, "Radiotherapy for life-threatening mediastinal hemangioma with Kasabach-Merritt syndrome," *Pediatric Blood and Cancer*, vol. 49, no. 5, pp. 739–744, 2007.

[4] G. W. Hall, "Kasabach-Merritt syndrome: pathogenesis and management," *British Journal of Haematology*, vol. 112, no. 4, pp. 851–862, 2001.

[5] B. Sevinir, "Çocukluk çağında hemanjiomlar ve klinik özellikleri," *The Journal of Current Pediatrics*, vol. 3, pp. 63–68, 2006.

[6] S. Vinay, S. K. Khan, and J. R. Braybrooke, "Lumbar vertebral haemangioma causing pathological fracture, epidural haemorrhage, and cord compression: a case report and review of literature," *Journal of Spinal Cord Medicine*, vol. 34, no. 3, pp. 335–339, 2011.

[7] C. Yaldız, K. Asil, Y. E. Aksoy, and D. Ceylan, "Spinal cord compression due to vertebral hemangioma mimicking a metastatic lesion: MRI and CT images," *Turkish Journal of Neurosurgery*, vol. 23, pp. 310–314, 2013.

[8] P. Wang, W. Zhou, L. Tao, N. Zhao, and X.-W. Chen, "Clinical analysis of Kasabach-Merritt syndrome in 17 neonates," *BMC Pediatrics*, vol. 14, article 146, 2014.

[9] L. Harper, J. L. Michel, O. Enjolras et al., "Successful management of a retroperitoneal kaposiform hemangioendothelioma with Kasabach-Merritt phenomenon using α-interferon," *European Journal of Pediatric Surgery*, vol. 16, no. 5, pp. 369–372, 2006.

[10] S.-M. Yuan, Z.-J. Hong, H.-N. Chen, W.-M. Shen, and X.-J. Zhou, "Kaposiform hemangioendothelioma complicated by Kasabach-Merritt phenomenon: ultrastructural observation and immunohistochemistry staining reveal the trapping of blood components," *Ultrastructural Pathology*, vol. 37, no. 6, pp. 452–455, 2013.

[11] Ş. Ozsoylu, "Megadose methylprednisolone for kasabach-Merritt syndrome," *Pediatric Hematology and Oncology*, vol. 10, no. 2, pp. 197–198, 1993.

[12] S. Ozsoylu, "Megadose methylprednisolone therapy for Kasabach-Merritt syndrome," *Journal of Pediatrics*, vol. 129, no. 6, pp. 947–948, 1996.

[13] J. W. Zheng, L. Zhang, Q. Zhou et al., "A practical guide to treatment of infantile hemangiomas of the head and neck," *International Journal of Clinical and Experimental Medicine*, vol. 6, no. 10, pp. 851–860, 2013.

[14] A.-P. Michaud, N. M. Bauman, D. K. Burke, J. M. Manaligod, and R. J. H. Smith, "Spastic diplegia and other motor disturbances in infants receiving interferon-alpha," *Laryngoscope*, vol. 114, no. 7, pp. 1231–1236, 2004.

[15] T. Uno, S. Ito, A. Nakazawa, O. Miyazaki, T. Mori, and K. Terashima, "Successful treatment of kaposiform hemangioendothelioma with everolimus," *Pediatric Blood and Cancer*, vol. 62, no. 3, pp. 536–538, 2015.

[16] J. W. Zheng, Q. Zhou, X. J. Yang et al., "Treatment guideline for hemangiomas and vascular malformations of the head and neck," *Head & Neck*, vol. 32, no. 8, pp. 1088–1098, 2010.

[17] E. Leong and S. Bydder, "Use of radiotherapy to treat life-threatening Kasabach-Merritt syndrome," *Journal of Medical Imaging and Radiation Oncology*, vol. 53, no. 1, pp. 87–91, 2009.

[18] S. Lindberg, P. Karlsson, B. Arvidsson, E. Holmberg, L. M. Lundberg, and A. Wallgren, "Cancer incidence after radiotherapy for skin haemangioma during infancy," *Acta Oncologica*, vol. 34, no. 6, pp. 735–740, 1995.

[19] R. M. Hatley, H. Sabio, C. G. Howell, F. Flickinger, and R. A. Parrish, "Successful management of an infant with a giant hemangioma of the retroperitoneum and Kasabach-Merritt syndrome with α-interferon," *Journal of Pediatric Surgery*, vol. 28, no. 10, pp. 1356–1359, 1993.

10

Thoracic Block Technique Associated with Positive End-Expiratory Pressure in Reversing Atelectasis

Luciana Carnevalli Pereira,[1] Ana Paula de Souza Netto,[1] Fernanda Cordeiro da Silva,[1] Silvana Alves Pereira,[2] and Cristiane Aparecida Moran[1]

[1]*University Nove de Julho (UNINOVE), São Paulo, Brazil*
[2]*Ana Bezerra University Hospital (HUAB/EBSERH) and Federal University of Rio Grande do Norte (UFRN/FACISA), RN, Brazil*

Correspondence should be addressed to Cristiane Aparecida Moran; crismoran@uol.com.br

Academic Editor: Larry A. Rhodes

A preschool four-year-old male patient had been admitted to the Mandaqui Hospital with a diagnosis of lobar pneumonia, pleural effusion, and right lung atelectasis. Treatment consisted of antibiotics and physiotherapy sessions, using a technique described in the literature as Insufflation Technique to Reverse Atelectasis (ITRA), which consists of a thoracic block of healthy lung tissue, leaving only the atelectasis area free, associated with the use of invasive or noninvasive mechanical ventilation with positive airway pressure for reversal of atelectasis. Two physiotherapy sessions were conducted daily. The sessions lasted 20 minutes and were fractionated into four series of five minutes each. Each series bilateral thoracic block was performed for 20 seconds with a pause lasting for the same time. Associated with the thoracic block, a continuous positive airways pressure was used using a facial mask and 7 cm H_2O PEEP provided via CPAP. *Conclusion.* ITRA technique was effective in reversing atelectasis in this patient.

1. Introduction

Despite the advances of mankind in recent years, high rates of infant mortality are still verified mainly in developing countries. Among the five main causes are the acute respiratory infections, responsible for the death of about three million children under five years per year [1, 2].

Among the acute respiratory infections, the community-acquired pneumonia represents the most severe form of acute respiratory infections, with an annual incidence of 150 million new cases, of which more than 11 million cases require hospitalization [2, 3].

In Brazil, about 48% of children with pneumonia are aged between one and four years; in these cases the bacterial causes gain more importance and are associated with increased risk of complications; family socioeconomic factors and child nutritional status also are involved. The main complications are pleural effusions and atelectasis, these being the main determinants of clinical worsening [2, 4, 5].

About 50% to 70% of pleural effusions in children are caused by infections secondary to pneumonia, which are discovered due to a chest X-ray for initial diagnosis and reversed with the same antibiotic treatment for community-acquired pneumonia. However, when there is no response to treatment, pleural effusion may have increased its volume and evolve into the so-called complicated pleural effusions and atelectasis [6, 7].

Atelectases are pulmonary changes due to bronchial obstruction caused by inflammation and are associated with functional consequences such as changes in oxygenation, decreased lung compliance, increased pulmonary vascular resistance, overexpansion of adjacent alveolar units, and lung injury. After the collapse of a segment or pulmonary lobe, the alveoli ventilation decreases, while the slightly decreased perfusion results in an area with low ventilation/perfusion (V/Q), causing consequent morbidities [8].

Scientific literature describes a technique known as ITRA, which is used to reverse atelectasis, Insufflation Technique to Reverse Atelectasis. The intervention consists in taking all the healthy lung tissue to an exhalation position and retaining them through thoracic block, leaving only the

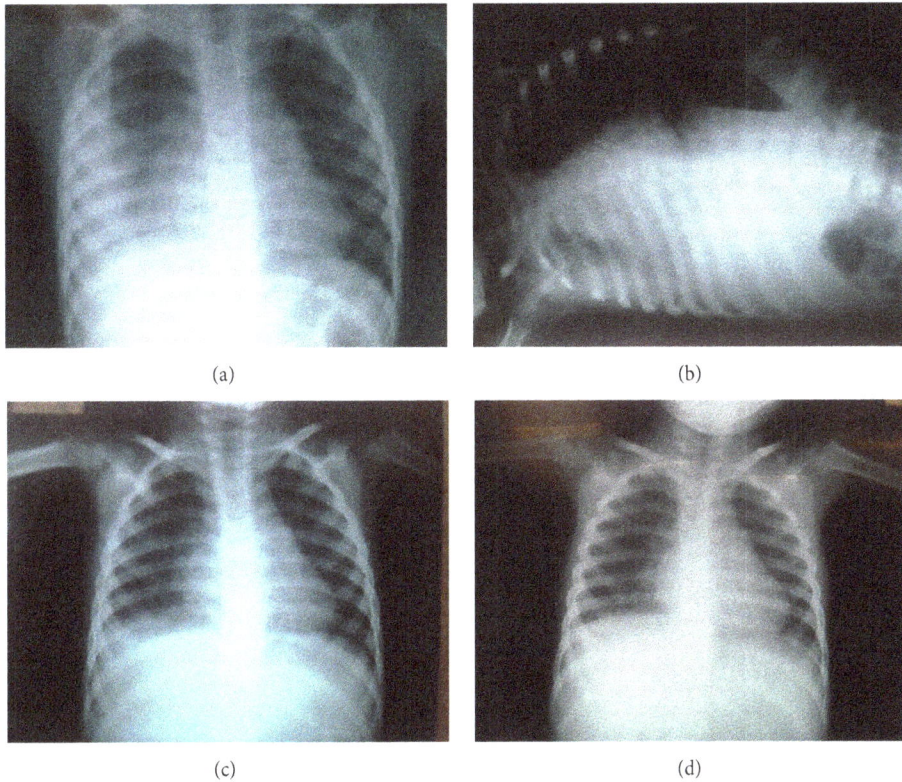

FIGURE 1: (a) Chest radiograph on the anteroposterior incidence, on day 1 of hospitalization and 15th day of clinical symptoms of pneumonia, showing the lobar pneumonia and a beginning of atelectasis in the right hemithorax. (b) Chest radiography on the incidence of Laurell on 1st day of admission showing pleural effusion in the right hemithorax. (c) Chest radiography on the posterior-anterior incidence on the 4th day of hospitalization, showing atelectasis improvement. (d) Chest radiography on the posterior-anterior incidence on the last day of hospitalization showing atelectasis reversal.

atelectasis area free, associated with the use of invasive or noninvasive mechanical ventilation with continuous positive airway pressure (CPAP). This positive pressure produces increased oxygenation, as it promotes the reexpansion of previously collapsed areas, decreases intrapulmonary pressure and increases the gas exchange surfaces, promotes the V/Q relation improvement, and decreases the work of breathing [8–10].

Although ITRA encourages the treatment of atelectasis in different ages [8–10], new studies that provide a better assessment of their effectiveness and a better prognosis in children shall be encouraged, because the pulmonary complications caused by community-acquired pneumonia are an important cause of morbidity in children aged zero to five years. This study aims to evaluate the efficiency of ITRA in reversing atelectasis.

2. Case Report

This case report was approved by the Committee of Research Ethics at University Nove de Julho, under the protocol number 40325.

A 4-year-old child, residing in the São Paulo city, proceeding from Medical Ambulatory Care, with a medical history of dry cough initiated on August 5, 2012. The patient had

been taken to the Primary Health Care Unit for three times, received antiallergic, and presented two fever's episodes (38°C and 38.5°C) and a vomit episode after cough. The patient was referred to the Mandaqui Hospital on August 20, 2012, and remained hospitalized with clinical and radiographic diagnosis of right lobar pneumonia with opacification of two-thirds of the right hemithorax and pleural thickening, being initiated on an antibiotic therapy with Crystalline Penicillin (200.000 U/kg/day), four times a day for 48 hours (Figures 1(a) and 1(b)).

During the assessment performed by the team of child surgery on August 21, a conservative treatment without the need for surgical intervention (thoracic drainage) was opted for. The ultrasonography performed on August 22, 2012, presented pleural effusion with septa in between and volume estimated at approximately 100 mL. After the pleural effusion diagnosis the patient underwent new antibiotic therapy, Ceftriaxone 600 mg two times a day (70 mg/kg/day) for 10 days and respiratory physiotherapy. Two daily sessions were performed during the period of hospitalization, except on weekends when there was no physiotherapist in attendance. During the 20-minute sessions, the ITRA was performed which consists of a thoracic block technique associated with the continuous positive airways pressure (CPAP), using a facial mask and 7 cmH$_2$O PEEP provided via CPAP [11, 12].

TABLE 1: Average parameters assessed during each physiotherapy session.

Variables	Before	During	After 10 min
Heart rate	122	110	111
Respiratory frequency	30	25	24
O_2 saturation	96%	97%	97%

This 20-minute sequence was fractionated in four series of five minutes each. During each series bilateral thoracic block was performed for 20 seconds with a pause lasting for the same time, and the healthy lung airflow was reduced by thoracic block [11]. The heart and respiratory rates were checked as well as the patient's O_2 saturation before and immediately after the application of the technique and 10 minutes after the end of the session. Table 1 presents the average behavior of clinical variables assessed.

After four days of the beginning of the sessions, a new radiography was performed and showed an image improvement (Figure 1(c)), remaining without complications until September 5, 2012 (Figure 1(d)), when the patient was discharged.

3. Discussion

The research demonstrated the reversal of atelectasis after thoracic-abdominal block's association with the CPAP technique known as ITRA, after 20 physiotherapy sessions. Despite the innovative name for Brazilian professionals, it consists of procedures routinely used by physiotherapists in hospitals in various clinical conditions [8–10].

The intervention of respiratory physiotherapy is still questioned regarding its benefits and efficiency in the treatment of respiratory disorders. Studies conducted using conventional physiotherapy techniques (tapping, percussion, postural drainage, and oropharyngeal aspiration assisted cough) showed no significant differences as to the period of hospitalization or course of the disease, when compared with the group of patients who did not undergo physiotherapy intervention [13, 14].

Also, in this context, studies conducted in order to prove the efficiency of the thoracic block in reversing atelectasis have only proved that the technique performance did not present significant differences between treated groups and control groups; on the other hand they observed that in the treated group the following can occur: respiratory rates increase, tidal volume reduction, minute volume preservation, and increased number of collapsed alveoli when compared with the control group [11, 12].

Considering the association of the thoracic block technique with an invasive or noninvasive mechanical ventilation apparatus, known in the literature as ITRA, research has achieved significant results in the reversal of atelectasis and, despite the fact that the control group had presented saturation decrease and transient bradycardia during block, the author considered that the ITRA had no adverse effects [9].

The blocking technique consists of changing the flow [15] and acting on the airway driving, without reaching the lung parenchyma, requiring change in volume to achieve the collapsed alveoli. This effect can be achieved by performing the ITRA due to the association of positive pressure, which produces an increased alveolar pressure, increased functional residual capacity, and consequently recruitment of alveolar units in this region [16, 17], a goal achieved in this study when the atelectasis has reversed without showing desaturation or transient bradycardia.

4. Conclusion

The use of the thoracic block technique associated with continuous positive airway pressure was efficient in this patient who had atelectasis as a complication of pneumonia and pleural effusion.

Conflict of Interests

The authors declare that there is no conflict of interests regarding the publication of this paper.

References

[1] K. Mulholland, "Global burden of acute respiratory infections in children: implications for interventions," *Pediatric Pulmonology*, vol. 36, no. 6, pp. 469–474, 2003.

[2] P. G. Amorim, A. M. Morcillo, A. T. Tresoldi, A. D. M. A. Fraga, R. M. Pereira, and E. C. E. Baracat, "Factors associated with complications of community-acquired pneumonia in preschool children," *Jornal Brasileiro de Pneumologia*, vol. 38, no. 5, pp. 614–621, 2012.

[3] B. G. Williams, E. Gouws, C. Boschi-Pinto, J. Bryce, and C. Dye, "Estimates of world-wide distribution of child deaths from acute respiratory infections," *The Lancet Infectious Diseases*, vol. 2, no. 1, pp. 25–32, 2002.

[4] F. E. Rodrigues, R. B. Tatto, L. Vauchinski et al., "Pneumonia mortality in Brazilian children aged 4 years and younger," *Jornal de Pediatria*, vol. 87, no. 2, pp. 111–114, 2011.

[5] A. G. L. Riccetto, M. P. Zambom, I. C. M. R. Pereira, and A. M. Morcillo, "Influence of social-economical and nutritional factors on the evolution to complications in children hospitalized with pneumonia," *Revista da Associação Médica Brasileira*, vol. 49, no. 2, pp. 191–195, 2003.

[6] P. Soares, J. Barreira, S. Pissara, T. Nunes, I. Azevedo, and L. Vaz, "Pediatric parapneumonic pleural effusions: experience in a university central hospital," *Revista Portuguesa de Pneumologia*, vol. 15, no. 2, pp. 241–259, 2009.

[7] E. Marchi, F. Lundgren, and R. Mussi, "Parapneumonic effusion and empyema," *Jornal Brasileiro de Pneumologia*, vol. 32, supplement 4, pp. S190–S196, 2006.

[8] C. Jonhston and W. B. Carvalho, "Atelectasias em pediatria: mecanismos, diagnóstico e tratamento," *Revista da Associação Médica Brasileira*, vol. 54, no. 5, pp. 455–460, 2008.

[9] S. Herry, "Technique Insufflatoire de Levée d'Atélectasie (TILA) en réanimation néonatale," *Kinésithérapie, La Revue*, vol. 7, no. 65, pp. 30–34, 2007.

[10] P. Pasquina, P. Merlani, J. M. Granier, and B. Ricou, "Continuous positive airway pressure versus noninvasive pressure support

ventilation to treat atelectasis after cardiac surgery," *Anesthesia and Analgesia*, vol. 99, no. 4, pp. 1001–1008, 2004.

[11] B. S. Sixel, D. A. Lemes, K. A. Pereira, and F. S. Guimarães, "Compressão manual torácica em pacientes com insuficiência respiratória aguda," *Fisioterapia Brasil*, vol. 8, no. 2, pp. 103–106, 2007.

[12] J. G. M. Lima, L. F. F. Reis, F. M. Moura, C. P. V. Souza, E. M. Walchan, and A. Bergmann, "Compressão manual torácica em um modelo experimental de atelectasia em ratos wistar," *Fisioterapia em Movimento*, vol. 21, no. 3, pp. 77–82, 2008.

[13] C. Perrotta, Z. Ortiz, and M. Roque, "Chest physiotherapy for acute bronchiolitis in paediatric patients between 0 and 24 months old," *Cochrane Database of Systematic Reviews*, no. 2, Article ID CD004873, 2005.

[14] M. K. Pupin, A. G. Riccetto, J. D. Ribeiro, and E. C. Baracat, "Comparação dos efeitos de duas técnicas fisioterapêuticas respiratórias em parâmetros cardiorrespiratórios de lactentes com bronquiolite viral aguda," *Jornal Brasileiro de Pneumologia*, vol. 35, no. 9, pp. 860–867, 2009.

[15] I. F. Ribeiro, A. P. L. Melo, and J. Davidson, "Fisioterapia em recém-nascidos com persistência do canal arterial e complicações pulmonares," *Revista Paulista de Pediatria*, vol. 26, no. 1, pp. 77–83, 2008.

[16] L. Bohé, M. E. Ferrero, E. Cuestas, L. Polliotto, and M. Genoff, "Indications of conventional chest physiotherapy in acute bronchiolitis," *Medicina*, vol. 64, no. 3, pp. 198–200, 2004.

[17] J. S. de Oliveira, T. F. Campos, R. de Oliveira Borja et al., "Análise do índice de percepção de esforço na avaliação das pressões respiratórias máximas em crianças e adolescentes," *Revista Brasileira de Crescimento e Desenvolvimento Humano*, vol. 22, no. 3, pp. 314–320, 2012.

11

A Case of Battery Ingestion in a Pediatric Patient: What Is Its Importance?

Elie Alam,[1] **Marc Mourad,**[1] **Samir Akel,**[2] **and Usamah Hadi**[1]

[1]*Department of Otolaryngology Head and Neck Surgery, American University of Beirut, P.O. Box 11-0236, Riad El Solh, Beirut 1107-2020, Lebanon*
[2]*Division of General Surgery, American University of Beirut, P.O. Box 11-0236, Riad El Solh, Beirut 1107-2020, Lebanon*

Correspondence should be addressed to Elie Alam; elie.elalam@gmail.com and Usamah Hadi; uhadi@dm.net.lb

Academic Editor: Bibhuti Das

This is a case of a two-year-old boy who has been suffering from food regurgitation and frequent vomiting over the past seven months which were progressively worsening with time. He was initially diagnosed with gastroesophageal reflux disease and treated accordingly but responded only minimally. Investigations and interventional procedures including a chest X-ray showed a metallic round object in the upper esophagus consistent with a button battery which was removed via a thoracotomy after an esophagoscopy was not successful. This child would not have developed such serious complications and would not have required major surgery had the foreign body been identified and removed early on.

1. Introduction

Pediatric foreign body ingestion is a problem encountered by many physicians including pediatricians, otolaryngologists, and emergency physicians frequently. Approximately 80% of cases of foreign body ingestions occur in children between the ages of six months and three years [1–3]. Button battery ingestion occurs at an estimate rate of ten in one million people per year, a small group of which are retained in the esophagus and later become complicated [1]. The aim of this report is to describe our case of a pediatric patient who ingested a button battery and was diagnosed late and to highlight the importance of having a high index of suspicion.

2. Case Report

This is the case of a two-year-old boy who was referred to our Emergency Department by his pediatric cardiologist for evaluation of his lung condition. The physician was performing a routine echocardiogram for the assessment of the child's preexistent foramen ovale, when he saw a round opacity in the thorax, suspicious of a foreign body. This finding necessitated further evaluation by a chest radiograph.

The patient was hemodynamically stable upon arrival and not in distress. He had normal oxygen saturation and a normal head and neck examination. Examination of the lungs revealed mild crackles over lung bases but with no evidence of stridor or hoarseness.

Upon questioning, the mother reported that he had been having vague upper respiratory symptoms with food regurgitation and frequent vomiting over the past seven months. She denied solid food dysphagia but reported mild daily drooling. These symptoms were progressively worsening over the past four months. He was initially diagnosed with gastroesophageal reflux disease and treated with prokinetics and proton pump inhibitors, to which he responded only minimally.

A chest radiograph was done in the emergency room showing the presence of a round metallic density over the topography of the upper esophagus showing irregular contour, with mild mass effect on the left aspect of the trachea (Figure 1). The lung fields appeared clear. Further evaluation by a CT scan showed the same round metallic object at the level of the upper esophagus (Figure 2). A barium swallow was performed and showed that the patient was swallowing without difficulty, with the foreign body apparently separate from the esophageal tract.

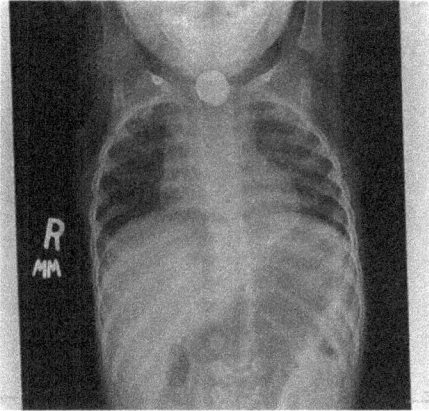

FIGURE 1

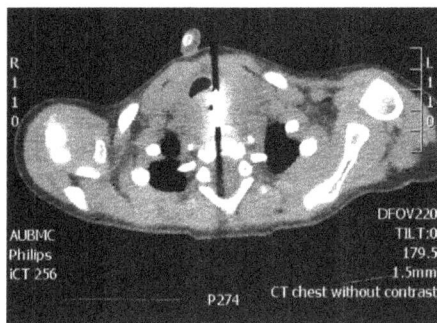

FIGURE 2

The decision was made to perform an esophagoscopy in the operating room to the attempt of foreign body removal. Intraoperatively, the foreign body was not seen but a hard mass was felt at the lateral esophageal wall, which was covered by granulation tissue. Multiple attempts to remove the foreign body were performed but unsuccessful. The decision was made to abort the surgery and proceed with an external approach and the patient was transferred to the pediatric intensive care unit.

Two days later, the patient was scheduled for a right posterolateral thoracotomy and an extrapleural approach for removal of foreign body with esophagostomy and esophagoplasty. The surgery was successful and was followed by a smooth uncomplicated course. The foreign body retrieved was a button battery.

Foreign body ingestion is a frequently occurring problem in pediatric age groups with 75% occurring at ages less than 4 years [4]. Esophageal foreign body impaction (EFBI) is a rare presenting pediatric complaint due to the fact that not all are present immediately following ingestion. The majority of ingested foreign bodies pass through the GI tract with no sequelae; however, those that do cause impaction do so in the upper esophagus, the most common site accounting for more than 75% of all cases [5, 6].

The presenting symptoms can range from being completely asymptomatic to being fatal. In between these ends of the spectrum, symptoms can include GI complaints including

vomiting, drooling, dysphagia, odynophagia, and respiratory complaints such as cough, stridor, and choking [1, 7, 8]. However, neither the symptoms upon presentation nor the location of impaction within the esophagus is predictive of the presence of esophageal injury [9].

The complications resulting from ingestion are mainly related to the duration of impaction. Moreover, the type of ingested foreign body affects the complication rate [1, 10]. Many studies have displayed findings that support this conclusion. Denney et al. showed that foreign bodies in situ for more than 24 hours were more likely to cause esophageal ulceration (46%) as compared to those in situ for less than 24 hours (23%) [9]. Similarly Miller et al. concluded that a higher rate of esophageal injury is seen in foreign body ingestion of over one week [11]. There is a wide range of complications that have been reported in the literature. These include mucosal abrasions and lacerations, perforations with mediastinitis, strictures, pulmonary edema, and esophageal diverticulum [1, 10, 12–16].

The child described here ingested a button battery. Previously injury was believed to occur secondary to leakage of alkaline material; however, recent studies proposed that the cause is the passage of a current through the tissue causing hydrolysis of tissue fluids. Moreover, lithium cells have been associated with worse outcomes. This is due to lithium being 3 V cells instead of 1.5 V cells and since they generate more current, more hydroxide is produced and is more rapid than other cells. In addition, studies have shown that the current generates hydroxide at the negative battery pole and as a result the esophageal injury can be predicted by the anatomic location and orientation of the battery [2, 3].

This case highlights the necessity of having high clinical suspicion and intervention early on. Studies have demonstrated that the worst anatomic area of impaction is in the esophagus. Furthermore, there is chance to have injury free removal of an esophageal battery if removed within 2 hours of ingestion [3]. The child described above would not have developed such serious complications and would not have required major surgery had the foreign body been identified and removed early on. As a result, physicians who are caring for children who present with respiratory or GI complaints should keep a high index of suspicion of foreign body ingestion especially if the child is nonverbal. In addition, new emerging technologies discuss battery coating which if swallowed decreases the external electrolytic currents which cause tissue injury. The authors conducted animal studies and reported significant decrease in tissue injury compared with uncoated control batteries [17]. More importantly, parents of young children should take extra caution in storing items which could be ingested by children around the house. Small items especially ones that have chemical composition such as batteries should be kept in areas out of reach of children to insure they never have access to them.

Conflict of Interests

The authors declare that there is no conflict of interests regarding the publication of this paper.

References

[1] W. Cheng and P. K. H. Tam, "Foreign-body ingestion in children: experience with 1,265 cases," *Journal of Pediatric Surgery*, vol. 34, no. 10, pp. 1472–1476, 1999.

[2] T. Litovitz, N. Whitaker, and L. Clark, "Preventing battery ingestions: an analysis of 8648 cases," *Pediatrics*, vol. 125, no. 6, pp. 1178–1183, 2010.

[3] T. Litovitz, N. Whitaker, L. Clark, N. C. White, and M. Marsolek, "Emerging battery-ingestion hazard: clinical implications," *Pediatrics*, vol. 125, no. 6, pp. 1168–1177, 2010.

[4] M. B. McNeill, S. L. W. Sperry, S. D. Crockett, C. B. Miller, N. J. Shaheen, and E. S. Dellon, "Epidemiology and management of oesophageal coin impaction in children," *Digestive and Liver Disease*, vol. 44, no. 6, pp. 482–486, 2012.

[5] L. B. Stack and D. W. Munter, "Foreign bodies in the gastrointestinal tract," *Emergency Medicine Clinics of North America*, vol. 14, no. 3, pp. 493–521, 1996.

[6] P. Nandi and G. B. Ong, "Foreign body in the esophagus: review of 2394 cases," *British Journal of Surgery*, vol. 65, no. 1, pp. 5–9, 1978.

[7] D. C. Little, S. R. Shah, S. D. St Peter et al., "Esophageal foreign bodies in the pediatric population: our first 500 cases," *Journal of Pediatric Surgery*, vol. 41, no. 5, pp. 914–918, 2006.

[8] D. Antoniou and G. Christopoulos-Geroulanos, "Management of foreign body ingestion and food bolus impaction in children: a retrospective analysis of 675 cases," *Turkish Journal of Pediatrics*, vol. 53, no. 4, pp. 381–387, 2011.

[9] W. Denney, N. Ahmad, B. Dillard, and M. J. Nowicki, "Children will eat the strangest things: a 10-year retrospective analysis of foreign body and caustic ingestions from a single academic center," *Pediatric Emergency Care*, vol. 28, no. 8, pp. 731–734, 2012.

[10] B. Tokar, A. A. Cevik, and H. Ilhan, "Ingested gastrointestinal foreign bodies: predisposing factors for complications in children having surgical or endoscopic removal," *Pediatric Surgery International*, vol. 23, no. 2, pp. 135–139, 2007.

[11] R. S. Miller, J. P. Willging, M. J. Rutter, and K. Rookkapan, "Chronic esophageal foreign bodies in pediatric patients: a retrospective review," *International Journal of Pediatric Otorhinolaryngology*, vol. 68, no. 3, pp. 265–272, 2004.

[12] E. J. Doolin, "Esophageal stricture: an uncommon complication of foreign bodies," *Annals of Otology, Rhinology and Laryngology*, vol. 102, no. 11, pp. 863–866, 1993.

[13] B. F. Gilchrist, E. R. Valerie, M. Nguyen, C. Coren, D. Klotz, and M. L. Ramenofsky, "Pearls and perils in the management of prolonged, peculiar, penetrating esophageal foreign bodies in children," *Journal of Pediatric Surgery*, vol. 32, no. 10, pp. 1429–1431, 1997.

[14] T. S. Sheen and S. Y. Lee, "Complete esophageal stricture resulting from a neglected foreign body," *The American Journal of Otolaryngology—Head and Neck Medicine and Surgery*, vol. 17, no. 4, pp. 272–275, 1996.

[15] C. C. Rao, W. L. McNiece, and G. Krishna, "Acute pulmonary edema after removal of an esophageal foreign body in an infant," *Critical Care Medicine*, vol. 14, no. 11, pp. 988–989, 1986.

[16] J. E. Kerschner, D. J. Beste, S. F. Conley, M. A. Kenna, and D. Lee, "Mediastinitis associated with foreign body erosion of the esophagus in children," *International Journal of Pediatric Otorhinolaryngology*, vol. 59, no. 2, pp. 89–97, 2001.

[17] B. Laulicht, G. Traverso, V. Deshpande, R. Langer, and J. M. Karp, "Simple battery armor to protect against gastrointestinal injury from accidental ingestion," *Proceedings of the National Academy of Sciences*, vol. 111, no. 46, pp. 16490–16495, 2014.

12

Multicentric Castleman's Disease in a Child Revealed by Chronic Diarrhea

Sarra Benmiloud, Sana Chaouki, Samir Atmani, and Moustapha Hida

Unit of Pediatric Hematology-Oncology, Department of Pediatrics, University Hospital Hassan II, Faculty of Medicine and Pharmacy, University Sidi Mohamed Ben Abdellah of Fez, Morocco

Correspondence should be addressed to Sarra Benmiloud; benmiloudsarra@yahoo.fr

Academic Editor: Josef Sykora

Multicentric Castleman's disease is a rare benign and unexplained lymphoproliferative disorder that is extremely uncommon in children. It presents with fever, systemic symptoms, generalized lymphadenopathy, and laboratory markers of inflammation. Its treatment is not standardized and its prognosis is poor. We report a novel case of multicentric Castleman's disease in a 13-year-old girl who had presented with chronic diarrhea as the only initial presenting symptom. The diagnosis of celiac or inflammatory bowel diseases was suspected, but two and a half years later, the diagnosis of multicentric Castleman's disease was brought following the appearance of abdominal mass whose biopsy revealed Castleman's disease in the plasma cell form. The outcome was favorable after treatment by corticosteroid, chemotherapy, and surgery. The occurrence of diarrhea as the initial symptom of multicentric Castleman's disease without lymph node involvement is very rare. This case report underlines the diagnostic difficulties and the long interval between onset and diagnosis when diarrhea occurs first.

1. Introduction

Multicentric Castleman's disease (MCD) is a poorly understood lymphoproliferative disorder that is rarely reported in children [1, 2]. It is characterised by peripheral lymphadenopathy with systemic symptoms and laboratory markers of inflammation. Its real incidence is unknown, and its prevalence is estimated to be less than 1/100,000. Most reported cases have been described in adult patients, with a peak of incidence in the third and fourth decade of life for localized forms and in the fourth and fifth decade of life for multicentric forms [1]. In children, Castleman's disease (CD) is predominantly diagnosed during the teenage years and it is usually a localized type with a slight predilection for girls [2]. The MCD is very rarely reported in children and represents only about 13% of Castleman's cases [2].

The point of special interest in our case is that clinical presentation is atypical and characterized by the occurrence of chronic diarrhea as the only initial presenting symptom. This case underlines also the diagnostic difficulties.

2. Case Report

A 13-year-old girl with no past medical history, complained for 2 years of chronic diarrhea with no other clinical signs, and this has necessitated several visits to pediatricians without improvement under symptomatic treatment. Due to the persistence of diarrhea associated with growth retardation (weight and height were at minus 2 standard deviations (SD)) with a bone age corresponding to 10 years; celiac disease was suspected; antitransglutaminase and antiendomysium antibodies were negative; jejunal biopsy with histological study was read as villous atrophy II. The patient was put on gluten-free diet for 6 months without improvement. The evolution was marked by the persistence of diarrhea and the appearance of an intermittent fever, ranging between 37.8 and 38.5°C, asthenia, anorexia, weight loss, night sweats, and a deterioration of the general state. Second gastric and duodenal biopsies with histological study were read to show a nonspecific chronic interstitial duodenitis. The search of Koch's bacillus in sputum and tuberculin skin test was

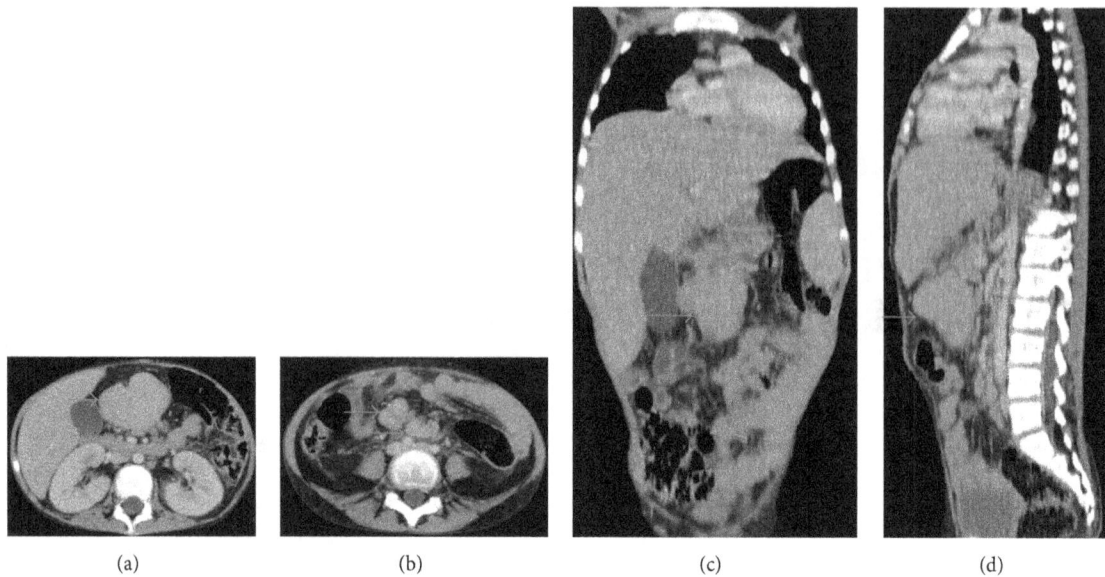

FIGURE 1: Thoracoabdominal-pelvic computed tomography injected in axial sections (a and b) with coronal (c) and sagittal (d) reconstructions demonstrating multiple adenomegalies and a mesenteric soft tissue mass.

negative. Six months later, the patient developed insidiously growing abdominal mass; lymphoma was suspected, so she was transferred to our department for evaluation.

Clinical examination at admission revealed a febrile patient at 38.5°C, in poor physical condition, pale, and with a growth retardation; her body weight was 24 Kg (minus 3 SD); and the body height was 138 cm (minus 3 SD). Abdominal palpation revealed a hepatomegaly (4 cm below the costal margin), a splenomegaly (2 fingerbreadth from the flange left costal), and a painless paraumbilical mass which was slightly mobile, measuring about 6 cm of diameter. The rest of the physical examination demonstrated lenticular inguinal and cervical lymph nodes. Abdominal ultrasound followed by thoracoabdominal-pelvic computed tomography revealed a hepatosplenomegaly, a multiple mesenteric lymph nodes (the largest measures 19 mm in diameter), and a soft tissue mass roughly rounded shape, well limited, enhanced moderately and homogeneously by the product of contrast and measuring $40 \times 65 \times 56$ mm in diameter. This mass has an intimate contact with the gallbladder without signs of invasion, and a contact with the antropyloric region of the stomach, with a significant infiltration of the surrounding fat (Figure 1). The chest X-ray was normal. The biological investigations revealed microcytic hypochromic anemia (hemoglobin = 7 g/dL) (normal range 10.5–13.5 g/dL), thrombocytosis (platelet count = 489,000/mm^3) (normal range 150000–450000/mm^3), and elevated inflammatory markers: erythrocytes sedimentation rate (ESR) = 145 mm in the first hour (normal range < 16 mm), c-reactive protein = 252 mg/L (normal range 0–6 mg/L), fibrinogen = 7.1 g/L (normal range 2–4 g/L), ferritin = 527.9 μg/L (normal range 20–250 μg/L), serum iron = 0.10 mg/L (normal range 0.6–1.9 mg/L), hypoalbuminemia (22 g/L) (normal range 33–50 g/L), an increase of

alpha 1 globulin (5.6 g/L) (normal range 1.2–4 g/L), alpha 2 globulin (14.4 g/L) (normal range 4–8 g/L), beta 2 globulin (6.7 g/L) (normal range 1–4 g/L), and hypergammaglobulinemia (37.5 g/L) (normal range 6–12 g/L). The insulin-like growth factor (IGF1) was low (26.5 ng/mL) (normal range 220–972 ng/mL) without abnormal secretion of growth hormone in the insulin stimulation test. The hepatic transaminases and lactate dehydrogenase were normal. The bacteriological, viral (Epstein Barr virus, cytomegalovirus, human immunodeficiency virus, hepatitis B and hepatitis C, and human herpes virus 8 (HHV8)), and parasite evaluation were negative. Immune and thyroid function tests were normal.

A scan-guided biopsy of the abdominal mass was performed. Microscopic examination revealed normal lymph node tissue architecture, with hyperplastic lymphoid follicles made of elements of variable size; in some areas they look like an onion bulb. In the interfollicular areas, a marked proliferation of plasma cells was identified. An immunestaining by the anti-CD20 and anti-CD3 shows a normal distribution of the lymphoid population. The anti-CD138 antibody shows a wealth of interfollicular tissue into mature plasma cells. These findings were compatible with the plasma cell form of CD. Because of the rarity of this disease, a study of the biopsy by another pathologist confirmed this result. The myelogram performed during general anesthesia was normal.

The patient received oral corticosteroid (prednisone) for a one month with a minimal response (20% the reduction of the size of the mass); thus she received chemotherapy based on 2 courses of VAMP (vinblastine, doxorubicin, methotrexate, and prednisone) that allowed a 62% reduction in the size of the mass, permitted to perform a total tumorectomy. The outcome was favorable with the disappearance of fever, night sweats, diarrhea, hepatosplenomegaly, and normalization of inflammatory markers. Currently we are at 26-month follow-up; the child is asymptomatic, starting to catch up the height and weight growth (minus 1.5 SD).

3. Discussion

This case illustrates the diagnostic difficulties when diarrhea occurs as the initial presenting symptom in MCD. This affection is characterised by peripheral lymphadenopathy (84%) with a mean of four sites involved and manifestations of multisystem involvement: fever, anorexia, weight loss, asthenia, weakness, night sweats, hepatosplenomegaly, skin rash, lung disorder, and kidney dysfunction. Sometimes, gastrointestinal symptoms may be encountered, such as diarrhea, vomiting or nausea, and less common, polyneuropathy, oedema, pleural or pericardial effusion, ascites, and so forth, [3, 4]. Typically there are also laboratory abnormalities: hypergammaglobulinemia, elevated inflammatory parameters, anemia, thrombocytosis, leucopenia, low serum albumin level, and, sometimes, elevated interleukin-6 (IL-6) [3]. MCD can be confused with malignant lymphoma; a definitive diagnosis requires an excisional biopsy. Histologically, MCD corresponds to the plasma cell type and is characterised by hyperplastic follicles, with marked proliferation of plasma cells in the interfollicular stroma, which is less vascular than in the hyaline-vascular variant.

The clinical course of MCD is variable; some patients may be largely asymptomatic or have spontaneous abatement of symptoms, but usually it may progress over several months or be episodic with recurrent exacerbations over a number of years [5]. The delay in diagnosis is often long because of clinical polymorphism and ignorance of the disease by pediatricians. In the case of our patient, it took two years and a half to make the diagnosis because we had diarrhea as the initial symptom without lymph node involvement. Initially, celiac or inflammatory bowel diseases were suspected with an impact on the growth of the child. But after the occurrence of an abdominal mass, lymphoma or CD was suspected. Reported gastrointestinal manifestations on CD in the literature are uncommon. The digestive tract may be secondarily involved and, in some cases, is responsible for the first manifestations of the disease. The gastrointestinal involvement was attributed to reactive amyloidosis or an intestinal lymphangiectasia [6, 7]. Rarely, there is colitis probably attributable to the immune dysregulation and cytokine induced intestinal epithelial cell apoptosis [8].

The aetiology of CD is unknown. Even if no underlying cause has been reported in children, it is generally believed that CD is an autoinflammatory disease resulting in an increase of IL-6 secretion. Several immunologic mechanisms have been proposed, including overproduction of IL-6 and HHV-8 infection [9, 10]. It is commonly thought to represent a defect in immune-regulation, resulting in an excessive proliferation of B lymphocytes and plasma cells in lymphoid organs. The opportunistic presence of HHV-8, favored by immune perturbations, and the direct pathogenic role of HHV-8, in association with dysregulation of cytokines, were suggested by demonstrating that HHV-8 is able to produce an IL-6 homologue, above all [10, 11]. This dysregulated overproduction of IL-6 by the affected lymph nodes is thought to be responsible for the systemic manifestations of the disease.

Treatment of MCD is not standardized. The optimal therapeutic approach is unknown. Diverse treatments are used, often in combination. MCD is too widespread to remove all affected nodes with surgery. Several types of treatment have been successful in some patients. Corticosteroid was used with amelioration of symptoms, but the effect is generally temporary with recurrence of symptoms likely on tapering or discontinuation of treatment [12]. In some cases, steroids alone can be sufficient for remission even though the treatment must often be prolonged [3]. In many cases, chemotherapy was used successfully in the symptomatic patients [3, 4]. Regimens against Hodgkin lymphoma are the most commonly used. These regimens use CVAD (cyclophosphamide, vincristine, doxorubicin, and dexamethasone) or CHOP (cyclophosphamide, doxorubicin, vincristine, and prednisolone). Radiation is sometimes used, but its role is uncertain except in localized form [13]. Adults with MCD have been successfully treated with agents including anti-IL-6 receptor antibody (tocilizumab), interferon-α, rituximab, and antivirals [1, 3, 4, 12]. Other treatments such as intravenous immunoglobulin, plasmapheresis, targeted agents (thalidomide and bortezomib), and autologous hematopoietic stem-cell transplantation have been used sporadically [4, 12]. In our case, we initially administered corticosteroids, but due to insufficient response, we gave the patient chemotherapy which allowed a good improvement with a regression of the size of the mass that was removed by surgery.

In MCD, despite treatment, the prognosis remains uncertain. The majority of children survive with persistence of disease. Death is either caused by infections or by the development of malignancy. About 20% of people with MCD develop lymphoma that usually grows fast and is hard to treat [3, 4, 12].

4. Conclusion

Pediatric MCD is a very rare benign lymphoproliferative disorder characterised by angiofollicular lymph-node hyperplasia. This affection is characterised by peripheral lymphadenopathy with manifestations of multisystem involvement and laboratory markers of inflammation. However, the diagnosis can be difficult because of the lack of clinical and radiological specificity. It is suggested by clinical presentation and confirmed by histology. The occurrence of chronic diarrhea as the only initial presenting symptom is atypical and can cause a delay diagnosis. MCD should be borne in mind in the differential diagnosis of patients with chronic diarrhea.

Conflict of Interests

The authors declare that there is no conflict of interests regarding the publication of this paper.

Acknowledgments

The authors would like to thank Pr Meryem BOUBBOU, radiologist, Pr Fouad Kettani, pathologist, Pr Saadia Zafad, hematologist-oncologist, and Pr Youssef BOUABDALLAH, pediatric surgeon, for their help in the management of this patient.

References

[1] B. Roca, "Castleman's disease. A review," *AIDS Reviews*, vol. 11, no. 1, pp. 3–7, 2009.

[2] N. Parez, B. Bader-Meunier, C. C. Roy, and J. P. Dommergues, "Paediatric Castleman disease: report of seven cases and review of the literature," *European Journal of Pediatrics*, vol. 158, no. 8, pp. 631–637, 1999.

[3] P. Farruggia, A. Trizzino, N. Scibetta et al., "Castleman's disease in childhood: report of three cases and review of the literature," *Italian Journal of Pediatrics*, vol. 37, article 50, 2011.

[4] N. Zhou, C. W. Huang, and W. Liao, "The characterization and management of castleman's disease," *Journal of International Medical Research*, vol. 40, no. 4, pp. 1580–1588, 2012.

[5] G. Frizzera, B. A. Peterson, E. D. Bayrd, and A. Goldman, "A systemic lymphoproliferative disorder with morphologic features of Castleman's disease: clinical findings and clinicopathologic correlations in 15 patients," *Journal of Clinical Oncology*, vol. 3, no. 9, pp. 1202–1216, 1985.

[6] S. F. Moss, D. M. Thomas, C. Mulnier, I. G. McGill, and H. J. F. Hodgson, "Intestinal lymphangiectasia associated with angiofollicular lymph node hyperplasia (Castleman's disease)," *Gut*, vol. 33, no. 1, pp. 135–137, 1992.

[7] A. Miura, I. Sato, and C. Suzuki, "Fatal diarrhea in a patient with Castleman's disease associated with intestinal amyloidosis.," *Internal Medicine*, vol. 34, no. 11, pp. 1106–1109, 1995.

[8] M. Yamamoto, K. Yoshizaki, T. Kishimoto, and H. Ito, "IL-6 is required for the development of Th1 cell-mediated murine colitis," *Journal of Immunology*, vol. 164, no. 9, pp. 4878–4882, 2000.

[9] S. Yamasaki, T. Iino, M. Nakamura et al., "Detection of human herpesvirus-8 in peripheral blood mononuclear cells from adult Japanese patients with multicentric Castleman's disease," *British Journal of Haematology*, vol. 120, no. 3, pp. 471–477, 2003.

[10] K. Yoshizaki, T. Matsuda, N. Nishimoto et al., "Pathogenic significance of interleukin-6 (IL-6/BSF-2) in Castleman's disease," *Blood*, vol. 74, no. 4, pp. 1360–1367, 1989.

[11] F. Sarrot-Reynauld, P. Morand, and M. Buisson, "Groupe français d'étude de la maladie de Castleman. Maladie de Castleman et infection par le virus HHV-8," *La Revue de Médecine Interne*, vol. 19, p. 413, 1998.

[12] F. van Rhee, K. Stone, S. Szmania, B. Barlogie, and Z. Singh, "Castleman disease in the 21st century: an update on diagnosis, assessment, and therapy," *Clinical Advances in Hematology and Oncology*, vol. 8, no. 7, pp. 486–498, 2010.

[13] G. M. Chronowski, C. S. Ha, R. B. Wilder, F. Cabanillas, J. Manning, and J. D. Cox, "Treatment of unicentric and multicentric Castleman disease and the role of radiotherapy," *Cancer*, vol. 92, no. 3, pp. 670–676, 2001.

13

An Interesting Fistula Tract Presenting with Recurrent Gluteal Abscess: Instructive Case

Gulsum Iclal Bayhan,[1] **Ozge Metin,**[2] **Burak Ardicli,**[3] **Ayse Karaman,**[3] **and Gonul Tanir**[2]

[1]*Department of Pediatric Infectious Disease, Yuzuncu Yil University, 65000 Van, Turkey*
[2]*Department of Pediatric Infectious Disease, Dr. Sami Ulus Maternity and Children's Training and Research Hospital,*
 06080 Ankara, Turkey
[3]*Department of Pediatric Surgery, Dr. Sami Ulus Maternity and Children's Training and Research Hospital, 06080 Ankara, Turkey*

Correspondence should be addressed to Gulsum Iclal Bayhan; gibayhan@gmail.com

Academic Editor: Isolina Riaño Galán

A fistula extending from the gluteus to penis is an extremely rare entity. In this paper, we have highlighted novel variant of congenital penile to gluteal fistula complicated with gluteal and penoscrotal abscess in a previously healthy boy. A fistulous tract extending from the gluteus to penis has been shown by fistulogram. Bleomycin has been used in fistula tract with successful results in our patient.

1. Introduction

A fistula extending from the gluteus to penis is an extremely rare entity. We report a patient with recurrent gluteal abscess having an unusual gluteal-penile fistula along the posteroanterior body axis.

2. Case

A 4.5-year-old boy presented to our hospital with complaint of recurrent abscess on the right hip since he was 7 months old. He had been diagnosed as having gluteal abscess accompanied with penile abscess previously on seven separate occasions and incision and drainage were performed. He was operated on for hypospadias by using Snodgrass technique at two years old. A month later, recurrent abscesses in the gluteal region had been excised; pathology reported chronic inflammation and congestion in fibroadipose tissue. During our hospital admission, abscesses on penile and gluteal sides were detected at the same time. Physical examination revealed discharging sinus surrounded with 2×2 cm induration on the right gluteus and discharging sinus on the penoscrotal junction. Abscess tract was palpated through to perineal region. Anorectum was normal.

Laboratory findings of the patient were as follows: white cell count was $11.9 \times 10^3/\mu L$ (normal range, 5.1–15.5 $\times$ $10^3/\mu L$), hemoglobin 9.5 g/dL, platelet count $460 \times 10^3/\mu L$, and C-reactive protein 32 mg/L (normal range, 0–8 mg/L). He was hospitalized and ceftriaxone was commenced after pus culture was obtained from both sites. Ultrasound examination revealed 31×22 mm lobulated contoured abscess forming dense content with the acoustic empowerment in the right gluteal region which reached to intergluteal region. Penoscrotal USG revealed 5×4 mm sized dense content abscess within the corpus cavernosum in the proximal part of the ventral penile adjacent to the left lateral side of the urethra. *Enterococcus* spp. had grown on his both pus cultures. Antibiotic treatment was switched to teicoplanin. The swellings in the gluteus and penoscrotal junction were gradually decreased in size with antibiotic treatment. A fistulography was performed and showed a long sinus tract extending from the region of the penoscrotal junction to the right gluteal region (Figure 1). There was no connection with the urinary and gastrointestinal tract.

Surgical treatment was required to be an extensive procedure with great risk of developing intraoperative damage to vital organs and nerves. Instead, sclerotherapy was administered to induce healing of the lesion. Penoscrotal sinus was

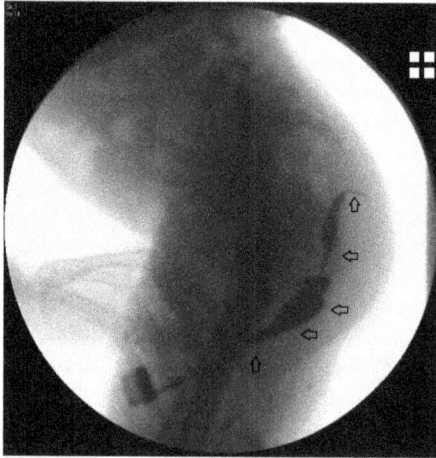

FIGURE 1: Fistulography of the patient. The opaque material was given from the mouth of the fistula at the level of the penoscrotal region. The opaque material extended superiorly to the inferior level of the coccyx and terminated under the skin.

catheterized and diluted bleomycin at a dose of 0.25 mg/kg was administered under general anesthesia. Postoperative recovery was uneventful, and the patient was discharged after 3 days. Six months later, the skin healed completely. The patient has been followed for one and half years and abscess was not repeated until now.

3. Discussion

The gluteal abscesses and fistula have been reported as complications of Crohn's disease, diverticulitis, colon carcinoma, and tuberculosis of lumbar vertebrae [1–3]. In our patient, recurrent abscesses history in both penoscrotal region and gluteus and the cultures from both abscess sides yielding the same microorganism suggested the possibility that there had been a fistula. In the case presented, initial diagnosis of a fistula could not be made till the fistulography was conducted. Despite the newer imaging modalities, a fistulography is still the best means of evaluating a sinus tract or fistula when an external communication is present. The fistulography allows visualization of the fistula tract and origin. Computed tomography is helpful if exact spatial delineation of the tract is necessary or a suspect of associated abscess exists. Because CT results in high radiation, it should be used carefully in young children in selected indications. Ultrasound examination is generally not useful since it is limited by bowel gas and surgical incisions [4, 5]. Magnetic resonance imaging (MRI) is reported as the golden standard in preoperative assessing and classifying of fistula, because MRI allows direct visualization of the tracts and abscesses through to high soft tissue resolution [6, 7].

Surgery has been the main therapy for any sinus and fistula tracts. Open surgical exploration and repair provide definitive management, avoid recurrence, and prevent infection. Although surgical excision has been considered as a mode of treatment by most of the surgeons, the patient may be faced with some conditions such as nerve injuries,

prolonged lymphatic drainage from the wound, recurrent lesions, wound infections, and unacceptable scar formations. Sclerotherapy using bleomycin is an established technique for the treatment of developmental vascular anomalies, also those which are at risk of developing intraoperative damage to vital organs and nerves, and lymphangiomas. Now sclerotherapy has been successfully used in the treatment of congenital sinus tracts [8–10]. Bleomycin is an antitumor agent and, besides its antineoplastic effect, bleomycin causes nonspecific inflammatory reaction leading to fibrosis in the surrounding tissues [10]. Bleomycin has been used in fistula tract with successful results in our patient. No procedure-related complications and no recurrence were observed in our patient.

In conclusion, the present case is a description of a novel fistula tractus. To the best of our knowledge, this is the first case with fistula deeply located and extending from the gluteus to penis in the literature. Clinicians should consider underlying congenital malformation in the differential diagnosis of recurrent perineal and/or gluteal abscess. Catheter-based bleomycin injection could be applied as a safe, minimally invasive, and effective option for complex gluteal fistula, which makes it a suitable and durable alternative to open surgery. Treatment of this entity is individualized according to the site of fistula and associated anomalies, as well as the condition of the distal urethra.

Conflict of Interests

The authors declare that there is no conflict of interests regarding the publication of this paper.

References

[1] G. Singh, B. Kaur, and S. Gupta, "Gluteal fistula—an unusual manifestation of carcinoma colon," Indian Journal of Gastroenterology, vol. 11, no. 4, p. 171, 1992.

[2] K. Puthezhath, B. Zacharia, and T. P. Mathew, "Gluteal abscess: diagnostic challenges and management," Journal of Infection in Developing Countries, vol. 4, no. 5, pp. 345–348, 2010.

[3] M. Hussien and D. G. Mudd, "Crohn's disease presenting as left gluteal abscess," International Journal of Clinical Practice, vol. 55, no. 3, pp. 217–218, 2001.

[4] E. S. Alexander, S. Weinberg, R. A. Clark, and R. D. Belkin, "Fistulas and sinus tracts: radiographic evaluation, management, and outcome," Gastrointestinal Radiology, vol. 7, no. 2, pp. 135–140, 1982.

[5] T. Nicholson, M. W. Born, and E. Garber, "Spontaneous cholecystocutaneous fistula presenting in the gluteal region," Journal of Clinical Gastroenterology, vol. 28, no. 3, pp. 277–279, 1999.

[6] G. N. Buchanan, S. Halligan, C. I. Bartram, A. B. Williams, D. Tarroni, and C. R. G. Cohen, "Clinical examination, endosonography, and MR imaging in preoperative assessment of fistula in ano: comparison with outcome-based reference standard," Radiology, vol. 233, no. 3, pp. 674–681, 2004.

[7] O. Baskan, M. Koplay, M. Sivri, and C. Erol, "Our experience with MR imaging of perianal fistulas," Polish Journal of Radiology, vol. 79, pp. 490–497, 2014.

[8] P. P. Nixon and A. E. Healey, "Treatment of a branchial sinus tract by sclerotherapy," *Dentomaxillofacial Radiology*, vol. 40, no. 2, pp. 130–132, 2011.

[9] L. Duman, I. Karnak, D. Akinci, and F. C. Tanyel, "Extensive cervical-mediastinal cystic lymphatic malformation treated with sclerotherapy in a child with Klippel-Trenaunay syndrome," *Journal of Pediatric Surgery*, vol. 41, no. 1, pp. 21–24, 2006.

[10] V. Erikçi, M. Hoşgör, M. Yıldız et al., "Intralesional bleomycin sclerotherapy in childhood lymphangioma," *Turkish Journal of Pediatrics*, vol. 55, no. 4, pp. 396–400, 2013.

14

Successful Treatment with Mycophenolate Mofetil and Tacrolimus in Juvenile Severe Lupus Nephritis

Tomoo Kise, Hiroshi Yoshimura, Shigeru Fukuyama, and Masatsugu Uehara

Division of Pediatric Nephrology, Okinawa Prefectural Nanbu Medical Center-Children's Medical Center, Arakawa 118-1, Haebaru, Okinawa 901-1193, Japan

Correspondence should be addressed to Tomoo Kise; tomookise@yahoo.co.jp

Academic Editor: Nan-Chang Chiu

Lupus nephritis (LN) of juvenile onset often has severe disease presentation. Despite aggressive induction therapy, up to 20% of patients with LN are resistant to initial therapy and up to 44% suffer a renal relapse. However, there is no consensus on an appropriate therapeutic regimen for refractory LN. We report a 13-year-old girl with recurrent LN who was not taking her medications. At age of 11 years, she was diagnosed with LN classified as International Society of Nephrology/Renal Pathology Society (ISN/RPS) class IV G (A) + V. She was treated with prednisolone and MMF after nine methylprednisolone pulses. Nineteen months later, she was admitted to the hospital with generalized edema. Her symptoms were nephrotic syndrome and acute renal dysfunction. She received three methylprednisolone pulses for 3 days, followed by oral prednisolone and MMF. Twenty-seven days after the three methylprednisolone pulses, her acute renal dysfunction was improved, but the nephrotic syndrome was not improved. A second biopsy showed diffuse lupus nephritis classified as the predominant finding of ISN/RPS class V. We added tacrolimus to the MMF. Four months after adding tacrolimus, the nephrotic syndrome improved. We conclude that adding tacrolimus to the treatment regimen for LN resistant to MMF is effective.

1. Introduction

Juvenile onset lupus nephritis (LN) often has very active and severe disease presentation. Several studies have shown that mycophenolate mofetil (MMF) is at least as effective as intravenous cyclophosphamide (IVCY) for active LN [1–3]. Despite aggressive induction therapy, up to 20% of patients with LN are resistant to initial therapy and up to 44% suffer a renal relapse [4]. However, there is no consensus on an appropriate therapeutic regimen for refractory LN.

Tacrolimus (Tac) is an immunosuppressive macrolide of the calcineurin inhibitors. Recently, the addition of Tac to treatment with MMF has been reported to be useful in refractory LN [5, 6]. We report a 13-year-old girl with recurrent LN (nephrotic syndrome and acute renal dysfunction), who was not taking her medications. Administration of three methylprednisolone pulses and doubling of the MMF dose improved the acute renal dysfunction but could not improve the patient's nephrotic syndrome. Tacrolimus was introduced to control disease activity.

2. Case Report

A 13-year-old girl was admitted to our hospital emergently with anasarca and renal dysfunction. At the age of 11 years, she was diagnosed with systemic lupus erythematosus (SLE) according to the American Rheumatism Association criteria, based on positive antinuclear antibody, positive anti-double stranded DNA (dsDNA) antibody, pancytopenia, and persistent proteinuria. Renal dysfunction was showed in serum creatinine of 0.8 mg/dL, blood urea nitrogen of 28 mg/dL, and an estimated glomerular filtration rate (eGFR) of 80 mL/min/1.73 m^2 using the Schwartz formula. Urine protein creatinine ratio was 9.01 g/g Cr. Urinary sediment showed 30–49 red blood cells/high power field (HPF), 5–9 white blood cells/HPF, hyaline cast, and granular cast. Renal biopsy showed diffused lupus nephritis classified as International Society of Nephrology/Renal Pathology Society (ISN/RPS) class IV G (A) + V associated with cellular crescents (60%), endocapillary hypercellularity, karyorrhexis, wire loop lesions, leukocyte infiltrates,

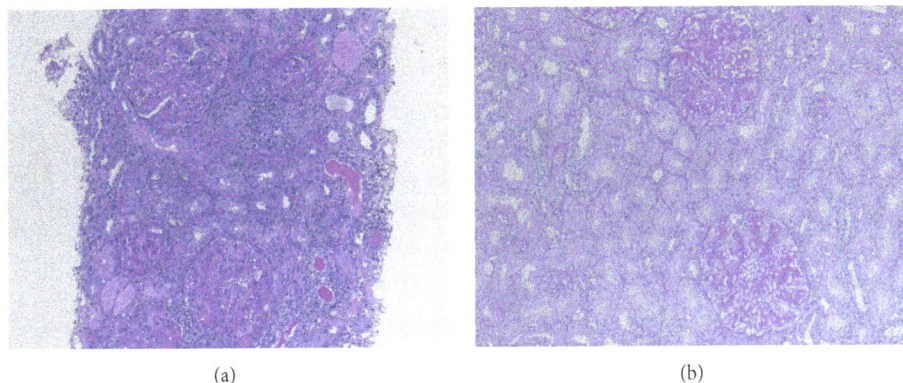

(a)   (b)

FIGURE 1: Renal biopsy findings. (a) Initial renal biopsy findings. Light microscopy reveals diffuse global mesangial proliferation. Renal interstitium is filtrated by lymphocytes. Tubular atrophy and tortuosity are shown. Periodic acid-Schiff (PAS) staining, ×200. (b) Second renal biopsy findings. Light microscopy revealed that the mesangial proliferation and the renal tubular lymphocyte infiltration are improved. Tubular atrophy and tortuosity are not shown. PAS staining, ×200.

and subepithelial immune deposits separated by spikes (Figure 1(a)). Immunofluorescence revealed "full-house" staining for C3, C1q, IgG, IgA, and IgM in the mesangial and endocapillary regions. She was treated with prednisolone at 30 mg/day (0.75 mg/kg/day, body weight 40.3 kg) and MMF at 1 g/day after nine methylprednisolone pulses (1000 mg/day) for 18 days. At 7 months after being diagnosed with LN, she became well, and prednisolone was reduced to 10 mg/day while maintaining MMF at 1 g/day. She had lost 2 kg in weight and her edema was relieved. Her urine protein creatinine ratio had decreased to 6 g/g Cr, and her serum albumin had increased to 2.6 g/dL.

Six months later, she was admitted to the hospital with generalized edema. At admission, she was found to have gained 8 kg in weight over the last three weeks. Vital signs were stable except for mild hypertension with blood pressure of 126/78 mmHg. There was the absence of extrarenal disease. Laboratory studies (Table 1) at admission showed hypoproteinemia (4.0 g/dL), hypoalbuminemia (1.5 g/dL), renal dysfunction (blood urea nitrogen 12 mg/dL, serum creatinine 0.9 mg/dL, and eGFR 74 mL/min/1.73 m^2), and hypocomplementemia (C3 50 mg/dL). Hemoglobin was 12.5 g/dL. The early morning urine-protein to creatinine ratio was 7.18 g/g Cr. Urinary sediment showed 5–9 red blood cells/HPF, 10–19 white blood cells/HPF, granular cast, and oval fat body. She admitted that she had not been taking her medicine. The patient received three methylprednisolone pulses (500 mg/day) for 3 days, followed by oral prednisolone increased to 30 mg/day from 10 mg/day, and MMF was increased to 2 g/day from 1 g/day. In addition to benzylhydrochlorothiazide, we administered furosemide at 40 mg/day to improve the anasarca. One month later, after administration of the three methylprednisolone pulses, the patient's serum creatinine improved to 0.5 mg/dL; eGFR was 116 mL/min/1.73 m^2. Her acute renal dysfunction was improved, but her nephrotic syndrome became worse (Table 1). Serum albumin was 1.8 g/dL, and immunoglobulin G decreased from 540 mg/dL on admission to 130 mg/dL. Hemoglobin was 13.6 g/dL. Urine-protein to creatinine ratio

was 7.97 g/g Cr. Urinary sediment showed 5–9 red blood cells/HPF, 10–19 white blood cells/HPF, granular cast, and oval fat body. We had to replenish gamma globulin. On the following day, a second renal biopsy was performed. Light microscopic examination showed 51 glomeruli, of which 3 were globally sclerotic. The remaining 48 glomeruli had global subepithelial spike formation (Figure 1(b)). Wire loop lesions, mesangial cell proliferation, karyorrhexis, hematoxylin bodies, and cellular crescents could not be seen in any glomeruli. Neither lymphocyte infiltration nor neutrophils were apparent in the glomeruli or interstitium. Immunofluorescence revealed staining for C3, C1q, IgG, and IgA in the mesangial and endocapillary regions. On the basis of these findings, we made a diagnosis of lupus nephritis classified as a predominant finding of ISN/RPS class V. Based on active renal lesions seen in the second biopsy, we administered tacrolimus (3 mg/day) in addition to oral prednisolone and MMF. We titrated the dose so that the tacrolimus blood concentration increased to 5 ng/mL. One month after the addition of tacrolimus, it was no longer necessary to replenish gamma globulin for augmentation of immunoglobulin G. By the end of 4 months of tacrolimus therapy, all laboratory findings and the patient's anasarca were improved (Table 1). We explained to the patient and her father the need for taking the medicine, and she was discharged.

Three months after discharge, she was free of edema, and her blood concentration of tacrolimus was maintained. In the outpatient department, she reported that she was "taking the medicine well."

3. Discussion

Adding tacrolimus to MMF and prednisolone in this patient with severe LN was effective. Bao et al. reported the effectiveness of the combination of MMF, tacrolimus, and prednisolone (multitarget therapy) as induction therapy for lupus nephritis [6]. Cortés-Hernández et al. and Lanata et al. reported that adding tacrolimus for MMF-resistant LN patients (classes III, IV, and V) was effective [4, 5]. Mok et al.

TABLE 1: Laboratory findings on admission, at 1 month after methylprednisolone pulses and at discharge.

	At admission	1 month from methylprednisolone pulses	1 month from addition of tacrolimus	At discharge (4 months from addition of tacrolimus)
White blood count ($\times 10^2/\mu L$)	51	193	85	82
Hemoglobin (g/dL)	12.5	13.6	10.2	11.5
Platelets ($\times 10^4/\mu L$)	30.9	37.3	28	29.9
Total protein (g/dL)	4.0	3.9	4.6	5.5
Albumin (g/dL)	1.5	1.8	2.4	3.0
Blood urea nitrogen (mg/dL)	12	18	18	12
Creatinine (mg/dL)	0.9	0.5	0.5	0.5
C3 (mg/dL)	50	63	88	111
Immunoglobin G (mg/dL)	540	130	218	371
dsDNA antibodies (IU/mL)	98	15	14	12
Urine-protein to creatinine ratio (g/gCr)	3.13	7.97	2.79	1.07
Urine sediment				
RBC/HPF	5–9	5–9	<1	<1
WBC/HPF	10–19	10–19	1–4	1–4
Cast	Granular (+)	Granular (+)	(−)	(−)
Oval fat body	(+)	(+)	(+)	(−)

reported that they administered triple-drug therapy of MMF, tacrolimus, and prednisolone to lupus nephritis patients for whom a regimen of two immunosuppressive regimens had been insufficient; the urine protein was improved in 75% of the patients [7].

The treatment of the MMF-resistant lupus nephritis include the multitarget therapy and various biologics that target B cells, T cells, or different cytokines [8]. Cyclophosphamide or cyclosporine is considered as treatment of class V LN with first choice [9]. On the other hand, for the treatment of class IV LN, cyclophosphamide or MMF is first choice. MMF is the prodrug of mycophenolic acid (MPA), which blocks antibody formation by polyclonally activated B-lymphocytes. MPA also blocks production of cytokines such as interleukin- (IL-) 2, IL-10, interferon- (IFN-) γ, and tumor necrosis factor-alpha (TNF-α) [7]. Tacrolimus blocks the phosphate activity of calcineurin and reduces IL-2 gene transcription of activated T cells. Blocking T cell activation also leads to reduction in the production of other proinflammatory cytokines that are important in regulating B cell activity [7]. These authors explained that, because the mechanism of action was different using tacrolimus, MMF, and steroids, the combination of these three drugs could control inflammatory, proliferative, vasculitic, and membranous lesions synchronously [6, 7].

The membranoproliferative class diagnosed in the initial biopsy was transformed to membranous lupus nephritis despite immunosuppressive treatment with MMF. The multitarget therapy was effective in our case of class V LN. There are few reports of such transformations. Dalton et al. stated that it was unclear whether treatment of their patient with MMF had contributed to the development of a membranous lesion or it had been inadequate treatment for the lesion as it developed [10].

In our patient, no adverse effects were observed during a treatment period of 6 months. In the four reports mentioned above [4–7], 62 adverse effects were noted in 62 patients: infection not requiring hospitalization, 16 cases; digestive symptoms (diarrhea, dyspepsia, and nausea), 9 cases; major infection requiring hospitalization, 7 cases; muscle symptoms, 6 cases; herpes infection, 5 cases; hypercholesterolemia, 4 cases; hypertension, 3 cases; hyperglycemia or diabetes mellitus, 3 cases; leukopenia, 2 cases; transient increase in serum creatinine, 2 cases; alopecia, 2 cases; tremor, 2 cases; and irregular menstruation, 1 case. None of these adverse effects led to protocol withdrawal. Mok et al. stated that the long-term risk of nephrotoxicity and adverse vascular effects could be minimized by using a lower dose of tacrolimus [7].

In conclusion, we believe that adding tacrolimus to MMF and prednisolone in patients with juvenile onset lupus nephritis is effective. Long-term observation is needed to determine whether this therapy continues to be tolerated and effective.

Conflict of Interests

The authors declare that no conflict of interests exists.

References

[1] T. M. Chan, F. K. Li, C. S. O. Tang et al., "Efficacy of mycophenolate mofetil in patients with diffuse proliferative lupus nephritis. Hong Kong-Guangzhou Nephrology Study Group," *The New England Journal of Medicine*, vol. 343, no. 16, pp. 1156–1162, 2000.

[2] E. M. Ginzler, M. A. Dooley, C. Aranow et al., "Mycophenolate mofetil or intravenous cyclophosphamide for lupus nephritis," *The New England Journal of Medicine*, vol. 353, no. 21, pp. 2219–2228, 2005.

[3] G. B. Appel, G. Conteras, M. A. Dooley et al., "Mycophenolate mofetil versus cyclophosphamide for induction treatment of lupus nephritis," *Journal of the American Society of Nephrology*, vol. 20, pp. 1103–1112, 2009.

[4] J. Cortés-Hernández, M. T. Torres-Salido, A. S. Medrano, M. V. Tarrés, and J. Ordi-Ros, "Long-term outcomes— mycophenolate mofetil treatment for lupus nephritis with addition of tacrolimus for resistant cases," *Nephrology Dialysis Transplantation*, vol. 25, no. 12, pp. 3939–3948, 2010.

[5] C. M. Lanata, T. Mahmood, D. M. Fine, and M. Petri, "Combination therapy of mycophenolate mofetil and tacrolimus in lupus nephritis," *Lupus*, vol. 19, no. 8, pp. 935–940, 2010.

[6] H. Bao, Z.-H. Liu, H.-L. Xie, W.-X. Hu, H.-T. Zhang, and L.-S. Li, "Successful treatment of class V+IV lupus nephritis with multitarget therapy," *Journal of the American Society of Nephrology*, vol. 19, no. 10, pp. 2001–2010, 2008.

[7] C. C. Mok, C. H. To, K. L. Yu, and L. Y. Ho, "Combined low-dose mycophenolate mofetil and tacrolimus for lupus nephritis with suboptimal response to standard therapy: a 12-month prospective study," *Lupus*, vol. 22, no. 11, pp. 1135–1141, 2013.

[8] G. J. Pons-Estel, R. Serrano, M. A. Plasín, G. Espinosa, and R. Cervera, "Epidemiology and management of refractory lupus nephritis," *Autoimmunity Reviews*, vol. 10, no. 11, pp. 655–663, 2011.

[9] H. A. Austin III, G. G. Illei, M. J. Braun, and J. E. Balow, "Randomized, controlled trial of prednisone, cyclophosphamide, and cyclosporine in lupus membranous nephropathy," *Journal of the American Society of Nephrology*, vol. 20, no. 4, pp. 901–911, 2009.

[10] K. Dalton, M. Smith, and J. M. Thurman, "The development of membranous lupus nephritis during treatment with mycophenolate mofetil for proliferative renal disease," *Nephrol Dial Transplant Plus*, vol. 3, no. 4, pp. 346–348, 2010.

Eikenella corrodens Sepsis with Cerebrospinal Fluid Pleocytosis in a Very Low Birth Weight Neonate

Christopher Sawyer, Dimitrios Angelis, and Robert Bennett

Division of Neonatology, Department of Pediatrics, Texas Tech University Health Sciences Center, Odessa, TX 79763, USA

Correspondence should be addressed to Dimitrios Angelis; d_agelis@hotmail.com

Academic Editor: Nan-Chang Chiu

We report a case of *Eikenella corrodens* sepsis associated with CSF pleocytosis in a very low birth weight neonate. A 1000-gram male neonate was born at 27-week gestation due to preterm labor. The patient presented with signs and symptoms of sepsis and was treated for suspected meningitis with intravenous ampicillin and gentamicin for 7 days, with cefotaxime added for three weeks. He had a normal brain MRI at discharge and normal development at 6 months of life. To our knowledge, this is the first case of *E. corrodens* sepsis and associated meningitis in a very low birth weight neonate.

1. Introduction

Eikenella corrodens is a gram negative rod which is a normal inhabitant of human gastrointestinal tract, including the oral cavity. *E. corrodens* is primarily an opportunistic pathogen capable of causing a wide range of diseases. Presented here is a case of neonatal sepsis in a 27-week gestational age male newborn associated with cerebrospinal fluid pleocytosis.

2. Case Presentation

A 1000-gram male neonate was born at 27-week gestation to a previously healthy mother. Routine prenatal labs were unremarkable except group B streptococcus (GBS) status, which was unknown. The mother presented in preterm labor and a male infant was delivered precipitously, at a referring hospital. Rupture of membranes occurred spontaneously one hour prior to delivery, with the amniotic fluid reported as clear. One hour prior to delivery the mother received prenatal steroids as well as one dose of ampicillin intravenously. From the maternal history, there was no reported fever, abdominal pain, weight loss, or other constitutional symptoms.

Following delivery, the baby developed respiratory distress and apnea. Initial resuscitation efforts included positive pressure ventilation and intubation at approximately 3 minutes of life. Apgar scores were 4 and 7, at 1 and 5 minutes,

respectively. An initial chest radiograph was suggestive of respiratory distress syndrome; 1 dose of surfactant was subsequently given and infant was placed on mechanical ventilation. Prior to transport, a blood culture was obtained and ampicillin and gentamicin were initiated for suspected neonatal sepsis. He remained on mechanical ventilation for 1 day and was subsequently extubated to nasal continuous positive airway pressure (nCPAP). Initial complete blood count, at about six hours of life, was significant for a low total white blood cell count with left shift. Specifically, WBCs were 4800/μL with a differential count: segmented PMN 19%, bands 30%, metamyelocytes 4%, lymphocytes 30%, and monocytes 17%. The I : T ratio was 0.64 (normal < 0.2). On admission, the platelets were 240,000/μL and the hemoglobin was 13 grams/dL. Initial CRP was 1.3 mg/dL (normal < 1 mg/dL) and the peak value, which occurred on day of life 2 (DOL 2), was 2.3 mg/dL.

On DOL 3 the initial blood culture obtained at the referring hospital grew *E. corrodens*. This finding triggered a complete evaluation for sepsis including a repeat blood culture as well as a lumbar puncture and urine culture. The cerebrospinal fluid (CSF) findings revealed pleocytosis and specifically CSF red blood cells (RBCs) 24800/μL and white blood cells (WBCs) 990/μL (58% segmented PMN, 2% bands, 35% lymphocytes, and 5% monocytes). However, gram stain and culture remained negative. The total protein and the glucose in CSF were within normal limits for the degree of prematurity. A blood culture was repeated for three consecutive days, 24 hours apart, all of which remained negative. The urine analysis was negative for white blood cells and the culture remained negative. Due to the initial blood culture, and after consultation with an infectious disease specialist, cefotaxime was added to the initial antibiotic regimen and the overall antibiotic regimen was readjusted as follows: ampicillin (100 mg/kg/dose every 12 hours), gentamicin (4.5 mg/kg/dose every 36 hours), and cefotaxime (50 mg/kg/dose every 12 hours). Ampicillin and gentamicin were discontinued after 7 days of treatment (ensuring that the subsequently obtained blood cultures remained negative) while he received a 3-week course of cefotaxime. Due to low birth weight, prematurity, use of prolonged course of antibiotics, and the presence of a central catheter, it was felt that the infant was at high risk for developing invasive fungemia and hence fluconazole prophylaxis was initiated at a dose of 3 mg/kg/dose every 72 hours intravenously. Fluconazole was discontinued upon completion of the antibiotic treatment and removal of the peripherally inserted central catheter. An echocardiogram was performed and ruled out endocarditis. The remaining hospital course was unremarkable. He was discharged home on DOL 60 (36-week corrected age), neurologically appropriate, and weighing 2300 grams. A brain MRI was obtained prior to discharge and was normal. At six-month follow-up, the patient was developmentally appropriate for age.

3. Discussion

Neonatal sepsis is a systemic infection that occurs early in an infant's life. Early onset sepsis (EOS) develops within 72 hours of life and is typically attributed to pathogens acquired perinatally. GBS and *E. coli* account for more than 70% of cases of EOS. On occasion, rare opportunistic pathogens are the cause of EOS. We describe here a case of EOS caused by *Eikenella corrodens* in an extremely preterm male neonate. *E. corrodens* is found in the oral cavity as well as the gastrointestinal tract of both humans and animals. It is a small, nonmotile, gram negative rod which occasionally can appear as coccobacillus. *E. corrodens* is known as the corroding bacteria, named for the phenomenon where colonies of the bacteria form characteristic pits on agar plates. *E. corrodens* is a facultative anaerobe and is generally only able to grow on blood or chocolate agar with 3–10% CO_2 [1]. The paucity of cases of neonatal infections involving *E. corrodens* could be partially explained by the difficulty in isolating and culturing the bacteria. Molecular techniques, such as DNA hybridization, have been also used for the identification of several pathogens of the oral cavity, including *E. corrodens* [2].

E. corrodens has been implicated in a variety of infections, including head and neck infections in those with local cancer, osteomyelitis (particularly secondary to bite wounds), endocarditis (a member of the HACEK group, predominantly found in intravenous drug users who lick their needles), meningitis, intra-abdominal infections, suppurative thyroiditis, and neonatal conjunctivitis [3–5]. In all these cases, antibiotic treatment is deemed necessary. *E. corrodens* is

commonly susceptible to penicillin, ampicillin, piperacillin, and both second- and third-generation cephalosporins. *E. corrodens* is commonly resistant to antistaphylococcal penicillins such as methicillin and nafcillin [6]. Additionally, beta-lactamase expression has been reported, raising the potential issue of resistance to penicillins. As a result, third-generation cephalosporins, such as cefotaxime, are good first-line antibiotics [7].

E. corrodens is a rare cause of neonatal sepsis. A literature review shows seven documented cases of neonatal sepsis since 1985 [8–13]. All cases described occurred in premature infants, where the presenting symptom was predominantly preterm labor and associated neonatal sepsis. The median gestational age of the reviewed cases was 30 weeks. In all the reviewed cases the outcome was favorable except in one case of a 24-week gestational age neonate that did not survive beyond the immediate neonatal period [13]. One possible risk factor for the development of maternofetal infection with *E. corrodens* is the presence of advanced periodontal disease in the mother. Periodontitis has been shown to cause bacteremias by oral bacteria, including some of the HACEK (*Haemophilus* species, *Actinobacillus, Cardiobacterium hominis, Eikenella corrodens,* and *Kingella*) group, either following surgical procedures or spontaneously, and is therefore associated with a variety of diseases that have significant impact in early childhood, as well as in adult life [14, 15]. Several studies have shown that periodontitis can have a significant impact on the placental-fetal unit, exacerbate a fetal inflammatory response, and lead to preterm delivery [16]. In our case, although we were not able to elicit a history of periodontitis, we could speculate that this could be a contributing factor given the presence of *E. corrodens* and preterm labor. The risk of maternofetal infection can also be associated with close contact with animals [8, 9].

Our patient exhibited symptoms and signs of sepsis and he was evaluated for associated meningitis although he did not present with typical neurologic symptoms such as seizures and severe apnea. His initial hospital course was complicated with respiratory depression requiring mechanical ventilation on day of life 0, with improvement afterwards. The organism was not isolated from the spinal fluid despite the significant CSF pleocytosis. Meningitis in this case was presumed based on the CSF analysis but not proven by CSF culture. A possible explanation for this result includes receiving multiple doses of antibiotics prior to CSF analysis and culture. Additionally, although *E. corrodens* has been shown to cause meningitis and brain abscesses in adults [3], as well as chronic meningitis in immunocompromised hosts [17], it has never been documented in neonates, to our knowledge. The CSF analysis showed an increased red blood cell count, a common finding when interpreting neonatal CSF samples [18]. It has been shown that in neonates almost 50% of CSF examinations return results with high red blood cell counts [19], interfering with the interpretation of these studies [20]. The patient had been diagnosed with a low grade intraventricular hemorrhage at birth, which could also have contributed to the presence of RBCs in the analysis that we performed, although sequelae of this finding were not confirmed on MRI prior to discharge.

Standard treatment of neonatal infections, specifically with ampicillin, provides coverage of *E. corrodens*. Furthermore, in the event of preterm labor and suspicion of chorioamnionitis, routine treatment with ampicillin prior to delivery may have eradicated the penicillin sensitive *E. corrodens* strains and have contributed to the negative blood and CSF cultures during evaluation of the neonate. In similar cases, different techniques, such as polymerase chain reaction or mass spectrometry, may be more helpful in identifying neonates with *E. corrodens* culture negative sepsis [21, 22].

4. Conclusion

E. corrodens is an opportunistic pathogen which can cause sepsis in both adults and children. It is usually associated with characteristic risk factors. Symptoms of neonatal sepsis caused by *E. corrodens* are nonspecific, making diagnosis on clinical grounds challenging. Culture proven cases attributed to *E. corrodens* have been rarely reported. Interestingly, there is a paucity of cases of CNS involvement of *E. corrodens* in neonatal literature. It is reassuring that the majority of strains of *E. corrodens* are susceptible to ampicillin, part of standard treatment in early onset sepsis. Typically, the pathogen is susceptible to cephalosporins also, which are frequently used to treat the infection and yield favorable results. Our patient presented with bacteremia in addition to presumed meningitis and was successfully treated with a three-week antibiotic regimen, including initially ampicillin and gentamicin and later a third-generation cephalosporin. Further research into what risks and events predispose to *E. corrodens* maternofetal infections could lead to both prevention and identification of this specific pathogen prior to culture results.

Conflict of Interests

The authors have no conflict of interests to disclose.

Authors' Contribution

Christopher Sawyer wrote the initial and revised drafts of the paper and approved the final paper as submitted. Dimitrios Angelis was the neonatologist attending who took care of the patient, wrote parts of the initial paper, and approved the final paper as submitted. Robert Bennett was the neonatologist attending that took care of the patient, reviewed and revised the paper, and approved the final paper as submitted.

References

[1] M. D. Decker, "Eikenella corrodens," *Infection Control*, vol. 7, no. 1, pp. 36–41, 1986.

[2] N. Buduneli, H. Baylas, E. Buduneli, O. Türkoğlu, T. Köse, and G. Dahlen, "Periodontal infections and pre-term low birth weight: a case-control study," *Journal of Clinical Periodontology*, vol. 32, no. 2, pp. 174–181, 2005.

[3] A. M. Emmerson and F. Mills, "Recurrent meningitis and brain abscess caused by *Eikenella corrodens*," *Postgraduate Medical Journal*, vol. 54, no. 631, pp. 343–345, 1978.

[4] M. S. Chhabra, W. W. Motley III, and J. E. Mortensen, "Eikenella corrodens as a causative agent for neonatal conjunctivitis," *Journal of AAPOS*, vol. 12, no. 5, pp. 524–525, 2008.

[5] Y. Yoshino, Y. Inamo, T. Fuchigami et al., "A pediatric patient with acute suppurative thyroiditis caused by *Eikenella corrodens*," *Journal of Infection and Chemotherapy*, vol. 16, no. 5, pp. 353–355, 2010.

[6] D. Sofianou and A. Kolokotronis, "Susceptibility of Eikenella corrodens to antimicrobial agents," *Journal of Chemotherapy*, vol. 2, no. 3, pp. 156–158, 1990.

[7] E. J. Goldstein, C. E. Cherubin, M. L. Corrado, and M. F. Sierra, "Comparative susceptibility of *Yersinia enterocolitica*, *Eikenella corrodens*, and penicillin-resistant and penicillin-susceptible *Streptococcus pneumoniae* to β-lactam and alternative antimicrobial agents," *Reviews of Infectious Diseases*, vol. 4, supplement, pp. S406–S410, 1982.

[8] B. L. Hu, J. M. Crewalk, and D. P. Ascher, "Congenital sepsis caused by *Eikenella corrodens*," *Open Journal of Pediatrics*, vol. 2, no. 2, pp. 175–177, 2012.

[9] A. R. Jadhav, M. A. Belfort, and G. A. Dildy III, "*Eikenella corrodens* chorioamnionitis: modes of infection?" *American Journal of Obstetrics & Gynecology*, vol. 200, no. 5, pp. e4–e5, 2009.

[10] F. Garnier, G. Masson, A. Bedu et al., "Maternofetal infections due to *Eikenella corrodens*," *Journal of Medical Microbiology*, vol. 58, no. 2, pp. 273–275, 2009.

[11] M. T. Andrés, M. C. Martín, J. F. Fierro, and F. J. Méndez, "Chorioamnionitis and neonatal septicaemia caused by Eikenella corrodens," *Journal of Infection*, vol. 44, no. 2, pp. 133–134, 2002.

[12] K. G. Jeppson and L. G. Reimer, "Eikenella corrodens chorioamnionitis," *Obstetrics and Gynecology*, vol. 78, no. 3, pp. 503–505, 1991.

[13] J. M. J. Sporken, H. L. Muytjens, and H. M. Vemer, "Intrauterine infection due to eikenella corrodens," *Acta Obstetricia et Gynecologica Scandinavica*, vol. 64, no. 8, pp. 683–684, 1985.

[14] N. B. Parahitiyawa, L. J. Jin, W. K. Leung, W. C. Yam, and L. P. Samaranayake, "Microbiology of odontogenic bacteremia: beyond endocarditis," *Clinical Microbiology Reviews*, vol. 22, no. 1, pp. 46–64, 2009.

[15] G. Pizzo, R. Guiglia, L. L. Russo, and G. Campisi, "Dentistry and internal medicine: from the focal infection theory to the periodontal medicine concept," *European Journal of Internal Medicine*, vol. 21, no. 6, pp. 496–502, 2010.

[16] Y. A. Bobetsis, S. P. Barros, and S. Offenbacher, "Exploring the relationship between periodontal disease and pregnancy complications," *Journal of the American Dental Association*, vol. 137, supplement, pp. 7S–13S, 2006.

[17] X.-Y. Dong and L. Gong, "Chronic meningitis caused by *Eikenella corrodens*," *Kaohsiung Journal of Medical Sciences*, vol. 29, no. 8, pp. 466–467, 2013.

[18] L. E. Nigrovic, S. S. Shah, and M. I. Neuman, "Correction of cerebrospinal fluid protein for the presence of red blood cells in children with a traumatic lumbar puncture," *Journal of Pediatrics*, vol. 159, no. 1, pp. 158–159, 2011.

[19] R. G. Greenberg, P. B. Smith, C. M. Cotten, M. A. Moody, R. H. Clark, and D. K. Benjamin, "Traumatic lumbar punctures in neonates: test performance of the cerebrospinal fluid white blood cell count," *Pediatric Infectious Disease Journal*, vol. 27, no. 12, pp. 1047–1051, 2008.

[20] K. Pacatte, "Analysis of cerebrospinal fluid in the neonate," *Neonatal Network*, vol. 27, no. 6, pp. 419–422, 2008.

[21] N. Laforgia, B. Coppola, R. Carbone, A. Grassi, A. Mautone, and A. Iolascon, "Rapid detection of neonatal sepsis using polymerase chain reaction," *Acta Paediatrica*, vol. 86, no. 10, pp. 1097–1099, 1997.

[22] O. Clerc, G. Prod'hom, L. Senn et al., "Matrix-assisted laser desorption ionization time-of-flight mass spectrometry and PCR-based rapid diagnosis of Staphylococcus aureus bacteraemia," *Clinical Microbiology and Infection*, vol. 20, no. 4, pp. 355–360, 2014.

16

Bilateral Symmetrical Herpes Zoster in an Immunocompetent 15-Year-Old Adolescent Boy

Alexander K. C. Leung[1] and Benjamin Barankin[2]

[1]*The Alberta Children's Hospital, The University of Calgary, Calgary, AB, Canada T2M 0H5*
[2]*Toronto Dermatology Centre, Toronto, ON, Canada M3H 5Y8*

Correspondence should be addressed to Alexander K. C. Leung; aleung@ucalgary.ca

Academic Editor: Andrea E. Scaramuzza

Herpes zoster is uncommon in immunocompetent children. The bilateral symmetrical occurrence of herpes zoster lesions is extremely rare. We report a 15-year-old immunocompetent Chinese adolescent boy who developed bilateral symmetrical herpes zoster lesions. To our knowledge, the occurrence of bilateral symmetrical herpes zoster lesions in an immunocompetent individual has not been reported in the pediatric literature.

1. Introduction

Herpes zoster, also known as shingles, is caused by reactivation of endogenous latent varicella-zoster virus (VZV) that resides in a sensory dorsal root ganglion [1]. Herpes zoster can develop any time after a primary infection with VZV (i.e., varicella or chickenpox) or varicella vaccination [1]. The activated virus travels back down the corresponding cutaneous nerve to the adjacent skin, causing typically a painful, unilateral vesicular eruption in a restricted dermatomal distribution. Herpes zoster is more common in persons with relative cell-mediated immunologic compromise such as elderly individuals or patients with an immunosuppressive illness or receiving immunosuppressive therapy. Immunocompromised individuals have a 20 to 100 times greater risk than immunocompetent individuals of the same age [2]. The bilateral symmetrical occurrence of herpes zoster lesions is extremely rare especially in immunocompetent children. We report a case of a 15-year-old immunocompetent Chinese adolescent boy with bilateral symmetrical herpes zoster lesions along T7, T8, and T9 dermatomes. To our knowledge, the occurrence of bilateral symmetrical herpes zoster lesions in an immunocompetent individual has not been reported in the pediatric literature.

2. Case Report

A 15-year-old Chinese boy presented with a bilateral and symmetrical painful eruption on the upper abdomen of 7 days' duration. The eruption was preceded by a 2-day history of malaise and low grade fever. He did not have the varicella vaccine but had chickenpox at 3 years of age. His past health was otherwise unremarkable. In particular, he did not have recurrent or chronic infections. The patient did not have recent weight loss and was not on any medications. There was no history of recent travel. He did not have exposure to venereal or other infectious diseases. The family history was noncontributory.

Physical examination revealed multiple vesicles/bullae on an erythematous base, distributed bilaterally and symmetrically in a band-like distribution along T7, T8, and T9 dermatomes (Figure 1). The rest of the physical examination was unremarkable. His weight was 76 kg (90th percentile) and height 178 cm (70th percentile). His vital signs were normal and he was not in distress. There was no lymphadenopathy in the axillary or groin area, no organomegaly, and no muscle wasting.

Laboratory investigations revealed hemoglobin of 12.8 g/dL and white blood cell count of 7.8×10^9/L with

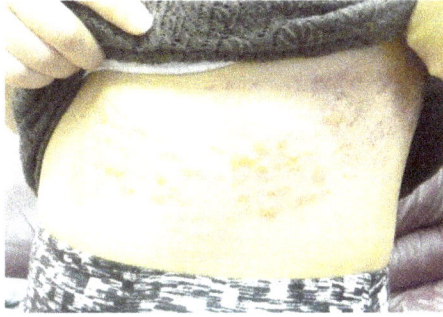

FIGURE 1: Bilateral, symmetrically distributed herpes zoster lesions along T7, T8, and T9 dermatomes.

a normal differential count. His immunoglobulin levels were normal. The patient was treated with acyclovir 800 mg five times a day for 7 days. The blistering and discomfort resolved in 14 days, and the secondary dyspigmentation took 3 months to completely fade.

3. Discussion

In herpes zoster, the onset of disease is usually heralded by pain within the dermatome and precedes the lesions by 48 to 72 hours. An area of erythema then follows and precedes the development of a group of vesicles in the distribution of the dermatome that corresponds to the infected dorsal root ganglion. The diagnosis of herpes zoster is mainly made clinically, based on the distinctive clinical appearance and symptomatology. Laboratory tests usually are not necessary unless the rash is atypical.

In herpes zoster, usually one or, less commonly, two or three adjacent dermatomes are affected. The lesions typically do not cross the midline [1]. In individuals with immunodeficiency, the lesions may involve multiple contiguous, noncontiguous, bilateral, or unusual dermatomes. Dissemination occurs in 2 to 10% of immunocompromised individuals but rarely in immunocompetent individuals [1, 3]. Our patient was immunocompetent based on the history (unremarkable past health, absence of recurrent infections, or weight loss), physical findings (no muscle wasting, absence of fever, lymphadenopathy, or organomegaly), laboratory tests (normal complete blood count and immunoglobulin levels), and excellent response to oral acyclovir with complete recovery. The patient was not tested for HIV because he did not have venereal exposure, and there was no sign suggestive of HIV or immunodeficiency.

The simultaneous occurrence of herpes zoster in two noncontiguous dermatomes involving different halves of the body, also termed herpes zoster duplex bilateralis, is distinct from disseminated VZV infection. Herpes zoster duplex bilateralis is rarely reported, especially in immunocompetent individuals [4–7]. It is estimated that herpes zoster duplex bilateralis accounts for less than 0.1% of all herpes zoster cases and occurs mainly in immunocompromised individuals [7].

The bilateral symmetrical occurrence of herpes zoster lesions, also known as herpes zoster duplex symmetricus,

is extremely rare, especially in immunocompetent individuals [8]. Presumably, such occurrence is related to a high VZV genome load in the dorsal root ganglia in the same dermatome bilaterally. A perusal of the literature revealed only 3 cases of herpes zoster occurring bilaterally in the same dermatome [8–10]. In 1947, Thomas reported a 33-year-old woman who had herpes zoster in the upper sacral areas, hips, and upper part of the buttocks bilaterally [9]. In 2003, Arfan-ul-Bari et al. described a 24-year-old otherwise healthy man who had herpes zoster lesions over the lower chest in a horizontal band-like distribution bilaterally [10]. In 2006, Brandon et al. reported a 39-year-old female who developed bilateral herpes zoster at the T8 dermatome level on the fourth day after bilateral thoracoscopic splanchnicectomy for chronic severe visceral pain [8]. Her past health included 6 years of chronic pancreatitis secondary to hyperlipidemia and associated insulin-dependent diabetes mellitus. To our knowledge, our patient represents the first immunocompetent patient who had bilateral symmetrical herpes zoster in the pediatric age group.

It is known that vaccine-associated herpes zoster is milder than herpes zoster after wild-type varicella [1]. As such, there is a need for prevention of VZV infection through universal childhood immunization [11].

4. Conclusion

The bilateral symmetrical occurrence of herpes zoster lesions is extremely rare, especially in immunocompetent individuals. We report a Chinese immunocompetent teenager who had bilateral symmetrical herpes zoster lesions. To our knowledge, the occurrence of bilateral symmetrical herpes zoster lesions in an immunocompetent individual has not been reported in the pediatric literature.

Conflict of Interests

Professor Alexander K. C. Leung and Dr. Benjamin Barankin have disclosed no relevant financial relationship. They have received no external funding for the preparation of this paper.

References

[1] A. K. C. Leung, W. L. M. Robson, and A. G. Leong, "Herpes zoster in childhood," *Journal of Pediatric Health Care*, vol. 20, no. 5, pp. 300–303, 2006.

[2] I. Staikov, N. Neykov, B. Marinovic, J. Lipozenčić, and N. Tsankov, "Herpes zoster as a systemic disease," *Clinics in Dermatology*, vol. 32, no. 3, pp. 424–429, 2014.

[3] R. E. Oladokun, C. N. Olomukoro, and A. B. Owa, "Disseminated herpes zoster ophthalmicus in an immunocompetent 8-year old boy," *Clinics and Practice*, vol. 3, no. 2, article e16, 2013.

[4] B. Brar, R. Gupta, and S. Saghni, "Bilateral herpes—zoster of widely separated dermatomes in a non-immunocompromised female," *Indian Journal of Dermatology, Venereology and Leprology*, vol. 68, no. 1, pp. 48–49, 2002.

[5] P. Gahalaut and S. Chauhan, "Herpes zoster duplex bilateralis in an immunocompetent host," *Indian Dermatology Online Journal*, vol. 3, no. 1, pp. 31–32, 2012.

[6] Y. Karmon and N. Gadoth, "Delayed oculomotor nerve palsy after bilateral cervical zoster in an immunocompetent patient," *Neurology*, vol. 65, no. 1, article 170, 2005.

[7] Y. Takaoka, Y. Miyachi, Y. Yoshikawa, M. Tanioka, A. Fujisawa, and Y. Endo, "Bilateral disseminated herpes zoster in an immunocompetent host," *Dermatology Online Journal*, vol. 19, no. 2, p. 13, 2013.

[8] E. L. Brandon, J. Akers, and D. Rapeport, "Development of bilateral herpes zoster following thoracoscopic splanchnicectomy," *Anaesthesia and Intensive Care*, vol. 34, no. 3, pp. 382–383, 2006.

[9] E. W. P. Thomas, "Bilateral zoster: report of a case," *The Lancet*, vol. 250, no. 6486, pp. 910–911, 1947.

[10] A. Arfan-ul-Bari, N. Iftikhar, and S. ber Rahman, "Bilateral symmetrical herpes zoster in an immuno-competent patient (herpes zoster duplex symmetricus)," *Journal of the College of Physicians and Surgeons Pakistan*, vol. 13, no. 9, pp. 524–525, 2003.

[11] A. K. C. Leung, J. D. Kellner, and H. D. Davies, "Chickenpox: an update," *Journal of Pediatric Infectious Diseases*, vol. 4, no. 4, pp. 343–350, 2009.

17

Severe IgG4-Related Disease in a Young Child:
A Diagnosis Challenge

Susana Corujeira,[1] **Catarina Ferraz,**[2] **Teresa Nunes,**[2] **Elsa Fonseca,**[3] **and Luísa Guedes Vaz**[2]

[1]*Pediatric Department, Centro Hospitalar São João, Alameda Professor Hernâni Monteiro, 4200-319 Porto, Portugal*
[2]*Pediatric Pulmonology Unit, Pediatric Department, Centro Hospitalar São João, Alameda Professor Hernâni Monteiro,*
 4200-319 Porto, Portugal
[3]*Pathology Department, Centro Hospitalar São João, Alameda Professor Hernâni Monteiro, 4200-319 Porto, Porto, Portugal*

Correspondence should be addressed to Susana Corujeira; susanamcorujeira@gmail.com

Academic Editor: Abraham Gedalia

Immunoglobulin G4-related disease (IgG4-RD) is an increasingly recognized syndrome that can appear with multiple organ involvement, typically with tumor-like swelling, lymphoplasmacytic infiltrate rich in IgG4-positive plasma cells, and elevated serum IgG4 concentrations. We report the case of a 22-month-old female child with failure to thrive and recurrent respiratory tract infections since 8 months of age. Physical examination was normal except for pulmonary auscultation with bilateral crackles and wheezes. Laboratory tests revealed elevated erythrocyte sedimentation rate, and elevated serum IgG and IgG4 with polyclonal hypergammaglobulinemia. Thoracic CT and MRI showed multiple mediastinal lymphadenopathies and a nodular posterior mediastinal mass in right paratracheal location with bronchial compression. Initial fine needle aspiration biopsy was compatible with reactive lymphadenopathy but after clinical worsening a thoracoscopic partial resection of the mass was performed and tissue biopsy revealed lymphoplasmacytic infiltrate and increased number of IgG4-positive plasma cells and a ratio of IgG4/IgG positive cells above 40%. Glucocorticoids therapy was started with symptomatic improvement, reduction in the size of the mass, and decrease of serum IgG4 levels after 6 weeks. There are very few reports of IgG4-RD in children. Long-term follow-up is necessary to monitor relapses and additional organ involvement.

1. Introduction

Immunoglobulin G4-related disease (IgG4-RD) is an increasingly recognized syndrome of unknown aetiology comprised of a collection of disorders that share specific pathologic, serologic, and clinical features. It is characterized by tumefactive lesions, a dense lymphoplasmacytic infiltrate rich in IgG4-positive plasma cells, storiform fibrosis, and elevated serum IgG4 concentrations [1–3]. The disease was initially recognized in the pancreas but has now been described in virtually every organ system: the biliary tree, salivary glands, periorbital tissues, kidney, lungs, lymph nodes, meninges, aorta, breast, prostate, thyroid, pericardium, and skin. The histopathological features bear striking similarities across the involved organs [1–9]. However, some organs, like the lymph nodes, show a distinct involvement and histopathological features [7, 10].

The clinical picture is highly heterogeneous and the symptoms are related to involvement of the specific target organ, often in the form of a mass lesion. The epidemiology and prevalence of the disease are poorly described and most epidemiologic studies focus on autoimmune pancreatitis. The majority of patients are men older than 50 years [1, 3, 5].

We report a case of a child with pulmonary manifestations of IgG4-RD.

2. Case Presentation

A 22-month-old girl was referred to our pulmonology clinic for recurrent respiratory tract infections. She was born after a 38-week gestation and anthropometric measures at birth were normal. She had history of gross motor development delay having sat at 10 months of age and walked independently at 20 months of age.

Recurrent respiratory tract infections started at 7 months of age and were associated with failure to thrive. These respiratory infections were frequently associated with fever and wheezing and treated with inhaled short-acting beta 2 agonists. Despite treatment with montelukast and weekly respiratory physiotherapy, she persisted with chronic morning cough.

On physical examination, there were bilateral crackles and wheezes on pulmonary auscultation and her weight and height were at the 10th percentile. There were no palpable lymph nodes and no abdominal masses.

Complete blood count revealed normal haemoglobin (12.2 g/dL), normal platelet count (256×10^9/L), and peripheral eosinophilia (0.72×10^9/L) and there was polyclonal hypergammaglobulinemia. Blood biochemistry with liver and renal function, iron metabolism, lactate dehydrogenase, and thyroid function tests were normal (serum total protein 80.4 g/L, AST 36 U/L, ALT 15 U/L, alkaline phosphatase 272 U/L, LDH 250 U/L, urea 20 mg/dL, creatinine 0.20 mg/dL, sodium 136 mEq/L, potassium 4.2 mEq/L, chlorides 104 meq/L, calcium 5.1 mEq/L, TSH 2.01 μUI/mL, and T4 1.17 ng/dL). C-reactive protein was normal (2.9 mg/L) and erythrocyte sedimentation rate was elevated (32 mm/hr). The serum angiotensin converting enzyme was normal (22 U/L).

Immunological testing presented with elevated serum immunoglobulin (Ig) G (1690 mg/dL), elevated IgG4 (805 mg/dL) and IgE (127 kU/L), normal IgA (61 mg/dL), normal IgM (107 mg/dL), normal complement levels, and normal neutrophil oxidative burst tests.

Thoracic CT scan showed multiple right mediastinal and hilar lymphadenopathies, a nodular posterior mediastinal mass (21×15 mm) in the right paratracheal region, and bronchovascular consolidation of the right lung base but also of the right upper and medial lobe. Thoracic MRI confirmed the presence of a complex nodular posterior mediastinal mass (34×22 mm) infiltrating the right hilum along with consolidation of areas in both of the upper lobes and the right lower lobe suggestive of atelectasis (Figure 1). Bronchofibroscopy examination revealed abundant purulent secretions in the right bronchial tree without visualization of bronchial compression. Bronchoalveolar lavage was negative for infectious aetiologies and cytological examination excluded malignancy and the presence of Cd1a positive cells. Fine needle aspiration biopsy was compatible with reactive lymphadenopathy.

One month later, she continued to have chronic cough and wheezing. A thoracoscopic partial resection was performed of a conglomerate of lymph nodes ($30 \times 25 \times 10$ mm). Tissue biopsy histopathological examination revealed follicular hyperplasia with germinal centers. A plasmacytic infiltrate was present in some areas. The number of IgG4-positive plasma cells was high, with 16 IgG4-positive plasma cells/high power field (HPF) and a ratio of IgG4/IgG positive cells over 40% (Figure 2). Histopathological examination of the biopsy

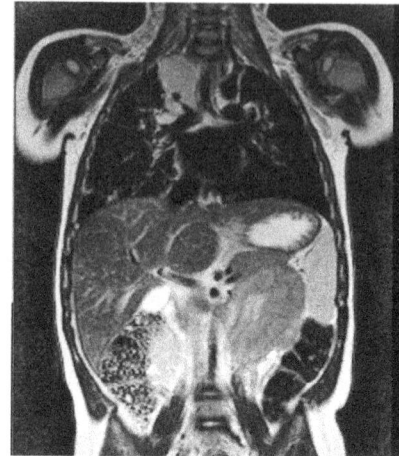

(a)

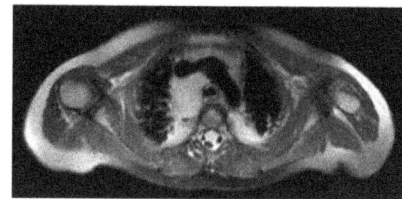

(b)

FIGURE 1: (a) Coronal T2 MRI: complex nodular posterior mediastinal mass infiltrating the right hilum; (b) axial T2 MRI: bilateral mediastinal and hilar lymphadenopathies.

sample excluded signs of malignancy and sarcoidosis due to the absence of noncaseating granulomas.

Immunodeficiency, infectious diseases, tuberculosis, cystic fibrosis, malignancy, lymphoma, sarcoidosis, and Castleman's disease were excluded.

After resection there was worsening of respiratory symptoms and two episodes of pulmonary infection treated with systemic antibiotic therapy. Thoracic MRI, repeated 4 months after resection, showed increase in the size of the right paratracheal mediastinal mass compared to its initial dimensions (30×19 mm) and was persistence of subsegmental bilateral atelectasis.

Glucocorticoid therapy was started (prednisone 2 mg per kilogram) with clinical improvement and decrease of serum IgG4 levels (226 mg/dL) after 6 weeks. Significant reduction of the mass size was confirmed by MRI which showed a small right tracheal nodular image (7 mm). Glucocorticoids were tapered over a period of six months. The patient has been clinically stable for 12 months after stopping therapy, with height and weight at the 50th percentile at 4 years old.

3. Discussion

Pulmonary involvement in IgG4-RD has been reported with a broad spectrum of intrathoracic findings. These manifestations appear to be rather heterogeneous resulting from involvement of the lung parenchyma, intrathoracic lymph nodes, mediastinum, and pleura [4, 9]. Lung parenchymal

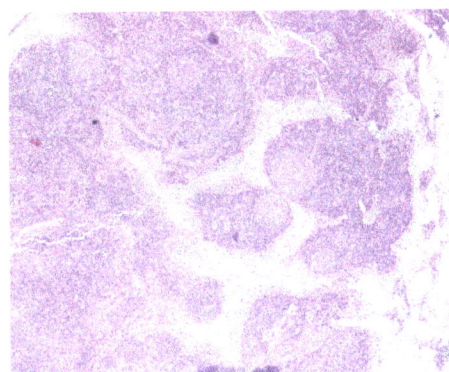

(a)

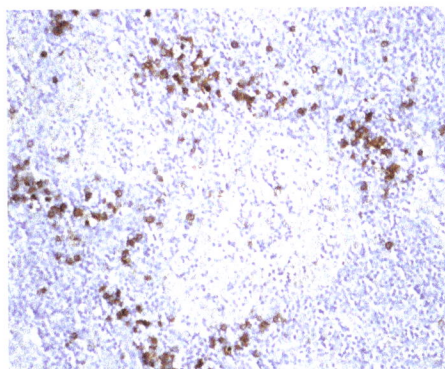

(b)

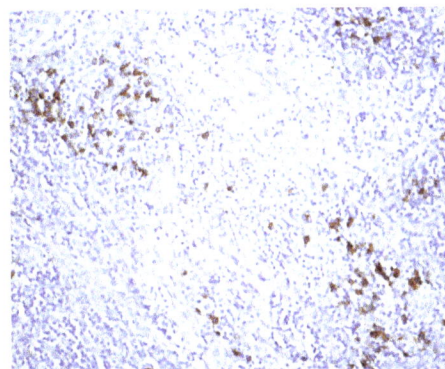

(c)

FIGURE 2: Mediastinal mass biopsy showed reactive lymph nodes presenting follicular hyperplasia with germinal centers and plasmacytic infiltrate ((a) H&E stain, 40x; (b) immunohistochemical stain for IgG, 400x; (c) immunohistochemical stain for IgG4, 400x).

involvement consists mainly of rounded opacities and interstitial lung disease. Airway disease can be caused by extrinsic compression of the central airways due to fibrosing mediastinitis and bronchiectasis. Pleural disease consisted of nodular lesions in the visceral or parietal pleura, pleural effusion, and pleuritis [5, 9]. The most common intrathoracic manifestation is mediastinal and hilar lymphadenopathy, which has been described in 40% to 90% of patients with IgG4-RD. Intrathoracic manifestations have been reported in the presence or absence of one or more extrapulmonary lesions, such as autoimmune pancreatitis [5, 8, 9, 11].

Lymphadenopathy can develop subsequent to the diagnosis of extranodal IgG4-RD or it can be the initial presentation of the disease [3–5]. When lymphadenopathy is generalized, constitutional symptoms are usually absent and lactate dehydrogenase level is normal. Differential diagnosis is broad and includes lymphoma, sarcoidosis, Castleman's disease, or disseminated malignancy [3, 5, 6].

In other patients with IgG4 –RD lymphadenopathy increased serum levels of IgG, IgG4, and IgE, polyclonal hypergammaglobulinemia, elevated sedimentation rate, and positive autoantibodies have also been reported [3, 7, 10]. Many patients have allergic features such as atopy, eczema, asthma, and modest peripheral blood eosinophilia [1, 3].

The majority of patients with IgG4-RD have elevated serum IgG4 concentration (>135 mg/dL). However, elevated IgG4 may also be observed in other diseases suggesting that high serum IgG4 is not a specific marker of IgG4-RD [1, 5, 7].

The diagnosis of IgG4-RD requires both characteristic histopathological features and increased number of IgG4 positive plasma cells or an elevated IgG4 : IgG ratio in tissue. The major histopathological features observed in several organs are a dense lymphoplasmacytic infiltrate, storiform fibrosis, obliterative phlebitis, and eosinophil infiltrate [1, 2, 5, 10]. However, the lymph nodes are an exception to this rule as storiform fibrosis and obliterative phlebitis may be inconspicuous or absent. Therefore, the histopathological diagnosis relies considerably on the number of IgG4 positive cells and on the ratio of IgG4 positive/IgG positive plasma cells [2, 5, 10]. Five histological patterns have been reported in the literature associated with IgG4-related lymphadenopathy: multicentric Castleman disease-like, follicular hyperplasia, interfollicular expansion, progressive transformation of germinal centers, and nodal inflammatory pseudotumor-like. Reactive follicular hyperplasia is a common histopathological finding in lymph nodes biopsies [2, 3, 5, 10, 12].

The appropriate cut-off point of the number of IgG4 positive plasma cells varies in different organs, but the presence of >10 IgG4 positive plasma cells/HPF on biopsy specimens has been proposed as diagnostic feature. However, IgG4 positive plasma cell count alone may not help to distinguish between IgG4-RD and other disorders [1, 2, 5, 7, 9]. The IgG4 positive/IgG positive plasma cell ratio of >40% is a comprehensive cut-off value in any organ and is very suggestive of the diagnosis [2, 5, 7].

The comprehensive clinical diagnostic criteria for IgG4-RD were fulfilled: (1) mediastinal and hilar lymphadenopathy, (2) elevated serum IgG4 concentrations, and (3) histopathologic examination with lymphoplasmacytic infiltration and >10 IgG4 positive plasma cells/HPF and IgG4 positive/IgG positive plasma cell ratio >40% [13].

There are very few reports of IgG4-RD in children and only one in a 15-year-old boy with lung involvement to our knowledge [14]. IgG4-related lymphadenopathy is often asymptomatic and may not require immediate treatment but our patient was very young and had significant lung disease with severe systemic repercussion and failure to thrive.

Benign/reactive lymph nodes are more common in children but are less frequently excised compared to adults.

Differential diagnostic is broad and although the findings have some distinctive features, in many circumstances, they may not be sufficiently distinctive as to exclude a diagnosis of IgG4-related lymphadenopathy.

Multiorgan disease may be evident at diagnosis but also can evolve metachronously over months to years. Spontaneous improvement is reported in a minority of cases but not in intrathoracic IgG4-RD [1, 5, 9].

No randomized treatment trials have been conducted, particularly in children. Glucocorticoids are the first line of therapy and most IgG4-RD patients respond favourably to this treatment. Most centers start with prednisolone at a dose of 0.6 mg per kilogram of body weight or 40 mg for 2 to 4 weeks and taper the dose over a period of 3 to 6 months, although some authors suggest to continue at a dose between 2.5 and 5 mg per day for up to 3 years [1, 5, 6, 9, 15].

Our patient had a good clinical response to glucocorticoids but durability of treatment response is unclear after prednisolone tapering and relapse is frequent. A major determinant of treatment responsiveness is the degree of fibrosis, which was absent in this case [1, 5]. Serial measurements of IgG4 concentrations have been proposed as indicator of disease activity but although IgG4 concentrations become lower with glucocorticoid treatment, they remain above normal value in most patients [1, 3, 5].

The natural history of IgG4-RD has not been well defined, particularly in paediatric patients. Long-term follow-up is necessary to closely monitor relapses and additional organ involvement. Other courses of steroid therapy may be needed and eventually immunosuppressive therapy.

Conflict of Interests

The authors declare that there is no conflict of interests regarding the publication of this paper.

References

[1] J. H. Stone, Y. Zen, and V. Deshpande, "IgG4-related disease," *The New England Journal of Medicine*, vol. 366, no. 6, pp. 539–551, 2012.

[2] V. Deshpande, Y. Zen, J. K. C. Chan et al., "Consensus statement on the pathology of IgG4-related disease," *Modern Pathology*, vol. 25, no. 9, pp. 1181–1192, 2012.

[3] A. Khosroshahi and J. H. Stone, "A clinical overview of IgG4-related systemic disease," *Current Opinion in Rheumatology*, vol. 23, no. 1, pp. 57–66, 2011.

[4] Y. Zen and Y. Nakanuma, "IgG4-related disease: a cross-sectional study of 114 cases," *The American Journal of Surgical Pathology*, vol. 34, no. 12, pp. 1812–1819, 2010.

[5] M. Guma and G. S. Firestein, "IgG4-related diseases," *Clinical Rheumatology*, vol. 26, no. 4, pp. 425–438, 2012.

[6] H. Pieringer, I. Parzer, A. Wöhrer, P. Reis, B. Oppl, and J. Zwerina, "IgG4- related disease: an orphan disease with many faces," *Orphanet Journal of Rare Diseases*, vol. 9, no. 1, article 110, 2014.

[7] K. Okazaki and H. Umehara, "Are classification criteria for IgG4-RD now possible? The concept of IgG4-related disease and proposal of comprehensive diagnostic criteria in Japan,"

International Journal of Rheumatology, vol. 2012, Article ID 357071, 9 pages, 2012.

[8] W. Cheuk, H. K. L. Yuen, S. Y. Y. Chu, E. K. W. Chiu, L. K. Lam, and J. K. C. Chan, "Lymphadenopathy of IgG4-related sclerosing disease," *The American Journal of Surgical Pathology*, vol. 32, no. 5, pp. 671–681, 2008.

[9] J. H. Ryu, H. Sekiguchi, and E. S. Yi, "Pulmonary manifestations of immunoglobulin G4-related sclerosing disease," *European Respiratory Journal*, vol. 39, no. 1, pp. 180–186, 2012.

[10] K. E. Grimm, T. S. Barry, V. Chizhevsky et al., "Histopathological findings in 29 lymph node biopsies with increased IgG4 plasma cells," *Modern Pathology*, vol. 25, no. 3, pp. 480–491, 2012.

[11] H. Hamano, N. Arakura, T. Muraki, Y. Ozaki, K. Kiyosawa, and S. Kawa, "Prevalence and distribution of extrapancreatic lesions complicating autoimmune pancreatitis," *Journal of Gastroenterology*, vol. 41, no. 12, pp. 1197–1205, 2006.

[12] T. Uehara, J. Masumoto, A. Yoshizawa et al., "IgG4-related disease-like fibrosis as an indicator of IgG4-related lymphadenopathy," *Annals of Diagnostic Pathology*, vol. 17, no. 5, pp. 416–420, 2013.

[13] H. Umehara, K. Okazaki, Y. Masaki et al., "Comprehensive diagnostic criteria for IgG4-related disease (IgG4-RD), 2011," *Modern Rheumatology*, vol. 22, no. 1, pp. 21–30, 2012.

[14] M. Pifferi, M. di Cicco, A. Bush, D. Caramella, M. Chilosi, and A. L. Boner, "Uncommon pulmonary presentation of IgG 4-related disease in a 15-year-old boy," *Chest*, vol. 144, no. 2, pp. 669–671, 2013.

[15] T. Kamisawa, K. Okazaki, S. Kawa et al., "Amendment of the Japanese consensus guidelines for autoimmune pancreatitis, 2013 III. Treatment and prognosis of autoimmune pancreatitis," *Journal of Gastroenterology*, vol. 49, no. 6, pp. 961–970, 2014.

18

Concurrence of Meningomyelocele and Salt-Wasting Congenital Adrenal Hyperplasia due to 21-Hydroxylase Deficiency

Heves Kırmızıbekmez,[1] Rahime Gül Yesiltepe Mutlu,[1] Serdar Moralıoğlu,[2] Ahmet Tellioğlu,[3] and Ayşenur Cerrah Celayir[2]

[1] *Pediatric Endocrinology, Zeynep Kamil Obstetrics and Pediatrics Education and Research Hospital, 34668 Istanbul, Turkey*
[2] *Pediatric Surgery, Zeynep Kamil Obstetrics and Pediatrics Education and Research Hospital, 34668 Istanbul, Turkey*
[3] *Department of Pediatrics, Zeynep Kamil Obstetrics and Pediatrics Education and Research Hospital, 34668 Istanbul, Turkey*

Correspondence should be addressed to Heves Kırmızıbekmez; heveskirmizibekmez@yahoo.com

Academic Editor: Mercedes Pineda

Congenital adrenal hyperplasia (CAH) is a group of inherited defects of cortisol biosynthesis. A case of classical CAH due to 21-hydroxylase deficiency (21-OHD) with early onset of salt waste and concurrence of meningomyelocele (MMC) was presented here. The management of salt-wasting crisis which is complicated by a postrenal dysfunction due to neurogenic bladder was described. Possible reasons of growth retardation in the one-year follow-up period were discussed. A significant regression of the phallus with proper medical treatment was also mentioned.

1. Introduction

Congenital adrenal hyperplasia (CAH) is a group of autosomal recessive disorders characterized by impaired cortisol synthesis leading to excessive corticotrophin stimulation of the adrenal cortex. More than 90% of CAH are caused by 21-hydroxylase deficiency (21-OHD), found in 1 : 10 000 to 1 : 15 000 live births. Potentially lethal adrenal insufficiency is characteristic of two-thirds to three-quarters of patients with the classical salt-wasting form of 21-OHD [1]. Accumulation of cortisol precursors that are diverted to androgens is the cause of virilisation in a female fetus. CAH is the most common cause of 46, XX Disorders of Sex Development (DSD). This case report defines the management of a patient with salt-wasting CAH and neurogenic bladder.

The most common cause of neurogenic bladder in children is neurospinal dysraphism [2]. MMC is the most common neural tube defect. It is characterized by a cleft in the vertebral column, with a corresponding defect in the skin so that the meninges and spinal cord are exposed. Nearly all patients with MMC have bladder dysfunction. This may adversely affect urinary continence and quality of life and can also lead to progressive deterioration of the upper urinary tract and chronic renal disease [3].

2. Case Report

A newborn was referred to our hospital for ambiguous genitalia on the first day of the birth. The weight was 3000 gr, the length was 50 cm, and the head circumference was 37 cm. The baby was born by caesarean section at the 37th week of the gestation. The parents were both healthy and no history of prenatal complication or medication was present. Parents were said to be nonconsanguineous; however, their family roots came from the same village.

Overall, the patient appeared healthy and the vital findings were normal and no dysmorphic finding was present. However, a MMC was found in the sacral area. The inspection of external genitalia revealed a phallus of 2.5×2 cm in size, no palpable gonad, and a single orifice at the base of the phallus (Figures 1 and 2). Bilateral ovaries, fallopian tubes, and a uterus were present in the pelvic ultrasonography. The initial findings were suggesting 46, XX DSD, most probably CAH.

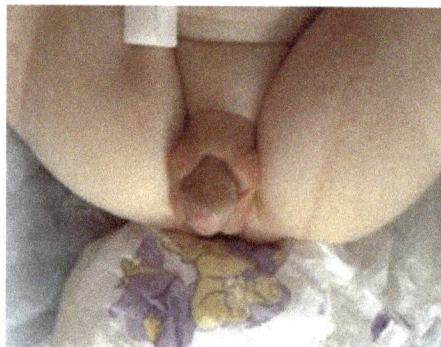

FIGURE 1: The external genitalia appeared to be significantly virilised (Prader stage 3).

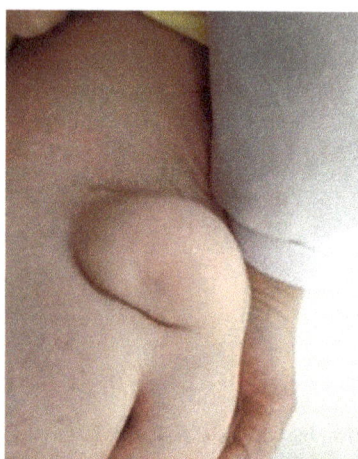

FIGURE 2: The meningomyelocele in the sacral area.

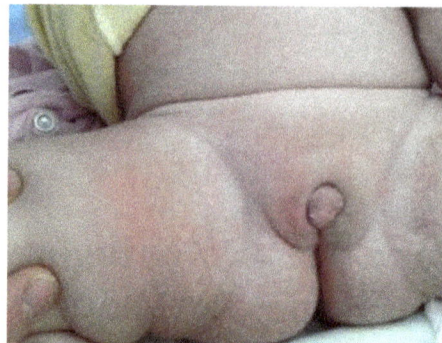

FIGURE 3: Regression of the phallus at the 7th month of the hormone replacement treatment (constructive operation has not yet been performed).

The patient's general status, vitals, feeding tolerance, glucose, and electrolyte levels were followed up carefully. On the 4th day, hypoactivity, poor feeding, and vomiting commenced. Electrolytes were suggesting salt waste. We stopped enteral feeding and before starting treatment we obtained blood samples for hormone tests. Fluid and electrolyte replacement began with saline and dextrose solutions (150 mL/kg/day, 100 mEq/L Na, and 10% dextrose). At the time, only methyl-prednisolone was available for an intravenous injection. At the beginning of the treatment we administered 5 mg of methyl-prednisolone and continued with divided equal doses every eight hours. Fludrocortisone was given (0.2 mg/day) for mineralocorticoid replacement. We also had to give 1 mg/day of table salt for a few days. On the 5th day, the patient's general appearance was better, vitals were normal, vomiting stopped, and electrolytes were improving. On the 6th day, feeding was well tolerated and electrolytes were normal. The amount of intravenous fluid and the dose of glucocorticoid treatment were reduced and continued with hydrocortisone tablets. Although the management of adrenal insufficiency was working properly, oliguria and declined renal functions occurred on the 7th day. Urine output was below 0.5 mL/kg/hr and creatinine level was 1.6 mg/dL. Physical examination revealed a "globe vesical,"

and urine output and renal functions improved after urinary catheterization.

The androgen levels were high as expected (Table 1). Adrenocorticotrophic hormone (ACTH) level was confirming that the baby had primary adrenal insufficiency and renin level had just started to increase due to the initiation of salt waste. The results of hormone studies and karyotype analyses (46, XX) further supported the diagnosis of salt-wasting CAH. 21OHD was confirmed by genetic analyses. A homozygous deletion of E1–E3 30 kb (P30L-I2G-8 bp del) in the CYP21 gene was detected. It was a previously known mutation, which has a genotype-phenotype correlation with salt-wasting CAH.

Committee on Disorders of Sex Development agreed on the decision to raise the patient as a girl and planned to perform the necessary constructive operations for female genitalia. The phallus was significantly regressed at the 7th month of the hormone replacement treatment. It was 1.5×1 cm in size, and a constructive operation has not yet been performed (Figure 3). Between 7th and 11th months, she was hospitalized four times because of urinary tract infection. The parents were asked to give hydrocortisone in double doses in case of fever and other systemic infection findings. Growth retardation was occurring, especially in this period (Figure 4). Fortunately, neuromotor development was normal and she could walk by the time she is 13 months old. She is also under supervision of a neurosurgeon, a pediatric urologist, and a pediatric nephrologist.

3. Discussion

Congenital adrenal hyperplasia is a group of inherited defects of cortisol biosynthesis. The condition can be classified into "salt-wasting," "simple virilising," and "nonclassical" forms. These are not different diseases but represent points on a spectrum of disease severity directly related to the degree of enzymatic compromise conferred by a given genetic defect [1]. Females with the classical form present with genital ambiguity. Males with the salt-wasting form who are not identified by neonatal screening present with failure to thrive, dehydration, hyponatremia, and hyperkalemia typically at 7

TABLE 1: Hormone profile of the patient before starting treatment.

Hormone	Result	Reference range	SI
Renin	**63 pg/mL**	3–33	**90.7 μU/mL**
Aldosterone	300 pg/mL	70–1840	**30 ng/dL**
ACTH	**>2000 pg/mL**	10–60	>444 pmol/L
Cortisol	14.7 pg/mL	4–20	406 nmol/L
17-OHP (**LC-MS/MS**)	**50.1 ng/mL**	0.07–0.77	**151.5 ng/mL**
Androstenedione	**>10 ng/mL**	0.2–2.9	**>3.5 pmol/L**
Total testosterone	**2330 ng/dL**	14–73	**807.8 pmol/mL**
DHEA-S	**1945 mcg/dL**	88–356	**52.9 nmol/L**

ACTH: adrenocorticotrophic hormone; 17-OHP: 17-hydroxy progesterone; DHEA-S: dehydroepiandrostenedione sulphate.

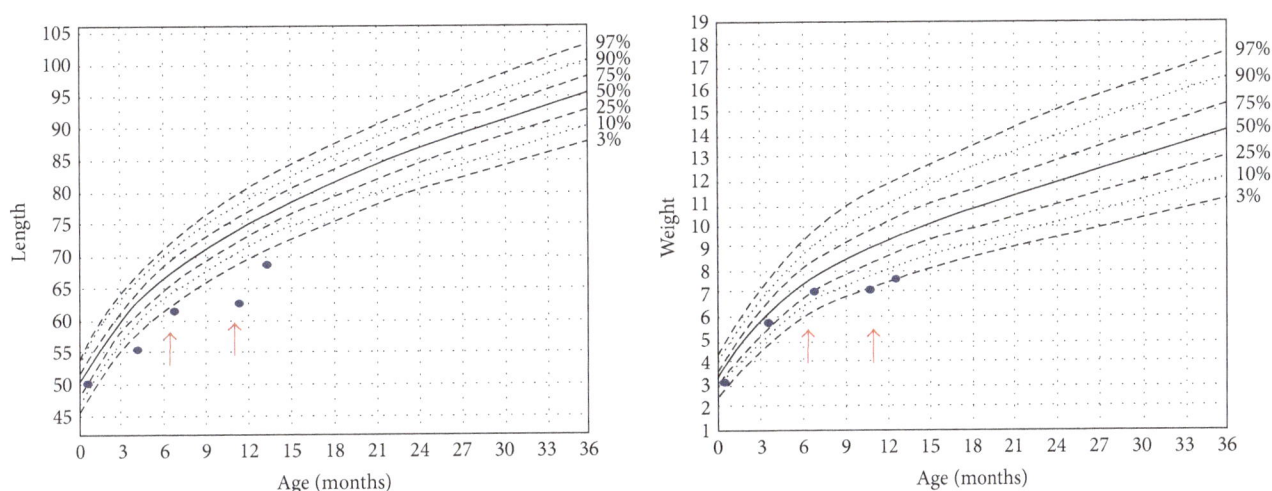

FIGURE 4: Growth retardation was occurring especially between 7th and 11th months.

to 14 days of life. Clinical findings of adrenal insufficiency occurred on the 4th day in this patient. Rapid progression to the salt-wasting crisis suggested a severe enzyme deficiency in the adrenal steroidogenesis pathway. Early onset of salt waste before the second week of life is a rare condition. This individual difference could also be due to varying sensitivity to aldosterone action in newborn infants. In the distal nephron, aldosterone, by binding to its receptor, tightly regulates the expression and the activity of several transport proteins implicated in sodium, potassium, and water homeostasis. A possible role of a partial and transient tubular unresponsiveness to mineralocorticoids, which is determined by genetic factors, might have effects on the timing of salt waste.

Approximately 95% of all disease-causing mutations in CYP21A2 gene are large deletions, large conversions, or one of eight point mutations (p.P30L, IVS2–13 C>G in intron 2 splice site (IVS-2), 8 bp deletion in exon 3, p.I172L, exon 6 cluster (p.I236N, p.V237E, and p.M239K), p.V281L, p.Q318X, and p.R356W) [4]. Large deletions or large conversions are typically associated with classical salt waste. This patient had a large homozygous deletion (P30L-I2G-8 bp del) in the CYP21 gene, causing severe 21OHD.

More than 90% of patients with 46, XX CAH assigned female in infancy. Evidence supports the current recommendation to raise virilised 46, XX infants with CAH as females [5]. There are no randomized controlled studies of either the best age or the best methods for feminizing surgery. Clitoral and perineal reconstruction are suggested in infancy for severely virilised (Prader stage 3) females [6]. However, an early surgery could not be performed in this patient, because of her neurogenic bladder and urinary tract infections. Meanwhile she was receiving the hormone replacement treatment properly, which provided a significant regression in the phallic structure. Both parents were quite pleased with the appearance of the external genitalia and urgent surgical intervention was not required. Deferring surgery might be an option for these patients until adolescence; however there is no evidence that either early or late surgery better preserves sexual function. Management should include the care for optimal psychosexual adjustment and increased quality of life.

Growth retardation of this patient was thought to be related to undernutrition due to frequent urinary tract infections. It was significant especially between 7th and 11th months, when she needed recurrent hospitalization. In this period hydrocortisone was used in double doses frequently, because of fever and other findings of infection. Fortunately, there was no cushingoid appearance or excessive weight gain.

This case report mainly aimed to attract attention to a concurring malformation, which might complicate the management of CAH. MMC leading to bladder dysfunction caused recurrent infections. This brought difficulties in achieving the optimal dose of glucocorticoid replacement. There are a few publications reporting congenital abnormalities concurring with CAH. Nabhan and Eugster determined upper-tract genitourinary malformations in 14 of 107 patients with CAH [7]. MMC is a common central nervous system birth defect. Various congenital and acquired abnormalities have been reported with MMC. A retrospective study [Baradaran et al.] was performed using the records of 390 patients with MMC. 17 cases of MMC with concurring congenital abnormalities, such as cardiac, musculoskeletal, and urological anomalies, were determined. Two of them had congenital adrenal hyperplasia patients with ambiguous genitalia [8]. So neural tube defects should be considered as a concurring abnormality in patients with CAH. This is one more reason why optimal care for children with CAH requires an experienced multidisciplinary team.

In conclusion, avoidance of a life-threatening crisis of adrenal insufficiency and maintaining normal height velocity and achieving normal adult height are important treatment goals in children with CAH. Long-term follow-up should include the regular monitoring of growth and bone age. Optimal health care requires monitoring of patients for signs of glucocorticoid excess as well as for signs of inadequate androgen suppression. This should remind us that management of CAH may become complicated by associating conditions.

Conflict of Interests

All authors have no financial interests or potential conflict of interests.

References

[1] M. G. Forest, "Recent advances in the diagnosis and management of congenital adrenal hyperplasia due to 21-hydroxylase deficiency," *Human Reproduction Update*, vol. 10, no. 6, pp. 469–485, 2004.

[2] S. B. Bauer, "Neurogenic bladder: etiology and assessment," *Pediatric Nephrology*, vol. 23, no. 4, pp. 541–551, 2008.

[3] A. Champeau and L. S. Baskin, "Urinary tract complications of myelomeningocele (spina bifida)," Up To Date, 2013.

[4] F. Baş, H. Kayserili, F. Darendeliler et al., "CYP21A2 gene mutations in congenital adrenal hyperplasia: genotype-phenotype correlation in Turkish children," *Journal of Clinical Research in Pediatric Endocrinology*, vol. 1, no. 3, pp. 116–128, 2009.

[5] P. A. Lee, C. P. Houk, S. F. Ahmed, I. A. Hughes, and International Consensus Conference on Intersex organized by the Lawson Wilkins Pediatric Endocrine Society and the European Society for Paediatric Endocrinology, "Consensus statement on management of intersex disorders. International Consensus Conference on Intersex," *Pediatrics*, vol. 118, no. 2, pp. e488–e500, 2006.

[6] P. W. Speiser, R. Azziz, L. S. Baskin et al., "Congenital adrenal hyperplasia due to steroid 21-hydroxylase deficiency: an Endocrine Society clinical practice guideline," *Journal of Clinical Endocrinology and Metabolism*, vol. 95, no. 9, pp. 4133–4160, 2010.

[7] Z. M. Nabhan and E. A. Eugster, "Upper-tract genitourinary malformations in girls with congenital adrenal hyperplasia," *Pediatrics*, vol. 120, no. 2, pp. e304–e307, 2007.

[8] N. Baradaran, H. Ahmadi, F. Nejat, M. El Khashab, and A. Mahdavi, "Nonneural congenital abnormalities concurring with myelomeningocele: report of 17 cases and review of current theories," *Pediatric Neurosurgery*, vol. 44, no. 5, pp. 353–359, 2008.

19

Successful Treatment of *Candida parapsilosis* Fungemia in Two Preterms with Voriconazole

Emel Altuncu,[1] **Hulya Bilgen,**[1] **Ahmet Soysal,**[2] **and Eren Ozek**[1]

[1]*Division of Neonatology, Department of Pediatrics, Faculty of Medicine, Marmara University, 34890 Istanbul, Turkey*
[2]*Division of Pediatric Infectious Disease, Department of Pediatrics, Faculty of Medicine, Marmara University, 34890 Istanbul, Turkey*

Correspondence should be addressed to Emel Altuncu; emelkayrak@yahoo.com

Academic Editor: Juan Manuel Mejía-Aranguré

Herein, we report two preterms with invasive candidiasis refractory to liposomal amphotericin B (AMB) treatment in spite of low MIC levels (MIC: 0.5 mcg/mL). Both of the patients' blood cultures were persistently positive for *C. parapsilosis* despite high therapeutic doses (AMB: 7 mg/kg per day). After starting voriconazole blood cultures became negative and both of the patients were treated successfully without any side effects. In conclusion, although it is not a standard treatment in neonatal patients, our limited experience with these patients suggests that voriconazole appears to be a safe antifungal agent to be used in critically ill preterm infants with persistent fungemia despite AMB treatment.

1. Introduction

Critically ill newborns are candidates for systemic fungal infections. Despite the administration of amphotericin B (AMB), invasive candidiasis is sometimes complicated by persistent fungemia and refractory invasive disease [1]. The problem has been augmented by the increasing prevalence of nonalbicans species that are often resistant to fluconazole and AMB. Recent studies have expanded our knowledge of newer antifungal agents such as the second generation triazoles and the echinocandins in older children have given us opportunity to extend the range of therapeutic alternatives; however, little is known about their usage in neonates [2].

This report represents effectiveness of voriconazole in two neonates with invasive candidiasis refractory to AMB therapy.

2. Case Presentations

Case 1 was a 570 g male premature infant born at the 24th week of gestation by Caesarian section (C/S) from a mother with chorioamnionitis with Apgar scores 8, 9, and 9 at the 1st, 5th, and 10th minutes of life, respectively. The infant was intubated and placed on mechanical ventilation and received surfactant because of respiratory distress syndrome (RDS).

An umbilical catheter was placed in the first hours of life. Systemic antibiotic therapy was initiated with ampicillin and gentamicin and they were stopped at the 7th day of life at the time of extubation.

On the 8th postnatal day, as the blood culture was positive for *Candida parapsilosis* the baby was placed on liposomal AMB (5.0 mg/kg/day) and the umbilical catheter was removed. Despite antifungal therapy, the patient developed persistent thrombocytopenia requiring platelet transfusions and liposomal AMB dosage was increased to 7 mg/kg/day. Cardiac, brain, and renal sonographic assessments and ocular examination of the infant were normal. At the 10th day of life, antifungal susceptibility test resulted in a low MIC (MIC: 0.5 mcg/mL) level for AMB. Despite higher AMB dosage and the removal of the central venous catheter, blood cultures remained positive for *C. parapsilosis* and at this point AMB was stopped and the systemic antifungal therapy was changed to voriconazole (8 mg/kg/day). The cultures obtained after 48 hours revealed negative blood/CSF/urine cultures for candida. Thrombocytopenia improved in a few days. The therapy was completed after 4 weeks without any side effects. Serial ultrasounds and fundoscopic examinations performed during and before treatment were normal. The infant was oxygen dependent at the corrected 36 weeks of age. His clinical course was also complicated by osteopenia of prematurity, anemia, apnea of prematurity, and clinical nosocomial sepsis. Retinopathy of prematurity (zone 2, grade 2) was detected during screening. The renal and liver function tests were within the normal limits during therapy. The patient was discharged on the 102nd day of life without any neurological and retinal sequelae. He is now 1 year old and his physical and neurological examination is normal.

Case 2 was a male premature infant born at 31 (+1) weeks of gestation via emergent C/S complicated by immune hydrops fetalis and fetal distress. His birth weight was 1750 g and the Apgar scores were 0, 1, and 4 at 1, 5, and 10 min, respectively. Urgent cardiopulmonary resuscitation was initiated and a silastic umbilical venous catheter was placed in the delivery room. The exchange/transfusion was performed with 0 Rh (−) packed red blood cells and whole blood in the delivery room.

The severely edematous baby was placed on mechanical ventilation and given two doses of surfactant six hours apart for RDS. The chest X-ray was remarkable for bilateral pleural effusions, pulmonary hypoplasia, and signs of fluid engorgement of the parenchyma. Pericardial effusion was detected during echocardiography which did not affect cardiac functions. Routine cultures of tracheal aspirates were negative at this time. Systemic ampicillin and gentamicin were started from birth. Albumin infusion and intravenous immunoglobulin were initiated immediately. Increasing doses of inotropes were required to maintain blood pressure in the normal range. The infant had renal and liver dysfunction and developed thrombocytopenia refractory platelet transfusions. The clinical course of the infant was complicated by grade 4 intracranial hemorrhage. During the first week of life, signs of acute renal failure (ARF) progressed and fluid overload was unresponsive to furosemide infusion. After the third exchange transfusion, ARF began to regress, urinary output gradually increased, and the infant began to lose weight. Throughout the first weeks, the infant required high settings on conventional mechanical ventilation.

Because of unimprovement in the respiratory status and persistent thrombocytopenia requiring frequent platelet transfusions, the antibiotic regimen was switched to cefepime, vancomycin, and fluconazole (FCZ) empirically on the 8th day. The other day it was reported that the blood culture yielded C. parapsilosis and FCZ was changed to liposomal AMB (7 mg/kg per day) (MIC 0.5 mcg/mL). Sonographic assessments including brain and abdominal sonographies and ocular examination for the potential seeding of the fungi were normal. Infected thrombus/vegetation in the mitral valve was detected by Doppler-echocardiography on the same day (postnatal 8th day). Because of the babies unstable condition, cardiac surgery was considered of high risk and treatment was continued with antifungal agents alone. As samples from blood cultures were repeatedly positive for C. parapsilosis and there were no reductions in the vegetations, AMB was ceased and intravenous administration of voriconazole (8 mg/kg/day) was started.

After 48 hours of voriconazole therapy, blood cultures became negative, thrombocytopenia improved, and the progression of cardiac vegetations stopped. At the 40th day of life,

he was extubated and enteral feeding was increased gradually. His clinical course was also complicated by osteopenia of prematurity, sepsis, and cholestasis, intracranial hemorrhage leading to hydrocephalus. Voriconazole was switched to its oral form after four weeks of therapy. The patient was discharged from the hospital on oral voriconazole therapy and therapy continued until the baby was one year of age. During the entire therapy, the liver and renal function tests were normal and no other side effects were detected. He is now 1 year old and has moderate neurological sequelae.

3. Discussion

Invasive candidiasis with non-albican species is the most frequent cause of death among neonatal infectious diseases and responds only to aggressive and prolonged antifungal therapy [1]. Amphotericin B or its liposomal formulations remain standard recommendations [3]. Due to treatment failures, the combination therapies with new antifungal agents, such as caspofungin and voriconazole, show promise in the treatment of candidiasis refractory to conventional therapy; however clinical experience with those new antifungals is limited in the newborn period [4]. Recently, Celik et al. reported that 12 newborns out of 17 with invasive fungal sepsis in whom the infection persisted despite conventional therapy had been cured successfully with voriconazole. In spite of cholestasis and liver function abnormalities drug was continued without permanent side effects [5].

Because of the persistent fungemia detected in our patients, antifungal therapy was changed to voriconazole. After the initiation of voriconazole, blood cultures became sterile within 48 hours of treatment.

Voriconazole, a triazole antifungal agent, acts via the inhibition of fungal ergosterol biosynthesis [4]. It is fungicidal against Aspergillus and active against all Candida species including Candida krusei and Candida glabrata [4]. It is available in both IV and oral formulations.

The first largest pediatric report of voriconazole was the evaluation of the drug in 58 children with proven or probable invasive fungal infection refractory to conventional therapies [6]. In their study, Walsh and colleagues described the efficacy (45% complete or partial response at the end of the therapy) and safety of the drug (less adverse reactions) in children [6]. Case reports also have documented the successful treatment of invasive neonatal candidiasis by voriconazole administered alone or in combination with other antifungals in a variety of conditions including those with meningitis [7], those with endocarditis [8], those with cutaneous aspergillosis [9, 10], and those with bloodstream infections [11, 12]. Turan et al. [13] reported 6 very low birthweight infants who had persistent candidemia despite antifungal treatment and who were treated successfully with voriconazole.

Generally, susceptibility studies indicate that most of the strains are susceptible to AMB as it was shown in our cases (MIC 0.5 mcg/mL). These cases reflect the difficulty in correlating data from in vitro susceptibility tests to microbiological improvement despite amphotericin B treatment. In both cases AMB had to be changed to voriconazole because of the persistence of positive blood cultures, although AMB dosage was increased from 5 to 7 mg/kg/day.

In conjunction with antifungal agents, aggressive surgical debridement, excision of localized infection, and removal of infected foreign bodies (such as intravenous catheters) are imperative to prevent or limit dissemination [14, 15]. Cardiac surgery in Case 2 was considered of high risk and we opted to treat him with antifungal agents alone. This therapeutic modality was reported successful in the neonatal age group with survival rates similar to those for combined medical and surgical treatment [15]. We have used IV therapy till the patient had to be in the hospital for other reasons and then completed the antifungal course with oral voriconazole therapy.

The adverse effects of voriconazole include fever, gastrointestinal symptoms, reversible visual disturbances, hepatitis, jaundice, and skin reactions [4]. In our cases, we did not observe any serious complications which might be attributable to voriconazole.

In conclusion, although it cannot be recommended as a standard treatment in neonatal patients based on the results of case reports with limited numbers, our experience with these patients suggests that voriconazole appears to be a safe antifungal agent to be used in critically ill preterm infants with persistent fungemia despite AMB treatment. Additionally, it has some advantages including wide spectrum of coverage without renal side effects and thrombocytopenia and a significant cost advantage over liposomal amphotericin. The oral preparation of the drug, for patients who need a longer duration of treatment, is another advantage.

Conflict of Interests

The authors declare that there is no conflict of interests regarding the publication of this paper.

References

[1] R. K. Devlin, "Invasive fungal infections caused by candida and malassezia species in the neonatal intensive care unit," *Advances in Neonatal Care*, vol. 6, no. 2, pp. 68–77, 2006.

[2] W. J. Steinbach and D. K. Benjamin, "New antifungal agents under development in children and neonates," *Current Opinion in Infectious Diseases*, vol. 18, no. 6, pp. 484–489, 2005.

[3] W. J. Steinbach, "Antifungal agents in children," *Pediatric Clinics of North America*, vol. 52, no. 3, pp. 895–915, 2005.

[4] C. Antachopoulos and T. J. Walsh, "New agents for invasive mycoses in children," *Current Opinion in Pediatrics*, vol. 17, no. 1, pp. 78–87, 2005.

[5] I. H. Celik, G. Demirel, S. S. Oguz, N. Uras, O. Erdeve, and U. Dilmen, "Compassionate use of voriconazole in newborn infants diagnosed with severe invasive fungal sepsis," *European Review for Medical and Pharmacological Sciences*, vol. 17, no. 6, pp. 729–734, 2013.

[6] T. J. Walsh, I. Lutsar, T. Driscoll et al., "Voriconazole in the treatment of aspergillosis, scedosporiosis and other invasive fungal infections in children," *Pediatric Infectious Disease Journal*, vol. 21, no. 3, pp. 240–248, 2002.

[7] Y.-Z. Shen, J.-R. Wang, and H.-Z. Lu, "Voriconazole in an infant with cryptococcal meningitis," *Chinese Medical Journal*, vol. 121, no. 3, pp. 286–288, 2008.

[8] J. A. Guzman-Cottrill, X. Zheng, and E. G. Chadwick, "Fusarium solani endocarditis successfully treated with liposomal amphotericin B and voriconazole," *Pediatric Infectious Disease Journal*, vol. 23, no. 11, pp. 1059–1061, 2004.

[9] R. P. Santos, P. J. Sánchez, A. Mejias et al., "Successful medical treatment of cutaneous Aspergillosis in a premature infant using liposomal amphotericin B, voriconazole and micafungin," *The Pediatric Infectious Disease Journal*, vol. 26, no. 4, pp. 364–366, 2007.

[10] K. Frankenbusch, F. Eifinger, A. Kribs, J. Rengelshauseu, and B. Roth, "Severe primary cutaneous aspergillosis refractory to amphotericin B and the successful treatment with systemic voriconazole in two premature infants with extremely low birth weight," *Journal of Perinatology*, vol. 26, no. 8, pp. 511–514, 2006.

[11] V. Kohli, V. Taneja, P. Sachdev, and R. Joshi, "Voriconazole in newborns," *Indian Pediatrics*, vol. 45, no. 3, pp. 236–238, 2008.

[12] K. M. Muldrew, H. D. Maples, C. D. Stowe, and R. F. Jacobs, "Intravenous voriconazole therapy in a preterm infant," *Pharmacotherapy*, vol. 25, no. 6, pp. 893–898, 2005.

[13] O. Turan, E. Ergenekon, I. M. Hirfanoğlu et al., "Combination antifungal therapy with voriconazole for persistent candidemia in very low birth weight neonates," *The Turkish Journal of Pediatrics*, vol. 53, no. 1, pp. 19–26, 2011.

[14] P. G. Pappas, C. A. Kauffman, D. Andes et al., "Clinical practice guidelines for the management of candidiasis: 2009 update by the Infectious Diseases Society of America," *Clinical Infectious Diseases*, vol. 48, no. 5, pp. 503–535, 2009.

[15] I. Levy, I. Shalit, E. Birk et al., "Candida endocarditis in neonates: report of five cases and review of the literature," *Mycoses*, vol. 49, no. 1, pp. 43–48, 2006.

20

Treatment for Retinopathy of Prematurity in an Infant with Adenoviral Conjunctivitis

Murat Gunay,[1] **Gokhan Celik,**[1] **and Rahim Con**[2]

[1]*Zeynep Kamil Maternity and Children's Diseases Training and Research Hospital, Department of Ophthalmology, 34668 Istanbul, Turkey*
[2]*Sanliurfa Obstetrics and Gynecology Hospital, Department of Ophthalmology, 63050 Sanliurfa, Turkey*

Correspondence should be addressed to Murat Gunay; drmurat301@yahoo.com.tr

Academic Editor: Mohammad M. A. Faridi

Retinopathy of prematurity (ROP) has been a major problematic disorder during childhood. Laser photocoagulation (LPC) has been proven to be effective in most of the ROP cases. Adenoviral conjunctivitis (AVC) is responsible for epidemics among adult and pediatric population. It has also been reported to be a cause of outbreaks in neonatal intensive care units (NICU) several times. We herein demonstrate a case with AVC who underwent LPC for ROP. And we discuss the treatment methodology in such cases.

1. Introduction

Retinopathy of prematurity (ROP) has been a leading cause of childhood blindness in developed and developing countries worldwide [1]. Cryotherapy, laser photocoagulation (LPC), and, later on, intravitreal bevacizumab injection (IVB) were administered for the treatment of the disease. Although LPC was the mainstay treatment option for most of ROP cases, IVB therapy has provided us with an alternative modality of treatment [2–4].

Adenoviral conjunctivitis (AVC), an acute ocular infection, includes findings such as photophobia, conjunctival injection, and excessive lacrimation [5]. The common form of AVC is epidemic keratoconjunctivitis which is responsible for several outbreaks among adult and pediatric population [6–8]. Various studies reported outbreaks due to adenovirus infections at neonatal intensive care unit (NICU). Also the association between AVC and ROP examinations has been previously published [9–11].

Our aim in this study was to introduce our clinical approach in LPC for ROP in a premature neonate infected with AVC.

2. Case Report

An infant with gestational age (GA) of 32 weeks and birth weight (BW) of 1440 g was firstly examined on postnatal 36 weeks for routine ROP screening in NICU of Zeynep Kamil Maternity and Children's Diseases Training and Research Hospital. Stage 1 zone II ROP without plus disease was noted in both eyes on fundus examination according to the International Classification of Retinopathy of Prematurity (ICROP) at first visit [12]. The child showed no other abnormalities in anterior and/or posterior segment. Five days later, the child presented with periorbital edema, redness, and tearing for which an ophthalmology consult was sought. There were 6 other infants at the same unit who presented with the same signs at the same time. The diagnosis of presumed AVC was made and the same medication was ordered for all affected neonates including topical antibiotic drops, artificial tear drops, and conjunctival irrigation with diluted povidone iodine. Because of not performing any laboratory investigations for the detection of adenovirus antigen, the diagnosis of presumed AVC was made empirically in all infants who had the same findings. All children who suffered from AVC were isolated in another room in NICU. Weekly

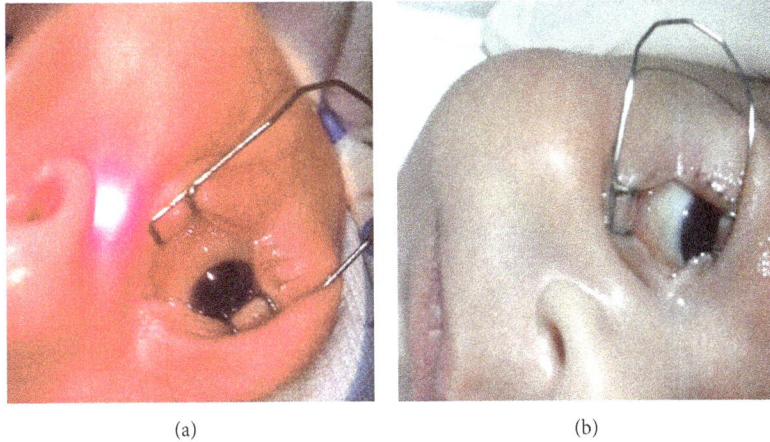

(a)   (b)

FIGURE 1: Edema of the inferior fornix conjunctiva and chemosis are easily seen before the first laser session in the right eye of the infant (a). Conjunctivitis is mostly resolved after medical therapy before the second laser session in the same eye (b).

examinations were performed for AVC during the follow-up period. Our case developed bilateral stage 3 zone II ROP with plus disease at postnatal 39 weeks. The child was still showing conjunctival chemosis, mild eyelid edema, pseudomembrane formation at tarsal conjunctiva, and mild corneal edema in both eyes; see Figure 1.

Laser treatment was considered in order to prevent the progression of ROP. A detailed informed consent was taken from the parents. 810 nm diode laser device (Iridex; Oculight SL, Mountainview, CA, U.S.A) was used for laser ablation. The laser was delivered to the avascular retina anterior to the ridge and posterior to the ridge which involved higher amount of fibrovascular component. Numbers of laser spots applied to right and left eyes were 620 and 605, at first laser session, respectively. LPC session ended due to increased conjunctival chemosis, conjunctival hemorrhage, and clouding of the ocular media. Topical drops were continued. And five days after the first laser session, the child was subjected to a second laser session to complete the ablation of the rest of avascular retinal zones. Totally 356 and 325 laser spots were delivered at second laser session, respectively.

The infant showed total recovery from AVC one week after the second laser session (Figure 1). ROP began to resolve and regressed after 3 weeks to a favorable outcome.

3. Discussion

There are several types of adenovirus infection in neonates including the most frequent ones as 4, 8, 11, 19, and 37. Outbreaks due to AVC in NICU centers remain an important comorbid factor particularly in infants with treatment requiring ROP [13]. As far as we know there was no information existing about the treatment approach in such cases in previous literature. Therefore, our aim in this report was to introduce a ROP case infected with AVC and discuss our treatment modality.

It has been previously stated that outbreaks of AVC in NICU were commonly manifested after ophthalmological examination procedures due to contaminated instruments [9, 11].

Low BW and patient care factors were also shown to be other causes of conjunctivitis among preterm infants [14]. Totally 7 newborns had infection with AVC in NICU during the study period and the current case was affected by the spread of this infection. Disposable types of equipment (eyelid speculum and depressor) are routinely used in our clinic for ROP examinations. However, several other factors such as inadequate hand hygiene, not excluding the infected staff members in NICU, and late isolation procedures of the infected infants in the same unit might also contribute to the spread of AVC [10].

Treatment requiring ROP can lead to blindness without timely intervention. Laser photocoagulation has been shown to be useful in ROP management. It prevents the progression of the disease and results in favorable outcomes [15]. The ETROP study indicated LPC for infants who had a high risk of progression for the disease [3]. Our newborn had stage 3 zone II high-risk prethreshold ROP at the time of the intervention as well as AVC related ocular findings. Laser application of the vascular retina posterior to the proliferative ridge tissue has been reported to lead an easier regression of ROP with favorable outcomes [15–17]. We performed a similar pattern of LPC in our case. However, we could not proceed to treatment due to increased chemosis of conjunctiva, hemorrhage from conjunctival membranes, and corneal haze in both eyes. We halted the procedure and rearranged a second laser session in order to complete laser ablation of the remaining avascular zones. Although divided laser sessions were mostly reported in aggressive posterior ROP (APROP) cases due to inadequate regression of the disease [18], gradual worsening of ocular surface findings in the present case compelled us to perform LPC in two laser sittings. Actually, this seemed to be an effective method in our case.

Several topical treatment methods have been applied for AVC, most of which are prophylactic including preservative-free antibiotic and artificial tears. Also some authors found povidone iodine 2.5% as an effective treatment in AVC [19]. We used the same treatment methodology during the course of AVC. And it resolves without any sequelae on ocular surface.

In conclusion, viral conjunctivitis related ocular surface findings may prevent laser ablation in a classical ROP case. Divided sessions of laser treatment may be an option in such cases. Also a more experienced surgeon in ROP treatment could handle the situation much more easily as well. Furthermore, immediate and careful treatment must be carried out for AVC conjunctivitis in an infant who has possibility for progression to treatment required ROP. Neonates with ROP and those who are infected with AVC in NICU should be subjected to immediate topical medication in order to perform an adequate LPC procedure.

Conflict of Interests

The authors declare that there is no conflict of interests regarding the publication of this paper.

References

[1] E. M. Lad, T. Hernandez-Boussard, J. M. Morton, and D. M. Moshfeghi, "Incidence of retinopathy of prematurity in the United States: 1997 through 2005," *The American Journal of Ophthalmology*, vol. 148, no. 3, pp. 451–458, 2009.

[2] Cryotherapy for Retinopathy of Prematurity Cooperative Group, "Multicenter trial of cryotherapy for retinopathy of prematurity: preliminary results," *Archives of Ophthalmology*, vol. 106, no. 4, pp. 471–479, 1988.

[3] Early Treatment For Retinopathy Of Prematurity Cooperative Group, "Revised indications for the treatment of retinopathy of prematurity: results of the early treatment for retinopathy of prematurity randomized trial," *Archives of Ophthalmology*, vol. 121, no. 12, pp. 1684–1694, 2003.

[4] H. A. Mintz-Hittner, K. A. Kennedy, and A. Z. Chuang, "Efficacy of intravitreal bevacizumab for stage 3+ retinopathy of prematurity," *The New England Journal of Medicine*, vol. 364, no. 7, pp. 603–615, 2011.

[5] I. F. Chaberny, P. Schnitzler, H. K. Geiss, and C. Wendt, "An outbreak of epidemic keratoconjunctivitis in a pediatric unit due to adenovirus type 8," *Infection Control and Hospital Epidemiology*, vol. 24, no. 7, pp. 514–519, 2003.

[6] J. Buffington, L. E. Chapman, M. G. Stobierski et al., "Epidemic keratoconjunctivitis in a chronic care facility: risk factors and measures for control," *Journal of the American Geriatrics Society*, vol. 41, no. 11, pp. 1177–1181, 1993.

[7] R. J. Cooper, R. Hallett, A. B. Tullo, and P. E. Klapper, "The epidemiology of adenovirus infections in Greater Manchester, UK 1982-96," *Epidemiology & Infection*, vol. 125, no. 2, pp. 333–345, 2000.

[8] H. Faden, R. J. Wynn, L. Campagna, and R. M. Ryan, "Outbreak of adenovirus type 30 in a neonatal intensive care unit," *The Journal of Pediatrics*, vol. 146, no. 4, pp. 523–527, 2005.

[9] S. Calkavur, O. Olukman, A. T. Ozturk et al., "Epidemic adenoviral keratoconjunctivitis possibly related to ophthalmological procedures in a neonatal intensive care unit: lessons from an outbreak," *Ophthalmic Epidemiology*, vol. 19, no. 6, pp. 371–379, 2012.

[10] Y. Ersoy, B. Otlu, P. Türkçüoğlu, F. Yetkin, S. Aker, and C. Kuzucu, "Outbreak of adenovirus serotype 8 conjunctivitis in preterm infants in a neonatal intensive care unit," *The Journal of Hospital Infection*, vol. 80, no. 2, pp. 144–149, 2012.

[11] S. S. Long, "Adenovirus and ophthalmologic examinations," *The Journal of Pediatrics*, vol. 146, no. 4, article A2, 2005.

[12] International Committee for the Classification of Retinopathy of Prematurity, "The International Classification of Retinopathy of Prematurity revisited," *Archives of Ophthalmology*, vol. 123, no. 7, pp. 991–999, 2005.

[13] E. Birenbaum, N. Linder, N. Varsano et al., "Adenovirus type 8 conjunctivitis outbreak in a neonatal intensive care unit," *Archives of Disease in Childhood*, vol. 68, no. 5, pp. 610–611, 1993.

[14] J. Haas, E. Larson, B. Ross, B. See, and L. Saiman, "Epidemiology and diagnosis of hospital-acquired conjunctivitis among neonatal intensive care unit patients," *The Pediatric Infectious Disease Journal*, vol. 24, no. 7, pp. 586–589, 2005.

[15] R. Axer-Siegel, I. Maharshak, M. Snir et al., "Diode laser treatment of retinopathy of prematurity: anatomical and refractive outcomes," *Retina*, vol. 28, no. 6, pp. 839–846, 2008.

[16] A. L. Ells, G. A. Gole, P. Lloyd Hildebrand, A. Ingram, C. M. Wilson,z and R. Geoff Williams, "Posterior to the ridge laser treatment for severe stage 3 retinopathy of prematurity," *Eye*, vol. 27, no. 4, pp. 525–530, 2013.

[17] M. O'Keefe, J. Burke, K. Algawi, and M. Goggin, "Diode laser photocoagulation to the vascular retina for progressively advancing retinopathy of prematurity," *British Journal of Ophthalmology*, vol. 79, no. 11, pp. 1012–1014, 1995.

[18] G. Sanghi, M. R. Dogra, D. Katoch, and A. Gupta, "Aggressive posterior retinopathy of prematurity: risk factors for retinal detachment despite confluent laser photocoagulation," *American Journal of Ophthalmology*, vol. 155, no. 1, pp. 159–164, 2013.

[19] Z. Ö. Tunay, O. Ozdemir, and I. S. Petricli, "Povidone iodine in the treatment of adenoviral conjunctivitis in infants," *Cutaneous and Ocular Toxicology*, 2014.

21

Klippel-Trenaunay Syndrome with Extensive Lymphangiomas

Sirin Mneimneh, Ali Tabaja, and Mariam Rajab

Pediatric Department, Makassed General Hospital, Lebanon

Correspondence should be addressed to Sirin Mneimneh; sirin.mneimneh@gmail.com

Academic Editor: Piero Pavone

Klippel-Trenaunay syndrome (KTS) is a rare disorder characterized by the triad of vascular malformations, venous varicosities, and bone and soft-tissue hypertrophy. We present a case of Klippel-Trenaunay syndrome with limb hypertrophy, port-wine stains, lymphangiomas, and venous varicosities in the limbs.

1. Introduction

Klippel-Trenaunay syndrome (KTS) was first described in 1900 by two French physicians, Klippel and Trenaunay [1]. The term describes a rare congenital syndrome of venous, lymphatic, and capillary malformations and soft tissue and bone hypertrophy [2].

63% of patients with KLS have the manifestation of the complete triad (port-wine stain, varicose veins, and hypertrophy of soft tissues/bones) [2]. Patients can be diagnosed with KTS with only one or more of the above-mentioned features since patient might not have all the features [3, 4].

Lymphangiomas are benign tumors of the lymphatic system. About 50% are present at birth and up to 90% become evident by the age of 2 years. Nearly 75% of the lesions are located on the head and neck (61%) or axilla (13%). The other 25% are distributed over the trunk (11%), extremities (11%), mediastinum (1%), and abdomen and genitalia (3%) [5].

We report a case of Klippel-Trenaunay with extensive lymphangioma throughout most of the body.

2. Case Report

A 20-month-old girl presented since birth with multiple soft truncal masses that involved the anterior aspect of the upper chest, abdomen (Figure 1), and right arm (Figure 2). The body was partly covered by a large port-wine stain capillary malformation (Figure 3). Extremities showed hypertrophy of the left thigh (Figure 4) and overgrowth of both feet, with syndactyly of the second and third toes of the right foot (Figure 5). The patient had dilated tortuous veins over the chest and the left leg (venous varicosities).

The patient had no dysmorphic features or facial malformations; on examination she had no murmur, no organomegaly, good muscle power, and no deficits with positive deep tendon reflexes along with normal developmental milestones and normal growth parameters. She was the product of a nonconsanguineous marriage to a gravida three mother with two previous healthy children, born by Cesarean section (due to fetal malformations).

Skeletal survey showed fused right second and third toes and hypertrophied soft tissue of these toes and of the right big toe. The patient also had fused left fourth and fifth toes and hypertrophied soft tissue of the left big toe (Figure 6).

MRI examination of the chest, abdomen, and pelvis showed extensive lymphangioma of the following (the lymphangioma appeared on T2 as high signal masses mostly cystic with multiple septation): right upper limb, upper part of the chest, upper portion of the left lower limb, left side of the pelvis, and the retroperitoneum (Figure 7). The liver is of normal size and signal showing no focal lesions. The pancreas has a normal acinar pattern with 12.3 mm hemangioma, and the Wirsung duct is of normal caliber. The spleen is of normal size and signal showing small hemangioma measuring 12 mm (Figure 8). The kidneys appear normal with no hydronephrosis.

The parents preferred to go abroad in order to do the surgical excision.

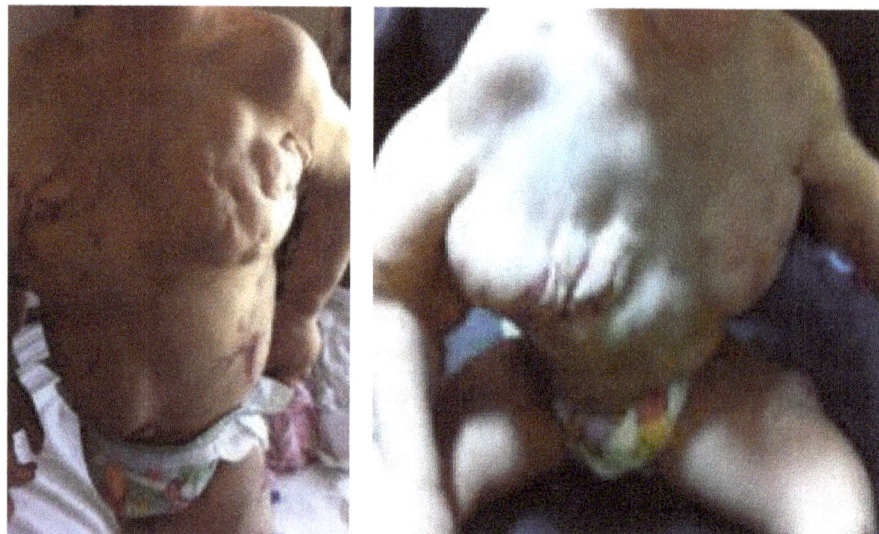

FIGURE 1: Focal overgrowth over the upper part of the chest.

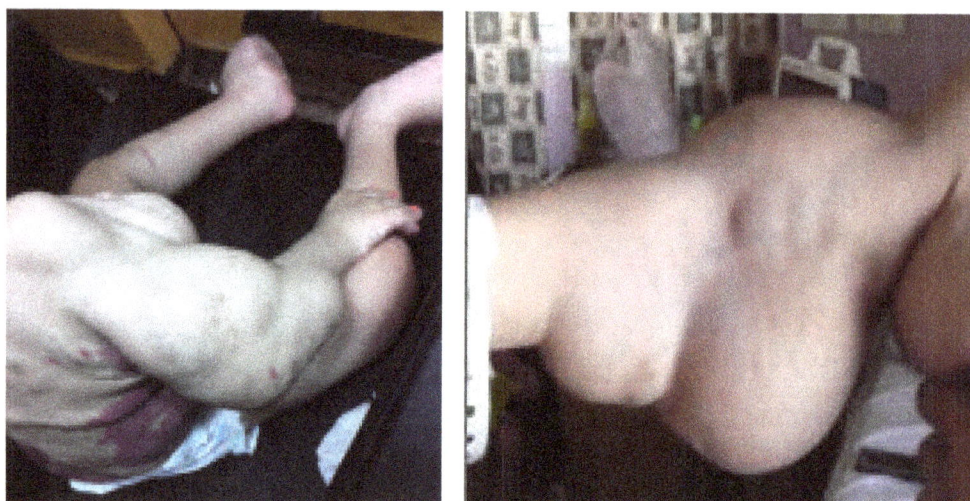

FIGURE 2: Multiple focal overgrowth of the right arm.

3. Discussion

Longitudinal growth results from complex multifactorial processes that take place in the broader context of different genetic traits and environmental influences. Overgrowth syndromes include a heterogeneous group of disorders that lead to excessive tissue proliferation, which is characterized by a phenotype of excessive visceral and somatic growth [6].

Klippel-Trenaunay syndrome is rare with uncertain origin with an incidence of approximately 1 : 100,000 live births [7]. It has no predilection for gender or race, and most of the cases are sporadic and appear at birth [8]. The French physicians Maurice Klippel and Paul Trenaunay first described this syndrome in 1900 when they associated vascular malformations with hypertrophy in the affected limb. Subsequently, Parkes Weber described arteriovenous fistulas in these patients [8].

The etiology of the disease is still under investigation. Some hypothesized that embryonic mesodermal changes resulting in increased angiogenesis lead to increased vascular flow causing tissue hypertrophy and vascular changes [9]. Others agree that the majority of cases of KTS are due to sporadic polygenic mutations [10]. The association between the angiogenic factor gene *AGGF1* and KTS appears to be significant [11].

KTS is characterized by the presence of capillary malformations associated with venous malformations or varicose veins and with bone or tissue hypertrophy [12].

Skin malformations in KTS are mostly capillary hemangiomas. Skin capillary malformations are diffuse or mostly located on the hypertrophic extremity side. Lower extremities are affected in about 95% of cases [3]. Changes can be limited to the skin only or can affect subcutaneous tissue, muscles,

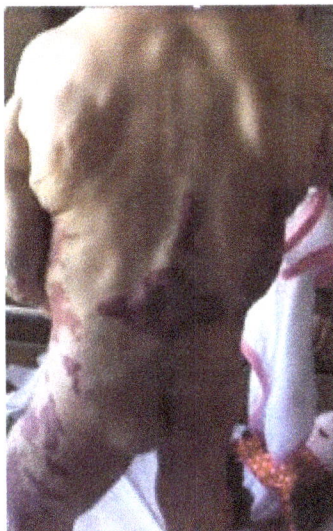

FIGURE 3: Port-wine stain over the back and thigh.

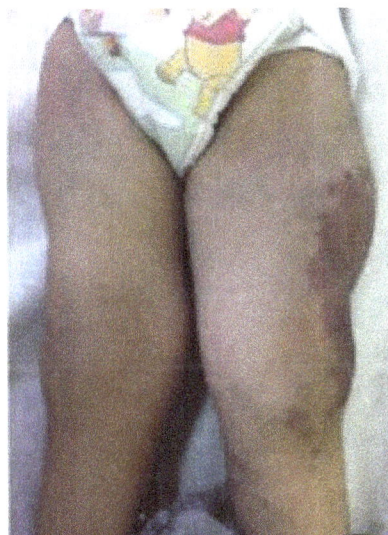

FIGURE 4: Hypertrophy of the left thigh.

and bones. 56% of patients have visceral vascular malformations including hemangiomas and/or lymphangiomas [13]. The spleen is rarely affected in patients with KTS and it can appear as splenomegaly, hemangioma, and/or lymphangioma of the spleen [14].

In a study at the Mayo Clinic, port-wine stains were seen in 98% of patients, varicosities or venous malformations in 72%, and limb hypertrophy in 67%. Atypical veins, including lateral veins and persistent sciatic veins, were present in 72% [15].

In a study of 144 patients, 95% had a cutaneous vascular malformation, 93% had soft tissue and bone hypertrophy, 76% had varicosities, and 71% had involvement limited to one extremity [16].

Sometimes lymphangiomas are associated with lymphangiomatosis located in the mediastinum, retroperitoneum,

axilla, or neck. Lymphangiomas are rarely unilocular or more often, as in this case, made of numerous septated cystic areas [17].

Our patient presented directly after birth with focal soft masses over the chest, hypertrophy of the soft tissues of lower extremities, associated with vascular malformation (port-wine stain) over the skin, and the hemangiomas in the internal organs. The extensive lymphangiomas make our case peculiar and distinguish it from other reported cases.

Complications are most often related to the underlying vascular pathological condition. Vascular malformations involving the gastrointestinal and genitourinary tract are a significant source of morbidity and even mortality. Involvement of the gastrointestinal tract occurs in 20% of the patients, can present at any age, and may go unrecognized in patients without overt symptoms.

Pulmonary embolism, cerebral aneurysm, and pulmonary vein varicosities are incidental findings and give rise to life-threatening complications [18].

Regular clinical and radiographic monitoring of the affected limbs, compression stockings for chronic venous insufficiency, intermittent pneumatic compression devices for reducing limb size, flash lamp-pumped pulsed dye laser for port-wine stains, and surgical correction of varicose veins are needed as required [19].

Surgical debulking often fails or worsens symptoms as venous and lymphatic channels are destroyed, leading to further swelling and poor wound healing. Overall, treatment is often not definitive and 50% of patients reexperience symptoms after surgery despite reported clinical and symptom severity improvement in many patients.

The main differential diagnosis includes the following.

Proteus syndrome is characterized by massive overgrowth and asymmetry. The types of skin lesions include linear verrucous epidermal nevi, intradermal nevi, hemangiomas, lipomas, and varicosities [20]. Macrodactyly and syndactyly can occur; although final height is normal, increased stature in childhood is common in addition to macrocephaly. Soft tissue hypertrophy, which may appear as gyriform changes, is mainly over the planter surface. Moderate mental deficiency occurs in approximately 50% of cases. Bone overgrowth, which is dysplastic, progressive, and irregular, is typical of Proteus syndrome and not observed in KTS; thus, its detection is an important tool in differentiating between the diseases. Our patient does not represent the typical skin lesions; her mental milestones are normal as well as her height, weight, and head circumference measurements.

Maffucci syndrome is characterized by multiple enchondromas, hemangiomas and, less often, lymphangiomas. Enchondromas are cartilaginous benign tumors that may develop most frequently in phalanges and long bones, but may also affect the tibia, fibula, humerus, ribs or cranium. Soft tissue tumors usually develop with the bone lesions [21].

Neurofibromatosis type I generally affects the skin, nervous system, bones, and endocrine glands by causing benign tumors. The diagnostic criteria for this disease were developed in 1987 and redefined in 1997 [22] and they are based on the presence of two or more of the following findings: a first-degree relative who has neurofibromatosis

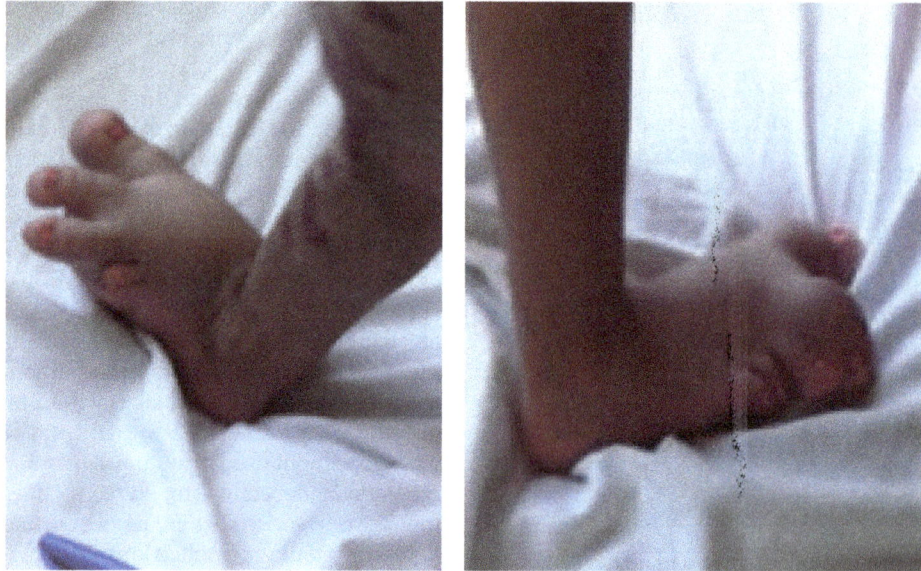

FIGURE 5: Syndactyly of the toes in both feet.

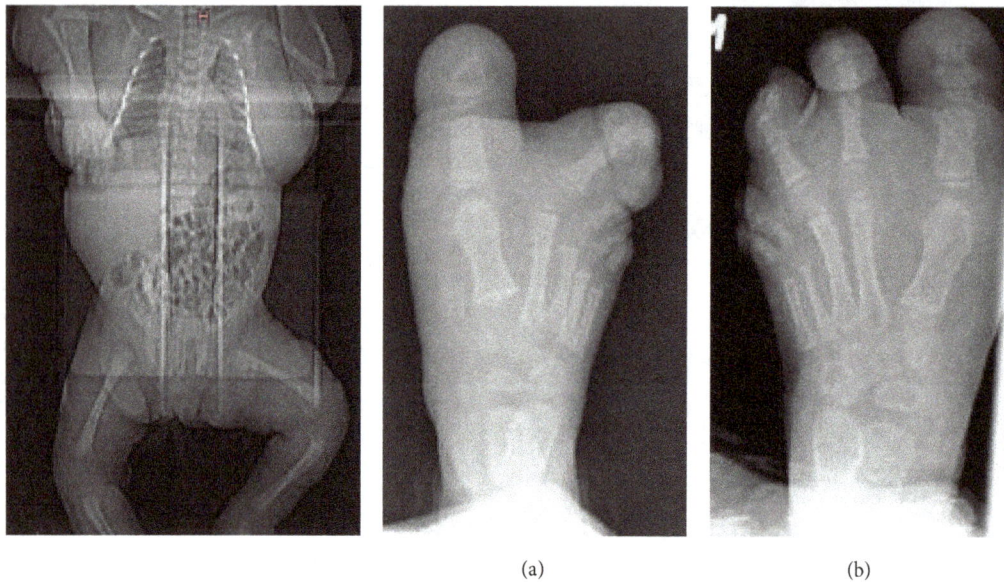

(a)   (b)

FIGURE 6: X-ray. (a) Right foot; (b) left foot.

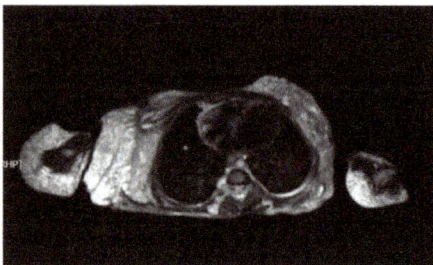

FIGURE 7: MRI of the chest (phase T2 sequence, with fat suppression), showed the lymphangioma in the upper part of the chest wall, in the right arm.

type I, "café-au-lait" spots, neurofibromas, freckles in the axillary or inguinal regions, optic gliomas, iris hamartomas, and distinctive bone lesions.

Sturge-Weber syndrome is a mesodermal phakomatosis characterized by a port-wine vascular nevus on the upper part of the face, leptomeningeal angiomatosis that involves one or both hemispheres, early onset seizure, choroidal vascular lesions associated with glaucoma, neurologic deterioration, and eventual neurodevelopmental delay [23].

Schnyder et al. [24] suggested that Klippel-Trenaunay, Parkes-Weber, and Sturge-Weber syndrome are variants with a common feature of local gigantism and hemangioma. Involvement of the head and neck with manifestations of

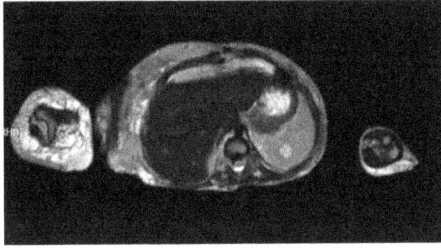

FIGURE 8: MRI of the abdomen showed the hemangioma in the spleen.

meningeal angiomatosis causing epileptic fits and choroidal hemangioma or glaucoma result in a presentation of Sturge-Weber syndrome. Local gigantism and hemangioma of the limbs with osteohypertrophy present as Klippel-Trenaunay or Parkes-Weber syndrome, depending on whether there are peripheral varices which cause KTS or arteriovenous anastomoses which would result in a picture of Parkes-Weber syndrome.

In summary, Klippel-Trenaunay syndrome is a rare disease of the vascular and lymphatic system or capillary malformation at birth associated with hypertrophy of the soft tissues/bones. Most cases are difficult to treat due to high rates of recurrence after surgical excision, but individualized intervention can help manage pain and help prevent serious complications.

Conflict of Interests

The authors declare that there is no conflict of interests regarding the publication of this paper.

References

[1] E. E. Huiras, C. J. Barnes, L. F. Eichenfield, A. N. Pelech, and B. A. Drolet, "Pulmonary thromboembolism associated with Klippel-Trenaunay syndrome," *Pediatrics*, vol. 116, no. 4, pp. e596–e600, 2005.

[2] A. G. Jacob, D. J. Driscoll, W. J. Shaughnessy, A. W. Stanson, R. P. Clay, and P. Gloviczki, "Klippel-Trenaunay syndrome: spectrum and management," *Mayo Clinic Proceedings*, vol. 73, no. 1, pp. 28–36, 1998.

[3] A. Lee, D. Driscoll, P. Gloviczki, R. Clay, W. Shaughnessy, and A. Stans, "Evaluation and management of pain in patients with Klippel-Trenaunay syndrome: a review," *Pediatrics*, vol. 115, no. 3, pp. 744–749, 2005.

[4] O. Kocaman, A. Alponat, C. Aygün et al., "Lower gastrointestinal bleeding, hematuria and splenic hemangiomas in Klippel-Trenaunay syndrome: a case report and literature review," *The Turkish Journal of Gastroenterology*, vol. 20, no. 1, pp. 62–66, 2009.

[5] J. E. Allanson, "Lymphatic circulation," in *Human Malformation and Related Anomalies*, R. E. Stevenson, J. G. Hall, and R. S. Goodman, Eds., pp. 293–304, Oxford University Press, New York, NY, USA, 1993.

[6] R. Visser, S. G. Kant, J. M. Wit, and M. H. Breung, "Overgrowth syndromes: from classical to new," *Pediatric Endocrinology Reviews*, vol. 6, no. 3, pp. 375–394, 2009.

[7] I. Lorda-Sanchez, L. Prieto, E. Rodriguez-Pinilla, and M. L. Martinez-Frias, "Increased parental age and number of pregnancies in Klippel-Trenaunay-Weber syndrome," *Annals of Human Genetics*, vol. 62, no. 3, pp. 235–239, 1998.

[8] C. D. A. De Leon, L. R. B. Filho, M. D. Ferrari, B. L. Guidolin, and B. J. Maffessoni, "Klippel-Trenaunay syndrome: case report," *Anais Brasileiros de Dermatologia*, vol. 85, no. 1, pp. 93–96, 2010.

[9] P. A. Baskerville, J. S. Ackroyd, and N. L. Browse, "The etiology of the Klippel-Trenaunay syndrome," *Annals of Surgery*, vol. 202, no. 5, pp. 624–627, 1985.

[10] C. E. U. Oduber, C. M. A. M. van der Horst, and R. C. M. Hennekam, "Klippel-Trenaunay syndrome: diagnostic criteria and hypothesis on etiology," *Annals of Plastic Surgery*, vol. 60, no. 2, pp. 217–223, 2008.

[11] Y. Hu, L. Li, S. B. Seidelmann et al., "Identification of association of common *AGGF1* variants with susceptibility for klippel-trenaunay syndrome using the structure association program," *Annals of Human Genetics*, vol. 72, no. 5, pp. 636–643, 2008.

[12] S. H. Cha, M. A. Romeo, and J. A. Neutze, "Visceral manifestations of Klippel-Trénaunay syndrome," *Radiographics*, vol. 25, no. 6, pp. 1694–1697, 2005.

[13] C. Maari and I. J. Frieden, "Klippel-Trénaunay syndrome: the importance of 'geographic stains' in identifying lymphatic disease and risk of complications," *Journal of the American Academy of Dermatology*, vol. 51, no. 3, pp. 391–398, 2004.

[14] R. Jindal, R. Sullivan, B. Rodda, D. Arun, M. Hamady, and N. J. W. Cheshire, "Splenic malformation in a patient with Klippel-Trenaunay syndrome: a case report," *Journal of Vascular Surgery*, vol. 43, no. 4, pp. 848–850, 2006.

[15] J. H. Lisko and F. Fish, "Klippel-Trénaunay syndrome," in *E-Medicine*, CME, 2006.

[16] I. Frieden, O. Enjolras, and N. Esterly, "Vascular birthmark and other abnormalities of blood vessels and lymphatics. Vascular malformations," in *Pediatric Dermatology in General Medicine*, L. A. Schachner and R. C. Hansen, Eds., pp. 1002–1019, McGraw-Hill, New York, NY, USA, 6th edition, 2003.

[17] M. Bezzi, A. Spinelli, M. Pierleoni, and G. Andreoli, "Cystic lymphangioma of the spleen: US-CT-MRI correlation," *European Radiology*, vol. 11, no. 7, pp. 1187–1190, 2001.

[18] G. Skourtis, O. Lazoura, P. Panoussis, and L. Livieratos, "Klippel-Trénaunay syndrome: an unusual cause of pulmonary embolism," *International Angiology*, vol. 25, no. 3, pp. 322–326, 2006.

[19] G. Gupta and D. Bilsland, "A prospective study of the impact of laser treatment on vascular lesions," *British Journal of Dermatology*, vol. 143, no. 2, pp. 356–359, 2000.

[20] K. L. Jones, "Systemic vasculature," in *Human Malformations and Related Anomalies*, R. E. Stevenson, J. G. Hall, and R. M. Goodman, Eds., pp. 266–267, Oxford University Press, New York, NY, USA, 1993.

[21] C. Biber, P. Ergun, U. Y. Turay, Y. Erdogan, and S. B. Hizel, "A case of Maffucci's Syndrome with pleural effusion: ten-year followup," *Annals of the Academy of Medicine, Singapore*, vol. 33, pp. 347–350, 2004.

[22] E. N. Washington, T. P. Placket, R. A. Gagliano, J. Kavolius, and D. A. Person, "Diffuse plexiform neurofibroma of the back: report of a case," *Hawaii Medical Journal*, vol. 69, no. 8, pp. 191–193, 2010.

[23] W. A. Sturge, "A case of partial epilepsy apparently due to a lesion of one of the vasomotor centers of the brain," *Transactions of the Clinical Society of London*, vol. 12, pp. 162–167, 1879.

[24] U. W. Schnyder, E. Landolt, and G. Martz, "Syndrome de Klippel-Trenaunay avec colombe irien atypique," *Journal of Human Genetics*, vol. 5, pp. 1–8, 1956.

22

A Case of Idiopathic Hypereosinophilic Syndrome Causing Mitral Valve Papillary Muscle Rupture

Tiffany Tamse,[1,2] **Avind Rampersad,**[1,2] **Alejandro Jordan-Villegas,**[1,3] **and Jill Ireland**[2]

[1]*Florida Hospital for Children, Orlando, FL 32803, USA*
[2]*University of Central Florida, Orlando, FL 32827, USA*
[3]*Orlando Health, Orlando, FL 32806, USA*

Correspondence should be addressed to Tiffany Tamse; tiffany.tamse.md@flhosp.org

Academic Editor: Hitoshi Horigome

Idiopathic Hypereosinophilic Syndrome (IHES) is a rare disease that can be difficult to diagnose as the differential is broad. This disease can cause significant morbidity and mortality if left untreated. Our patient is a 17-year-old adolescent female who presented with nonspecific symptoms of abdominal pain and malaise. She was incidentally found to have hypereosinophilia of 16,000 on complete blood count and nonspecific colitis and pulmonary edema on computed tomography. She went into cardiogenic shock due to papillary rupture of her mitral valve requiring extreme life support measures including intubation and extracorporal membrane oxygenation (ECMO) as well as mitral valve replacement. Pathology of the valve showed eosinophilic infiltration as the underlying etiology. The patient was diagnosed with IHES after the exclusion of infectious, rheumatologic, and oncologic causes. She was treated with steroids with improvement of her symptoms and scheduled for close follow-up. In general patients with IHES that have cardiac involvement have poorer prognoses.

1. Introduction

Hypereosinophilic Syndrome (HES) is a rare disease in childhood, usually occurring between 20 and 50 years of age, with the true prevalence unknown [1]. The Idiopathic HES variant is even less common. Cardiovascular involvement in IHES is not uncommon and poses the highest risk for morbidity and mortality. This case report of a 17-year-old female describes a course of cardiogenic shock resulting from an acute papillary muscle rupture secondary to eosinophilic infiltration. No cases have been reported in the pediatric literature and very few have been reported in the adult literature of papillary rupture [2]. It is important to recognize that, despite being a rare occurrence, marked hypereosinophilia in a child should be worked up thoroughly at presentation.

2. Case Report

This is a 17-year-old female with a history of depression, anxiety, chronic abdominal pain, and heavy and painful menses for which she takes an oral contraceptive pill. She presented with a two-week history of worsening abdominal pain, described as a constant dull ache located in the pelvic region and accompanied by nausea with bilious emesis, and mild chest pain. She had been seen in her primary care physician's office four days prior to admission and given hyoscyamine for her pain with minimal relief. No associated menstrual symptoms were noted.

The patient admits to smoking 5–7 cigarettes daily but denies any drug or alcohol use. Her last sexual encounter was 6 months prior to admission and she denies any prior pregnancy or sexually transmitted infections.

She presented to the Emergency Department and vital signs showed tachycardia and elevated blood pressure. Her cardiac examination was normal and there was no prior history of any murmur. Her abdominal exam showed diffuse tenderness in the lower quadrants and pelvic area, without distension. Cervical motion tenderness was elicited and white discharge was noted on pelvic exam. Wet prep was negative for trichomonas, yeast, and clue cells. Laboratory values were significant for leukocytosis of 30,850 and eosinophilia of

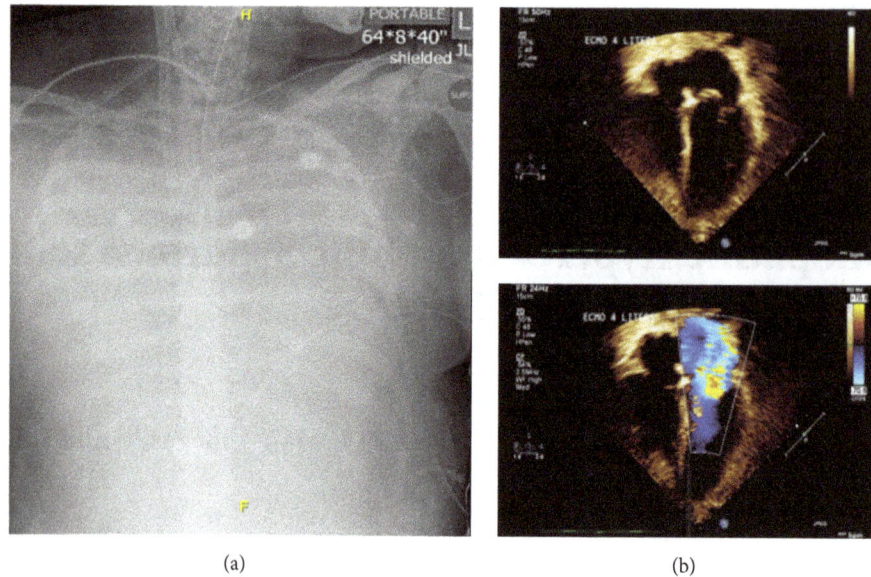

(a)   (b)

FIGURE 1: (a) Chest X-ray showing complete opacification of the thorax suspicion for complete lung consolidation secondary to edema. (b) Echocardiogram images showing flail mitral valve from a ruptured cord and severe mitral regurgitation.

52.4%. Computed tomography (CT) of the abdomen showed thickening and edema of the wall of the duodenum and proximal jejunum, ascites in the upper abdomen, and appearance of a collapsed hemorrhagic cyst/corpus luteum in the left adnexa. The patient was given intravenous doxycycline, cefotetan, and analgesia prior to admission.

Gynecology was consulted and treatment was directed towards a ruptured ovarian cyst. No surgical intervention was recommended and plan was to treat patient for a possible culture negative pelvic inflammatory disease. Repeat complete blood count was unchanged with eosinophilia and leukocytosis and clinically patient was improving.

On day two of admission she had an acute decompensation with bilious emesis and severe hypotension. She became hypoxic and was transferred to the pediatric intensive care unit, for suspected septic shock, where she was emergently intubated and started on inotropic support. She was taken to the operating room for an exploratory laparotomy. The small bowel was edematous and thickened throughout the proximal jejunum with full thickness enteritis. Areas of serosal erosion and adherent omentum as well as an area of pale bowel with lymphadenopathy were noted. A diverting jejunostomy was performed to allow the inflamed bowel to decompress and a specimen was sent to pathology.

She continued to decompensate and was started on high frequency oscillatory ventilation with nitric oxide. Her chest X-ray showed worsening interstitial and alveolar edema (Figure 1(a)). At this time the patient went into multiorgan dysfunction syndrome, due to increased level of support, she was placed on VA ECMO. Cardiac echocardiography demonstrated severe mitral regurgitation from a nonfunctioning valve, moderate left atrial enlargement (Figure 1(b)). The patient was taken to the operating room for replacement of the mitral valve and intraoperatively there was noted to be papillary muscle avulsion of the anterior leaflet without

evidence of vegetation. She was separated from ECMO support but developed acute renal failure requiring one week of hemodialysis. She was extubated on day ten of hospitalization and kidney function recovered completely. Neurologically she has remained without any deficits noted.

Pathology specimens, peripheral smear, bone marrow, bowel, and heart valve all demonstrated marked eosinophilic infiltration (Figures 2 and 3). Workup was negative for vasculitis, collagen vascular, infectious, and myeloproliferative diseases (Table 1).

She was diagnosed with IHES and received a single dose of ivermectin before she was started on solumedrol. She was discharged to inpatient rehabilitation on day 27 and then returned for ostomy reversal 5 days later.

3. Discussion

HES is defined as an absolute eosinophil count of greater than $1,500/mm^3$ that is associated with end organ damage that cannot be explained by another cause aside from the eosinophilia [3]. Historically there was a requirement of 6 months of hypereosinophilia but this is no longer the case as patients have presented with significant end organ damage warranting the diagnosis and treatment [3, 4].

HES among the pediatric population has a heterogeneous presentation, most commonly with fever, arthralgias, and rash [5]. Other nonspecific symptoms include fatigue, cough, dyspnea, and rhinitis. The disease can affect about every organ system through eosinophilic infiltration of the tissue causing varying degrees of damage and can be life threatening [4]. The major basic proteins in the cells are thought to play a role in the pathogenesis of this disease [6].

IHES, which we believe our patient has, is a diagnosis of exclusion and can only be made once all secondary causes of hypereosinophilia have been excluded. There must be

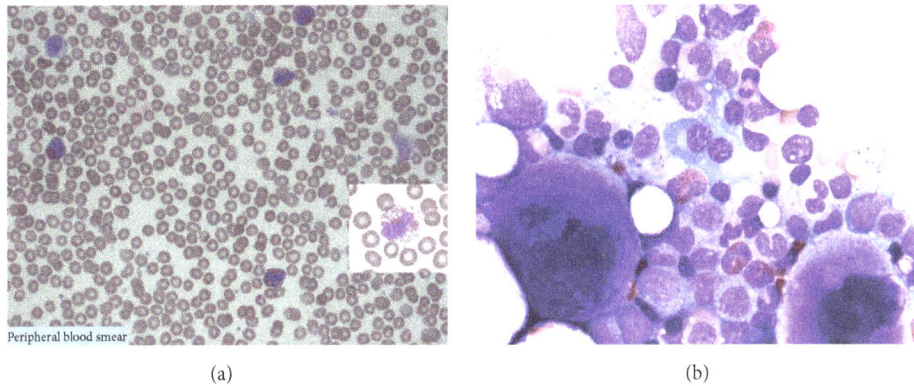

FIGURE 2: (a) Peripheral smear: marked eosinophilia (most eosinophils show intact cytoplasmic granules). (b) Bone marrow biopsy: normocellular marrow with mild megakaryocytic hyperplasia, eosinophilia, and no increase in blasts. No monoclonal B-cells or immunophenotypically abnormal T-cells are detected.

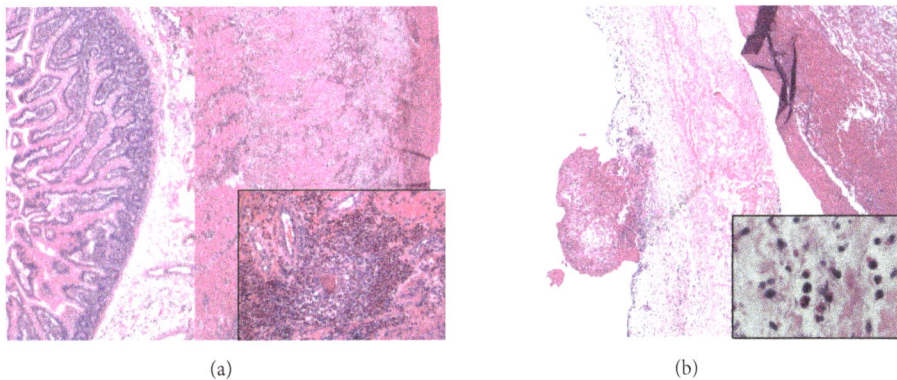

FIGURE 3: (a) Jejunum: diffuse marked eosinophilic infiltrate associated with ischemic tissue damage. (b) Mitral valve: benign endomyocardial tissue demonstrating myocardial necrosis and fibrinous endocarditis with mixed inflammatory infiltrate comprising of eosinophils, lymphocytes, and histiocytes.

an absence of eosinophil blasts in the blood and bone marrow [7].

There may be a different underlying pathogenesis in IHES of pediatric patients as compared to adult patients. There is only a slight male predominance in the pediatric population, whereas adult males have a predominance of 9 : 1 [5]. Also although chromosomal abnormalities and acute leukemia account for many pediatric cases for HES, rarely the FLP1L1-PDGFRA fusion gene is found, which is commonly seen in adults [1].

Cardiac involvement carries the highest morbidity and mortality and classically occurs in stages. Degranulated eosinophils in peripheral blood smears can indicate endocardial disease [6]. Eosinophils infiltrate the tissue and release toxic mediators. This causes endocardial damage and platelet thrombi leading to mural thrombi and risk for emboli. Over time fibrous thickening of the endocardial lining leads to a restrictive cardiomyopathy. The tricuspid and mitral valves can be effected leading to regurgitation [3]. Our patient had evidence of fibrinous endocarditis with mixed inflammatory infiltrate of eosinophils, lymphocytes, and histiocytes. There

was also intravascular debris demonstrating partially degenerated eosinophils.

Eosinophilic colitis with low ESR, as was present in our patient, is a common GI manifestation, as well as hepatitis, hepatosplenomegaly, cholangitis, and pancreatitis [7, 8]. Pathologic investigation of the bowel sample from our patient demonstrated diffuse marked eosinophilic infiltration associated with ischemic tissue damage and an ill-defined granulomatous reaction. Additionally, there was focal fibrinous necrosis of the small vessels as well as intravascular thrombi and eosinophilic perivasculitis.

Neurologically the disease can present as hemiplegia (focal deficits), peripheral neuropathy, or an altered behavior or cognitive dysfunction. Most patients with IHES with neurologic involvement also have an associated endocarditis with emboli being a source of the CNS complications. Neurotoxins have also been found in eosinophils which may account for the diffuse altered mental status [9].

Dermatologic manifestations include mucocutaneous ulcers, pruritic papules, and nodules as well as a reported case of recurrent vesicular rash with necrotic crusting lesions [10].

TABLE 1

Infectious	
HIV 1/2 Ag/Ab	Nonreactive
Hepatitis A, hepatitis B, and hepatitis C	Nonreactive
Bartonella henselae PCR	Negative
Toxocara	Negative
Strongyloides	Negative
Tropheryma whipplei PCR	Negative
Blood/fungus cultures	Negative
Urine cultures	Negative
Immunologic	
ANA (blood and abdominal fluid)	Negative
DSDNA/SSA Ab	Negative
Smith/RNP Ab	Negative
ANCA	Negative
C3	39 mg/dL
C4	2 mg/dL
IgG	345 mg/dL
IgA	111 mg/dL
IgM	143 mg/dL
IgE	191 kU/L
CD4 helper cells	34.3%
CD8 suppressor cells	26.4%
Total CD3	66.2%
Total B-cells	28.9%
Natural killer cells	3.2%
CD4/CD8 ratio	1.3
T-cell interpretation	Normal total B-cells (CD19)
Other	
Beta hCG (urine)	Negative
Cortisol	13.4 µg/dL
Tryptase	2.6 µg/L
Genetic analysis	
PDGFRa (4q12) FISH	Normal
PDGFRb (5q33) FISH	Normal
FGFR1 (8p11) FISH	Normal
BCR/ABL1/ASS1 t(9,22) FISH	Normal
KIT (c-KIT) mutation	Not detected
Next-Gen Sequencing myeloid disorders profile* (NeoTYPE analysis)	No evidence of mutation in any of genes tested. Low probability of myeloid neoplasm diagnosis (<10%)

*Myeloid disorders profile: ABL1, ASXL1, ATRX, BCOR, BCORL1, BRAF, CALR, CBL, CBLB, CBLC, CDKN 2A, CEBPA, CSF3R, CUX1, DNMT3a, ETV6, EZH2, FBXW7, FLT3, GATA1, GATA2, GNAS, HRAS, IDH1, IDH2, IKZF1, JAK2 Exon 12 + 14, JAK3, KDM6A, KIT, KRAS, MLL, MPL, MYD 88, NOTCH 1, NPM1, NRAS, PDGFRA, PHF 6, PTEN, PTPN11, RAD21, RUNX1, SETBP1, SF3B1, SMC1A, SMC3, SRSF2, STAG2, TET2, TP53, U2AF1, WT1, and ZRSR2.

Pulmonary presentation includes chronic cough, pulmonary infiltrates, fibrosis, and embolus. Hematologic insults including idiopathic thrombocytopenic purpura have been reported [4].

The differential for causes of hypereosinophilia is vast and a thorough investigation is indicated [6]. Workup for IHES should follow serial eosinophil counts. Blood and stool studies should be done to exclude parasitic infections. Peripheral smear initially and then bone marrow biopsy should be performed to rule out a malignancy. The vasculitides may be ruled out by ANCA, ANA, complements, ESR, and RF. HIV and Bartonella serology may be performed to rule out these diseases if at risk. Chest X-ray and CT of chest and abdomen may reveal pathology. At persistent eosinophil levels above 1,500, an ECHO must be performed and followed. Troponins may also be helpful in detecting asymptomatic endocarditis from eosinophilic infiltration [8].

The goal of treatment is to keep absolute eosinophil counts below 1,500. If patients are asymptomatic they may be observed but with serial echocardiograms and close follow-up. First-line treatment for IHES is corticosteroids [11]. Our patient responded to a 2-week methylprednisolone course with return of her eosinophils to below 500. Duration of therapy depends on response and control of symptoms and the steroids are tapered to the lowest efficacious dose. Some patients may need lifetime treatment. Interferon alpha, which inhibits proliferation of eosinophil precursors, is 2nd line for nonresponders to steroids. Hydroxyurea, vincristine, and other chemotherapeutic drugs are 3rd line [8]. Imatinib has primary use in patients with PDGFRA/B mutations but has also been useful even when no mutation is found, although this may be due to multiple variations of the mutations that may not have been detected [3]. Mepolizumab has been used for the FIP1L1-PDGFRA mutations as well. Bone marrow and peripheral stem cell transplantation for refractory causes is under investigation.

Surgery including heart valve replacement for severe mitral regurgitation is not uncommon although it is usually not as emergent as in our patient whose regurgitation was caused by papillary muscle rupture. Endocardial decortication and heart transplant may also be warranted but not as commonly [12]. Splenectomy for the disease has also been reported [3].

If untreated, the morbidity and mortality can reach 80% at 3 years for the IHES. With treatment the survival rate increases to 80% at 5 years and 42–60% at 10 years [8]. Poor prognostic factors include cardiac involvement, higher WBC count at presentation, and myelodysplastic features, while patients with good steroid response and elevated IgE levels have a better prognosis.

Abbreviations

IHES: Idiopathic Hypereosinophilic Syndrome
HES: Hypereosinophilic Syndrome
ECMO: Extracorporal membrane oxygenation.

Conflict of Interests

The authors declare that they have no conflict of interests regarding this paper.

Authors' Contribution

Tiffany Tamse was involved directly in patient care, conducted a literature search of the topic of IHES, drafted the initial paper, and approved the final paper as submitted. Avind Rampersad was involved directly in patient care, reviewed and revised the paper, and approved the final paper as submitted. Alejandro Jordan-Villegas was involved directly in patient care, reviewed and revised the paper, and approved the final paper as submitted. Jill Ireland was involved directly in patient care, conducted a literature search of the topic of IHES, helped to draft parts of the initial paper, and approved the final paper. All authors approved the final paper as submitted and agree to be accountable for all aspects of the work.

References

[1] M. Rapanotti, R. Caruso, E. Ammatuna et al., "Molecular characterization of paediatric idiopathic hypereosinophilia," *British Journal of Haematology*, vol. 151, no. 5, pp. 440–446, 2010.

[2] S. Madhwal, J. Goldberg, J. Barcena et al., "Unusual cause of acute mitral regurgitation: idiopathic hypereosinophilic syndrome," *Annals of Thoracic Surgery*, vol. 93, no. 3, pp. 974–977, 2012.

[3] J. Gotlib, "World Health Organization-defined eosinophilic disorders: 2014 update on diagnosis, risk stratification, and management," *American Journal of Hematology*, vol. 89, no. 3, pp. 325–337, 2014.

[4] M. Van Grotel, M. de Hoog, R. R. de Krijger, H. B. Beverloo, and M. M. van den Heuvel-Eibrink, "Hypereosinophilic syndrome in children," *Leukemia Research*, vol. 36, no. 10, pp. 1249–1254, 2012.

[5] J. James, "Pediatric hypereosinophilic syndrome (HES) differs from adult HES," *Pediatrics*, vol. 118, supplement 1, pp. S49–S50, 2006.

[6] M. A. Alfaham, S. D. Ferguson, B. Sihra, and J. Davies, "The idiopathic hypereosinophilic syndrome," *Archives of Disease in Childhood*, vol. 62, no. 6, pp. 601–613, 1987.

[7] A. M. Shah and M. Joglekart, "Eosinophilic colitis as a complication of the hypereosinophilic syndrome," *Postgraduate Medical Journal*, vol. 63, no. 740, pp. 485–487, 1987.

[8] J. Kanthila and N. Bhaskaranand, "Idiopathic hypereosinophilic syndrome in children: 3 cases with review of literature," *Indian Journal of Pediatrics*, vol. 80, no. 2, pp. 124–127, 2013.

[9] K. A. Kumar, A. Anjaneyulu, and J. M. K. Murthy, "Idiopathic hypereosinophilic syndrome presenting as childhood hemiplegia," *Postgraduate Medical Journal*, vol. 68, no. 804, pp. 831–833, 1992.

[10] T. J. Fischer, C. Daugherty, C. Gushurst, G. M. Kephart, and G. J. Gleich, "Systemic vasculitis associated with eosinophilia and marked degranulation of tissue eosinophils," *Pediatrics*, vol. 82, no. 1, pp. 69–75, 1988.

[11] V. Prasad, L. Rajam, and A. Borade, "Cardiogenic shock with hypereosinophilic syndrome," *Indian Pediatrics*, vol. 46, no. 9, pp. 801–803, 2009.

[12] A. Tang, J. Karski, J. Butany, and T. David, "Severe mitral regurgitation in acute eosinophilic endomyocarditis: repair or replacement?" *Interactive Cardiovascular and Thoracic Surgery*, vol. 3, no. 2, pp. 406–408, 2004.

23

Liver Transplant in a Patient under Methylphenidate Therapy: A Case Report and Review of the Literature

Hoi Y. Tong,[1] Carmen Díaz,[2] Elena Collantes,[3] Nicolás Medrano,[1] Alberto M. Borobia,[1] Paloma Jara,[2] and Elena Ramírez[1]

[1]Department of Clinical Pharmacology, Hospital Universitario La Paz, IdiPaz, School of Medicina, Universidad Autónoma de Madrid, Paseo de la Castellana 261, 28046 Madrid, Spain
[2]Pediatric Hepatology Department, Hospital Universitario La Paz, IdiPaz, Paseo de la Castellana 261, 28046 Madrid, Spain
[3]Pathological Anatomy Department, Hospital Universitario La Paz, IdiPaz, Paseo de la Castellana 261, 28046 Madrid, Spain

Correspondence should be addressed to Elena Ramírez; elena.ramirez@inv.uam.es

Academic Editor: Seyed Mohsen Dehghani

Background. Methylphenidate (MPH) is widely used in treating children with attention-deficit-hyperactivity disorder. Hepatotoxicity is a rare phenomenon; only few cases are described with no liver failure. *Case.* We report on the case of a 12-year-old boy who received MPH for attention-deficit-hyperactivity disorder. Two months later the patient presented with signs and symptoms of hepatitis and MPH was discontinued, showing progressive worsening and developing liver failure and a liver transplantation was required. Other causes of liver failure were ruled out and the liver biopsy was suggestive of drug toxicity. *Discussion.* One rare adverse reaction of MPH is hepatotoxicity. The review of the literature shows few cases of liver injury attributed to MPH; all of them recovered after withdrawing the treatment. The probable mechanism of liver injury was MPH direct toxicity to hepatocytes. In order to establish the diagnosis of MPH-induced liver injury, we used CIOMS/RUCAM scale that led to an assessment of "possible" relationship. This report provides the first published case of acute MPH-induced liver failure with successful hepatic transplantation. *Conclusions.* It is important to know that hepatotoxicity can occur in patients with MPH treatment and monitoring the liver's function is highly recommended.

1. Introduction

Methylphenidate hydrochloride (MPH) is a chain substituted amphetamine derivative that primarily acts as norepinephrine-dopamine reuptake inhibitor. The Food and Drug Administration (FDA) first approved MPH on 1955; however, it was not until the 1990s when MPH saw a dramatic increase in its prescription. In the PATS study almost one-third of the children revealed some side effects, mainly weight loss and neurological effects [1]. A few scattered and sporadic cases of hepatotoxicity with MPH treatment have been reported and usually referred to transient elevation of liver enzymes. This report describes a case of irreversible methylphenidate-induced liver failure.

2. Case Presentation

A 12-year-old boy with no relevant medical history was treated with MPH at an appropriate dose of 30 mg daily for attention-deficit-hyperactivity disorder (ADHD), and no other treatment was received in the previous months. After two months of treatment, the patient presented with a 2-day history of generalized itching, malaise, fatigue, and anorexia and with no fever. At that time, MPH was discontinued. Initial aminotransferases (alanine aminotransferase, ALT; aspartate aminotransferase, AST), total bilirubin, and alkaline phosphatase were elevated, while hepatitis panel (HBsAg, anti-HBcore, anti-HAV, anti-HIV, CMV IgM, and syphilis) was negative, and the patient's health continued to worsen in the next two months and finally he developed signs of liver failure and was transferred to Spain for hepatic transplantation. When the patient arrived, his liver function continued to deteriorate, and laboratory test on the first day determined the following levels: ALT of 155 U/L, AST of 310 U/L, and total serum bilirubin of 28.7 mg/mL, coagulation disorders (prothrombin activity of 13% and international normalized ratio of 4.9). After two days, the patient developed encephalopathy, with hyperammonemia (178 μcg/dL), he was translated to intensive care unit (Table 1). Alternative diagnoses were ruled out through immunological test (antinuclear antibodies, ANA; smooth muscle antibody; LKM antibody) negatives. Alpha-fetoprotein was negative. Infectious origin through microbiological test revealed the following: Enterovirus was negative; Herpes simplex virus IgM, negative; CMV IgG, positive; CMV IgM, negative; Epstein-barr VCA IgM, negative; anti-EBNA IgG, positive; Parvovirus IgM, negative; Parvovirus IgG, positive; IgM, negative; Adenovirus, negative; the hepatitis panel (HBsAg, anti-HB core, anti-HVA, anti-HVC, and anti-HVE), negative; anti-HIV, negative; Toxoplasma IgG, positive; Toxoplasma IgM, negative; and Syphilis, negative. Serum ceruloplasmin was 15.4 mg/dL (normal ranges 20–60 mg/dL) and serum copper was 68 mcg/dL (normal ranges 50–150 mcg/dL). Abdominal ultrasound revealed a decreased hepatic size, the caudate lobe was prominent, and there were images of periportal fibrosis, the bile duct was of normal caliber. On the 4th hospitalization day in Spain, successful liver transplantation was performed. Liver biopsy reported parenchyma showing conserved architecture with bridging perivenular submassive necrosis; periportal hepatocytes showed pseudoacinar change and cholangiolar reaction. In the best preserved areas, the hepatocytes had intrahepatic and canalicular cholestasis. The portal tract had normal morphology with no evidence of inflammatory or thrombotic phenomenon. At any level acute or chronic inflammatory infiltrates, abscesses, or eosinophils were not observed (Figure 1). Patient gradually improved over the next weeks and the liver function showed a normalization trend, and MPH has not been restarted and for the next 2 years the patient has been well controlled with no further hepatic alteration events.

3. Discussion

ADHD is a common neurobehavioral disorder and one of the most prevalent chronic health problems in childhood [1]. The current estimated prevalence of ADHD is 2–6% among preschool-age children and 3–7% for school-age children [2]. Recently, practice guidelines support the benefits of treatment with both behaviour therapy and MPH, which is the most commonly prescribed psychostimulant [3]. Common side effects of MPH include loss of appetite and anxiety, and the most worrying side effect was a small but significant impact on the cardiovascular system including increases in blood pressure and heart rate as well as sudden cardiac death [4, 5]. However, one known but rare adverse effect of MPH is hepatotoxicity. Only few case reports of liver injury attributed to MPH have been published, possibly due to the fact that most of the patients generally develop mild, asymptomatic,

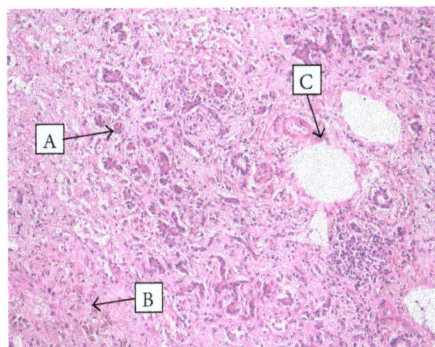

A: periportal area with hepatic regeneration
B: centrilobular zone with necrosis
C: periportal zone

FIGURE 1: Liver biopsy.

and reversible elevation of liver chemistries. The first case of hepatotoxicity due to MPH was described in 1972. In the case of a 67-year-old woman with MPH treatment, laboratory test showed elevated aminotransferases and alkaline phosphatase and MPH was discontinued and her liver's enzymes normalized [6].

The mechanism of hepatotoxicity associated with most drugs is idiosyncratic, which implies that drug-induced liver injury (DILI) develops in only a small proportion of subjects exposed to a drug in therapeutic doses, and must be consider the interaction between genetic and environmental risk factors making DILI unpredictable for most hepatotoxins. Thereby, we have found two case reports whose mechanism of hepatotoxicity of MPH could be idiosyncratic. They were patients with normal liver function previously. In one case after 5 weeks and in the other case after 3 months of onset of MPH therapy, elevated levels of aminotransferases and bilirubin were presented and alternative diagnostics were excluded. MPH was discontinued and liver's enzymes decreased [7, 8].

Allergy idiosyncratic hepatotoxicity is another possible mechanism of DILI, characterized by the presence of fever, skin reactions, eosinophilia, and formation of autoantibodies [9]. The other two cases in the literature can support this possible causal mechanism of MPH-induced hepatotoxicity. First, for the case of a 19-year-old black woman who had been injected intravenously with MPH and was admitted for jaundice, fever, and pain in the right upper abdomen, laboratory data showed elevated liver enzymes; a liver biopsy was performed revealing portal inflammation with lymphocytes, plasma cells, and eosinophils. Autoantibodies were not reported. Patient gradually got better the next 2 weeks and was given injection of MPH intravenously for two days after recovery and liver enzymes again showed a significant increase, proving positive rechallenge effect which strengthens the link of hepatotoxicity due to MPH [10]. The other case was reported by Lewis et al. a 57-year-old Caucasian male with a history of orthotopic liver transplantation 4 years before because of chronic hepatitis C, had maintained stable treatment and the liver's enzymes had been normal after transplantation. On routine laboratory evaluation that

TABLE 1: Laboratory results of liver function.

(a)

Date	Episode	ALT (normal, <35) UI/L	AST (normal, <45) UI/L	Total bilirubin (normal, 0–1.2) mg/dL	Alkaline phosphatase (normal, 30–355) UI/L	Prothrombin activity (80–120) %
18/12/10	Control	13	21	0.3	56	101
26/02/11	Jaundice, Coluria, acholia MPH was discontinued	423	857	4	339	71
04/04/11	Worsening coagulopathy	182	361	12.2	304	36

(b)

Date	Episode	ALT (normal, 30–65) UI/L	AST (normal, 15–37) UI/L	GGT (normal, 5–85) UI/L	Total bilirubin (normal, 0.2–1.4) mg/dL	Alkaline phosphatase (normal, 42–362) UI/L	Prothrombin activity (80–120) %
04/05/11	Arrived to Hospital Universitario La Paz	138	310	29	28.7		13
05/05/11	Onset of NAC	141	332	21	36.9	275	17
06/05/11	Encephalopathy medium-severe intensity with hyperammonemia	122	269	29	27		27
07/05/11		119	238	29	27.4		19
08/05/11	Hepatic transplantation	110	243	30	26.9		21
08/05/11	After hepatic transplantation	480	792	44	10.8		41
09/05/11		534	996	48	6.9		51
10/05/11		389	373	43	3.9		97
11/05/11		348	213	135	5.4		105
12/05/11		356	185		5.4		94
13/05/11		310	124	494	5.6		102
14/05/11		259	78	511	4.7		108
15/05/11		269	104	737	4.9		109
16/05/11		260	93	703	4.1		118
17/05/11		377	193	1106	4.7		109
18/05/11		459	194	1099	4.4		113
19/05/11		478	188	1139	3.9		107
20/05/11	Discharge from ICU	338	86	946	3		115
21/05/11		279	64	939	2.7		105
22/05/11		206	39	782	2.4		104
23/05/11		165	30	745	2.3	260	99
24/05/11		127	25	629	2		95
26/05/11		111	35	604	1.8		103
28/05/11		93	33	522	1.6		97
31/05/11		75	36	417	1.4		108
03/06/11		82	39	351	1.2	192	119
07/06/11	Discharge from the hospital	61	22	305	1.3	189	113
10/06/11		42	25	262	2.13	220	105
20/06/11		23	20	152	1.14	188	104

NAC: N-acetylcysteine.

discovered elevation of ALT, AST, and bilirubin, the only new medication that began 1 month earlier was MPH for depressive symptoms. Immunologic tests reported positive ANA, positive anti-SMA, negatives antimitochondrial antibody and anti-LKM, and elevated serum IgG immunoglobulins. A liver biopsy showed severe lobular and periportal necroinflammatory infiltrate with predominance of lymphocytes, plasma cells, and eosinophils, consistent with autoimmune hepatitis. MPH therapy was discontinued and liver's enzymes returned to previous levels [11].

MPH is a drug whose toxicity is increased by adrenergic agonist drugs [12]. A study in mice proved that when MPH is given as a single dose of 75 to 100 mg/Kg, it produced hepatic necrosis in male mice and when coadministered with beta-2 adrenoreceptors drugs can produce important potentiation of the liver injury by the increase in the MPH concentration [13]. In the literature, the cardiovascular effects of the sympathomimetic amines (increase in the heart rate, blood pressure, and blood vessel contraction) [14] have been described as well as cases of ischemic events (myocardial infarction and stroke) and sudden death in children and adults taking ADHD stimulants [4, 15]. For this reason we cannot discard that the overall low flow of blood in the liver could be another mechanism of MPH-induced liver injury.

In our case, we think that the mechanism of liver injury was MPH direct toxicity to hepatocytes as an idiosyncratic reaction, and we cannot support that the liver failure was due to autoimmune hepatitis, because of the negative findings of immunological test (ANA, smooth muscle antibody, and LKM antibody) and the absence of inflammatory damage or infiltration by plasma cells, lymphocytes, or eosinophils in the explanted liver [16]. And we do not have data on ischemia hepatopathy. In order to establish the diagnosis of DILI [17] we used CIOMS/RUCAM scale [18] that led to the assessment of "possible" relationship.

All cases reported were mild and recovered after withdrawing MPH, but in contrast, the case of our patient was severe and he was referred for liver transplantation. Our review of possible MPH-induced liver injury indicates a spectrum of presumed hepatotoxicity ranging from mild elevation of aminotransferases with spontaneous recovery after withdrawal of MPH to severe fulminant hepatitis requiring liver transplantation.

In conclusion, drug-induced liver injury (DILI) represents a frequently adverse drug reaction. Drugs account for 20–40% of all instances of fulminate hepatic failure. Approximately 75% of the idiosyncratic drug reactions result in liver transplantation or death [19]. It is important to know that although rarely but subacute liver failure can occur in patients with MPH treatment and must be taken into account by clinicians. This is the first case report of liver transplantation due to MPH therapy. This case has been reported to the National Pharmacovigilance Agency of Spain (registered as number 3433).

Abbreviations

ADHD: Attention-deficit-hyperactivity disorder
ALT: Alanine aminotransferase
ANA: Antinuclear antibody
Anti-HBc: Hepatitis B core antibody
Anti-HBs: Hepatitis B surface antibody
Anti-SMA: Anti-smooth muscle antibody
Anti-VHA: Hepatitis A antibody
Anti-VHB: Hepatitis C antibody
Anti-VHE: Hepatitis E antibody
AST: Aspartate aminotransferase
CMV: Cytomegalovirus
DILI: Drug-induced liver injury
FDA: U.S. Food and Drug Administration
LKM: Liver-kidney microsome antibodies
MPH: Methylphenidate hydrochloride.

Disclosure

The authors have indicated they have no financial relationships relevant to this paper to disclose.

Conflict of Interests

The authors have no conflict of interests relevant to this paper to disclose.

References

[1] L. Greenhill, S. Kollins, H. Abikoff et al., "Efficacy and safety of immediate-release methylphenidate treatment for preschoolers with ADHD," *Journal of the American Academy of Child and Adolescent Psychiatry*, vol. 45, no. 11, pp. 1284–1293, 2006.

[2] L. L. Greenhill, "Stimulant medication treatment of children with attention deficit hyperactivity disorder," in *Attention Deficit Hyperactivity Disorder: State of Science. Best Practices*, P. S. Jensen and J. R. Cooper, Eds., pp. 9–27, Civic Research Institute, Kingston, NJ, USA, 2002.

[3] Subcommittee on Attention-Deficit/Hyperactivity Disorder, Steering Committee on Quality Improvement and Management et al., "ADHD: clinical practice guideline for the diagnosis, evaluation, and treatment of attention-deficit/ hyperactivity disorder in children and adolescents," *Pediatrics*, vol. 128, no. 5, pp. 1007–1022, 2011.

[4] R. Arcieri, E. A. P. Germinario, M. Bonati et al., "Cardiovascular measures in children and adolescents with attention-deficit/ hyperactivity disorder who are new users of methylphenidate and atomoxetine," *Journal of Child and Adolescent Psychopharmacology*, vol. 22, no. 6, pp. 423–431, 2012.

[5] J. Martinez-Raga, C. Knecht, N. Szerman, and M. I. Martinez, "Risk of serious cardiovascular problems with medications for attention-deficit hyperactivity disorder," *CNS Drugs*, vol. 27, no. 1, pp. 15–30, 2013.

[6] C. R. Goodman, "Hepatotoxicity due to methylphenidate hydrochloride," *New York State Journal of Medicine*, vol. 72, no. 18, pp. 2339–2340, 1972.

[7] E. L. Torres, V. G. del Valle, K. Pachkoria, R. Cueto, and M. I. Lucena, "Hepatotoxicidad por metilfenidato en el tratamiento del trastorno por déficit de atención con hiperactividad," *Casos Farmacoterápicos*, vol. 3, no. 4, pp. 269–270, 2005.

[8] M. K. Bernhard, B. Hugle, and A. Merkenschlager, "Elevated liver enzymes under therapy with methylphenidate in a boy

with T-cell leukemia," *Journal of Pediatric Neurology*, vol. 7, no. 3, pp. 297–299, 2009.

[9] S. Russmann, G. A. Kullak-Ublick, and I. Grattagliano, "Current concepts of mechanisms in drug-induced hepatotoxicity," *Current Medicinal Chemistry*, vol. 16, no. 23, pp. 3041–3053, 2009.

[10] H. Mehta, B. Murray, and T. A. LoIudice, "Hepatic dysfunction due to intravenous abuse of methylphenidate hydrochloride," *Journal of Clinical Gastroenterology*, vol. 6, no. 2, pp. 149–151, 1984.

[11] J. J. Lewis, J. C. Iezzoni, and C. L. Berg, "Methylphenidate-induced autoimmune hepatitis," *Digestive Diseases and Sciences*, vol. 52, no. 2, pp. 594–597, 2007.

[12] S. M. Robert, R. P. DeMott, and R. C. James, "Adrenergic modulation of hepatotoxicity," *Drug Metabolism Reviews*, vol. 29, no. 1-2, pp. 329–353, 1997.

[13] S. M. Roberts, R. D. Harbison, L. Roth, and R. C. James, "Methylphenidate-induced hepatotoxicity in mice and its potentiation by β-adrenergic agonist drugs," *Life Sciences*, vol. 55, no. 4, pp. 269–281, 1994.

[14] T. E. Wilens, P. G. Hammerness, J. Biederman et al., "Blood pressure changes associated with medication treatment of adults with attention-deficit/hyperactivity disorder," *The Journal of Clinical Psychiatry*, vol. 66, no. 2, pp. 253–259, 2005.

[15] S. E. Nissen, "ADHD drugs and cardiovascular risk," *The New England Journal of Medicine*, vol. 354, no. 14, pp. 1445–1448, 2006.

[16] A. Suzuki, E. M. Brunt, D. E. Kleiner et al., "The use of liver biopsy evaluation in discrimination of idiopathic autoimmune hepatitis versus drug-induced liver injury," *Hepatology*, vol. 54, no. 3, pp. 931–939, 2011.

[17] M. García-Cortés, M. I. Lucena, R. J. Andrade, R. Camargo, and R. Alcántara, "Is the Naranjo probability scale accurate enough to ascertain causality in drug-induced hepatotoxicity?" *Annals of Pharmacotherapy*, vol. 38, no. 9, pp. 1540–1541, 2004.

[18] C. Bénichou, "Criteria of drug-induced liver disorders. Report of an international consensus meeting," *Journal of Hepatology*, vol. 11, no. 2, pp. 272–276, 1990.

[19] N. Mehta, L. Ozick, and E. Gbadehan, "Drug-induced hepatotoxicity," Medscape reference, January 2013, http://emedicine.medscape.com/article/169814-overview.

24

Chronic Lipoid Pneumonia in a 9-Year-Old Child Revealed by Recurrent Chest Pain

A. Hochart,[1] **C. Thumerelle,**[1] **L. Petyt,**[2] **C. Mordacq,**[1] **and A. Deschildre**[1]

[1]*Département de Pneumologie Pédiatrique, Hôpital Jeanne de Flandre, CHRU Lille, 59 037 Lille, France*
[2]*Département d'Imagerie Médicale, Hôpital Calmette, CHRU Lille, 59 037 Lille, France*

Correspondence should be addressed to A. Hochart; audrey.hochart@gmail.com

Academic Editor: Pannee Visrutaratna

Lipoid pneumonia in children is a rare disorder due to accumulation of fatty oily material in the alveoli and usually associated with an underlying condition. In absence of obvious context, diagnosis remains difficult with nonspecific clinical and radiological features. We report the first case of voluntary chronic aspiration of olive oil responsible for exogenous lipoid pneumonia, in a previously healthy 9-year-old boy. Clinical presentation was atypical; LP was revealed by isolated chest pain. We discuss radiological and bronchial alveolar lavage characteristics suggestive of lipoid pneumonia. *Conclusion.* Lipoid pneumonia is a disease to be reminded of in children, which can occur with original findings in terms of etiology and clinical presentation.

1. Introduction

Lipoid pneumonia (LP) is a rare inflammatory disease of the lung due to accumulation of fatty oily material in the alveoli. The first description was nearly a century ago [1] but LP remains difficult to diagnose in the absence of obvious context.

Pediatric cases of exogenous LP happen especially with certain risk factors such as aspiration of large amounts of oily materials [2], mineral oil being the most frequent. This aspiration of fatty material induces a pulmonary inflammatory reaction with nonspecific clinical and radiologic features, similar to bacterial pneumonia, complicating or delaying the diagnosis.

We report a case of LP revealed by isolated chest pain, due to a voluntary chronic aspiration of olive oil in a child.

2. Observation

A 9-year-old boy was admitted in our pediatric department with recurring episodes of right chest pain. For one month, he had been complaining of intermittent spontaneous right chest pain happening once or twice a week. There was no other associated sign (no respiratory distress, fever, cough, or hemoptysis) and no history of thoracic trauma.

The child had no respiratory medical history and did not receive any medication. He was followed in a psychiatric unit for behavioral disorders with continuation of a normal schooling. Environment was healthy.

On examination, his vitals were normal (oxygen saturation at 100% on room air, respiratory rate at 20/min). Chest auscultation and other clinical examinations were normal. Blood cells count, C-reactive protein, liver, renal, N-Terminal-Pro-B-Type Natriuretic Peptide, and troponin values were within normal limits. Cardiac evaluation was normal (electrocardiogram and transthoracic echocardiography). Chest X-ray revealed right upper and lower infiltrations (Figure 1). Chest CT showed airspace consolidations in the posterior segment of the right upper lobe and apical segment of the right lower lobe. These consolidations were characterized by very low density similar to fat tissue (Figure 2(a)).

Serological tests were positive for *Chlamydia pneumoniae* (IgM and IgG) and negative for *Mycoplasma pneumoniae*, toxocariasis, and ascariasis. Tuberculin skin test was negative. Based on the result of chlamydial serology, clarithromycin was introduced.

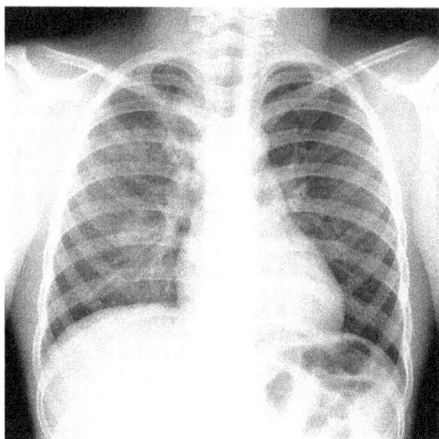

FIGURE 1: Initial chest X-ray: right upper and lower lobe infiltrations.

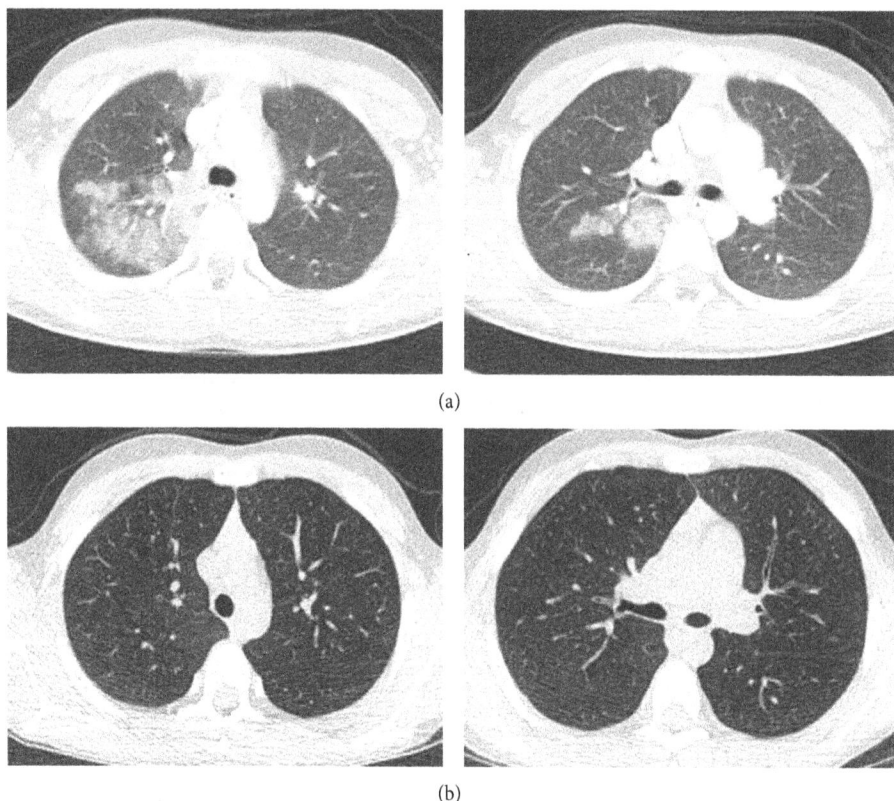

(a)

(b)

FIGURE 2: (a) Initial chest CT with upper and lower right lobe consolidations, characterized by low density (−129 HU within the lower lobe consolidation). (b) Chest CT two months later showed complete recovery.

However the diagnosis of chlamydial infection was questioned because of the unusual clinical presentation (chest pains without fever and cough), the absence of biological inflammation, and the CT scan aspect of the consolidation (very low density). For these reasons, a bronchoscopy was performed during hospitalization and showed no abnormality. The bronchoalveolar lavage (BAL) was negative for all microorganisms (bacterial culture, viral real-time PCR) but showed evidence of inflammation with a high total cell count (2900×10^6 cells/L) and increased lymphocytes (35%) and neutrophils (13%). Thirty percent of macrophages stained positive for lipid (lipid-laden alveolar macrophage (LLAM)). Exogenous LP was evoked.

The child improved during hospitalization and was discharged at day 3 without any residual pain. During the next week follow-up, the child and his family were asked about potential lipid aspiration, and we discovered the boy usually drank large amounts of olive oil when frustrated due to his behavioral disorders. Total eviction of oil was performed. One month later, the child had normal physical examination and did not report any pain. Chest CT showed complete recovery at 2 months (Figure 2(b)). The diagnosis of exogenous LP related to voluntary olive oil aspiration was retained.

3. Discussion

LP is an uncommon condition, due to accumulated lipids in the alveoli triggering a local inflammatory reaction. Exogenous forms are the most common, due to voluntary or accidental aspiration or inhalation of mineral, vegetable, or animal oil into the peripheral lung. Mineral oil, the most common incriminated substance, cannot be metabolized by pulmonary enzymes but is phagocytized by alveolar macrophages transforming in LLAM. The presence of LLAM triggers a granulomatous reaction in the alveoli, and chronic inflammation can lead to progressive pulmonary fibrosis [2].

In children, the main triggers of LP are accidental aspiration of mineral or vegetable oils, especially iatrogenic aspiration (laxative substances, oily nasal drops) [3, 4], and aspiration related to high-fat diet such as ketogenic diet [5]. Therefore, exogenous LP is usually associated with an underlying condition, such as severe gastroesophageal reflux, swallowing disorders, anatomical abnormalities of the pharynx and esophagus, cerebral palsy, or neuromuscular disorders [6]. These aspirations rarely occur in healthy patients. Psychological disorders responsible for LP are not described in children.

Excluding acute accidental aspiration of massive amount of lipids, diagnosis is difficult for chronic forms. Clinical symptoms are nonspecific; they vary from asymptomatic to severe presentation, depending on the duration of exposure, the type, and amount of aspirated fat. A previous study of exogenous LP in 28 children reported as main features: tachypnea (96%), cough (86%), and fever (82%) [2]. Other symptoms were dyspnea, lack of weight gain, and recurrent respiratory infections. On examination, main characteristics were crackles and wheezing, but 46% of children had a normal auscultation [2]. In adults, hemoptysis and chest pain have been also reported [6, 7]. Isolated chest pain as in our case is an unusual presentation of LP in children.

Without any obvious context, radiological characteristics and BAL are helpful to the diagnosis. High-resolution CT abnormalities of LP are consolidations, ground glass opacities, air-space nodules, and crazy-paving pattern [3, 8]. Lesions involve preferentially the upper right lobe with central and posterior distribution. The most typical CT finding is the unusual low density (−30 to −150 HU) within the consolidation area, suggesting the presence of fat [8]. The BAL is the reference method for diagnosis with presence of high count of LLAM. BAL fluid may have a macroscopic milky aspect with halo of supernatant fat. Cytological examination of our patient's BAL showed LLAM and marked inflammation with lymphocytes and neutrophils in relation with the local granulomatous reaction.

Except for the discontinuation of exposure, no other treatments are consensual in LP. In a prospective study of

10 children, Sias et al. demonstrated the potential role of multiple therapeutic BALs which facilitated the removal of LLAM implicated in the development of pulmonary fibrosis in chronic form [9]. Corticosteroids have also been tried in severe presentation and may be effective on the inflammatory response and would possibly prevent pulmonary fibrosis [9].

Prognosis of exogenous LP is usually good after the discontinuation of exposure. Complications such as pulmonary fibrosis, infection, or excavation can occur especially in case of persistent chronic exposure but have also been described in acute forms despite treatment [6].

Abbreviations

LLAM: Lipid-laden alveolar macrophage
LP: Lipoid pneumonia.

Conflict of Interests

No competing financial interests exist.

Acknowledgments

The authors thank Mr. David CHAVANEL and Mr. Samuel MEIGNAN for assistance and preparation of the manuscript.

References

[1] G. F. Laughlen, "Studies on pneumonia following naso-pharyngeal injections of oil," *The American Journal of Pathology*, vol. 1, pp. 407–414, 1925.

[2] S. M. D. A. Sias, A. S. Ferreira, P. A. Daltro, R. L. Caetano, J. D. S. Moreira, and T. Quirico-Santos, "Evolution of exogenous lipoid pneumonia in children: clinical aspects, radiological aspects and the role of bronchoalveolar lavage," *Jornal Brasileiro de Pneumologia*, vol. 35, no. 9, pp. 839–845, 2009.

[3] G. Zanetti, E. Marchiori, T. D. Gasparetto, D. L. Escuissato, and A. Soares Souza Jr., "Lipoid pneumonia in children following aspiration of mineral oil used in the treatment of constipation: high-resolution CT findings in 17 patients," *Pediatric Radiology*, vol. 37, no. 11, pp. 1135–1139, 2007.

[4] H. P. Bandla, S. H. Davis, and N. E. Hopkins, "Lipoid pneumonia: a silent complication of mineral oil aspiration," *Pediatrics*, vol. 103, no. 2, p. E19, 1999.

[5] P. Buda, A. Wieteska-Klimczak, A. Własienko et al., "Lipoid pneumonia—a case of refractory pneumonia in a child treated with ketogenic diet," *Pneumonologia i Alergologia Polska*, vol. 81, no. 5, pp. 448–452, 2013.

[6] A. Gondouin, P. Manzoni, E. Ranfaing et al., "Exogenous lipid pneumonia: a retrospective multicentre study of 44 cases in France," *European Respiratory Journal*, vol. 9, no. 7, pp. 1463–1469, 1996.

[7] E. Marchiori, G. Zanetti, C. M. Mano, and B. Hochhegger, "Exogenous lipoid pneumonia. Clinical and radiological manifestations," *Respiratory Medicine*, vol. 105, no. 5, pp. 659–666, 2011.

[8] E. Marchiori, G. Zanetti, C. M. Mano, K. L. Irion, P. A. Daltro, and B. Hochhegger, "Lipoid pneumonia in 53 patients after aspiration of mineral oil: comparison of high-resolution

computed tomography findings in adults and children," *Journal of Computer Assisted Tomography*, vol. 34, no. 1, pp. 9–12, 2010.

[9] S. M. A. Sias, P. A. Daltro, E. Marchiori et al., "Clinic and radiological improvement of lipoid pneumonia with multiple bronchoalveolar lavages," *Pediatric Pulmonology*, vol. 44, no. 4, pp. 309–315, 2009.

25

Prolonged Ileus in an Infant Presenting with Primary Congenital Hypothyroidism

Caroline Chua,[1] Shilpa Gurnurkar,[2] Yahdira Rodriguez-Prado,[1] and Victoria Niklas[3]

[1]*Division of Neonatology, Department of Pediatrics, University of Central Florida College of Medicine,
 Nemours Children's Hospital, Orlando, FL 32827, USA*
[2]*Division of Endocrinology, Department of Pediatrics, University of Central Florida College of Medicine,
 Nemours Children's Hospital, Orlando, FL 32827, USA*
[3]*Division of Neonatology and Newborn Services, Olive View UCLA Medical Center, Los Angeles, CA 91342, USA*

Correspondence should be addressed to Caroline Chua; caroline.chua@nemours.org

Academic Editor: Anibh Martin Das

Congenital hypothyroidism (CH) is the most common endocrine disorder affecting the newborn. Universal newborn screening (NBS) has virtually eliminated the static encephalopathy and devastating neurodevelopmental syndrome known as cretinism. This report describes the presentation of an infant referred by the primary pediatrician to our hospital at 12 days of age for confirmatory testing after the NBS was consistent with CH. The infant had hypoglycemia secondary to lethargy and poor feeding and required transfer to the neonatal intensive care unit for worsening abdominal distension despite normalization of serum thyroid function tests following hormone replacement. In particular, the recalcitrant ileus and secondary bowel obstruction resulted in an additional diagnostic workup and lengthened hospital day. Our report highlights the acute gastrointestinal consequences of hypothyroidism despite evidence of effective treatment. We believe that the preclinical detection and immediate therapy for CH have lessened the prevalence of this presentation in general practice, and hence practitioners are less likely to be familiar with its natural history and management.

1. Introduction

Congenital hypothyroidism (CH) is the most common endocrine disorder presenting in the newborn period with a prevalence of approximately 1 in 2500 births [1]. The failure to recognize and treat CH may result in static encephalopathy and neurodevelopmental disability, known historically as cretinism. The advent of universal screening programs has virtually eliminated the devastating consequences of untreated CH and lessened experience with the acute manifestations of disease and early disease treatment. Most newborns present with primary congenital hypothyroidism due to thyroid dysgenesis (85%) or dyshormonogenesis (15%) secondary to defective embryogenesis of the thyroid gland or inborn error of hormone synthesis [2]. Secondary CH results from a deficiency of TSH, which, in neonates, is most often associated with other pituitary hormone deficiencies due to a developmental anomaly of the pituitary gland.

With the advent of universal NBS across the United States as well as in most industrialized countries, infants rarely present with clinical symptoms of CH but come to medical attention after detection by an abnormal screening result. Hence, the clinical features of CH such as prolonged jaundice, large anterior and posterior fontanelles, macroglossia, goiter, and a history of poor feeding and constipation are now rarely seen [3, 4]. Generally, the clinical features of hypothyroidism are expected to resolve once the thyroid hormone levels are biochemically normalized. The acute systemic effects of CH such as lethargy, ileus, and changes in skin and hair may be variably present following birth or develop prior to disease reporting and recognition by NBS services. Indeed as was the case for the infant presented here, ileus and functional bowel obstruction may persist for weeks beyond the normalization of serologic thyroid function tests. We would like to raise awareness of the acute gastrointestinal consequences of hypothyroidism, as early detection and immediate therapy for CH have lessened the development of its clinical manifestations in the newborn population. While early treatment improves the neurodevelopmental outcome for infants with CH, the acute systemic consequences of hypothyroidism may also be present and could lead to unexpected management challenges for pediatric health care providers.

2. Case Presentation

The infant was a former 39-week gestational age female born weighing 2835 grams (10th–50th percentile) after cesarean section delivery for fetal distress to a mother whose prenatal course was unremarkable. Specifically, the mother did not have a history of thyroid disease. The infant required routine care in the delivery room, did well in the nursery, and was discharged home on day 3 of life tolerating full breast milk feeds, voiding and stooling normally. The primary care pediatrician received the results of the abnormal NBS on day 12 of life and referred the infant to our hospital for confirmatory testing of thyroid function.

Physical examination revealed a sleepy infant that aroused with exam. Her neurologic exam was nonfocal. Heart rate was 122, respiratory rate 31, and blood pressure 63/43 and oxygen saturation was 100% while the infant was breathing room air. Weight was 2555 grams, a decrease of nearly 10% from birth weight. The skin was yellowish, soft, and slightly dry to touch. A soft, uniform, mobile, and thyroid gland measuring 3 cm × 1.5 cm was palpable in the anterior neck. Chest exam revealed bilateral breath sounds that were clear to auscultation with a cardiac exam demonstrating a regular rate and rhythm without murmur. The abdomen was distended with visible bowel loops and decreased bowel sounds in all quadrants. The extremities had normal tone and movement and were warm and well perfused, without evidence of edema.

Laboratory investigation revealed a thyroid stimulating hormone (TSH) level of $500\,\mu IU/mL$ (normal 1.8–7.97 $\mu IU/mL$) and free thyroxine (FT_4) of <0.1 ng/dL (normal 0.9–2.2 ng/dL), thus confirming primary CH. A CBC and complete metabolic panel were normal except for a total bilirubin level that was 15 mg/dL (normal < 2 mg/dL) with an unconjugated fraction of <0.1 (normal) and blood glucose of 50 mg/dL (normal > 55 mg/dL). Thyroid ultrasound revealed a diffusely enlarged thyroid gland with increased vascularity. The right lobe measured 2.8 × 1.3 × 1.3 cm and the left lobe measured 2.6 × 1.1 × 1.3 cm with 0.4 cm of thickness at the isthmus. A thyroid uptake study was consistent with a normally sited and formed thyroid gland although uptake was increased, 46% at 4 hours (normal 8–25%) and 25% uptake at 24 hours (normal 8–25%). An abdominal radiograph revealed a distended proximal bowel and normal caliber distal bowel and stool seen throughout the colon (Figure 1). Serial studies of blood glucose were consistent with borderline hypoglycemia (32–53 mg/dL) and poor feeding necessitated the transfer of the infant to the neonatal intensive care unit for further evaluation and management.

On hospital day (HD) 6, the TSH had decreased to 115 $\mu IU/mL$ and the FT_4 had normalized to 1.6 ng/dL. On HD 12, the TSH had normalized to 10.3 $\mu IU/mL$ and the FT_4

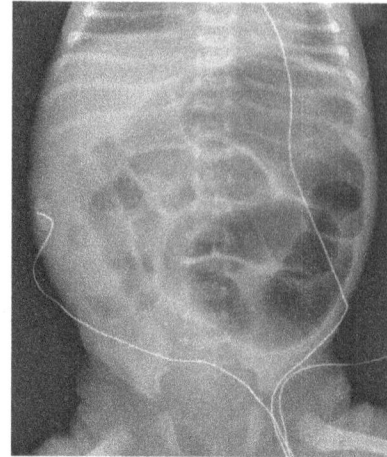

Figure 1: Abdominal radiograph obtained on HD 2 demonstrated dilation of the proximal bowel with normal caliber distal bowel and a paucity of air in the rectum.

was 3.3 ng/dL. However, during these 1st two weeks of hospital stay, the infant had recurrent feeding intolerance with emesis and abdominal distention despite improvement in the thyroid function tests. The infant was made NPO on several occasions, receiving a nasogastric tube for decompression and parenteral nutrition. Enteral levothyroxine was changed to IV form. Serial abdominal radiographs continued to reveal diffusely distended loops of bowel (Figure 2) prompting a surgical consult and a recommendation for a contrast enema. The contrast enema showed no transition zone but was notable for a diminished rectosigmoid index (Figure 3) and raised concern for Hirschsprung's disease, prompting a suction rectal biopsy. The rectal biopsy revealed ganglion cells and Hirschsprung's disease was ruled out. A regimen of rectal irrigation and glycerin suppositories was initiated to foster consistent distal bowel evacuation and decompression. Expressed breast milk feeds were reinitiated on HD 14 advancing to full enteral feeds by HD 16. Parenteral thyroid hormone replacement was discontinued and alternating doses of 25 mcg and 37.5 mcg of oral levothyroxine were given. The infant was discharged home on HD 19 with twice-daily glycerin suppositories to aid bowel evacuation. The discharge weight was 3038 grams with a follow-up weight 5 days after discharge of 3227 grams (weight gain 38 grams/day). The infant was tolerating ad lib feeds and stooling consistently with normal TSH (7.23 $\mu IU/mL$) and FT_4 (1.6 nmol/L) levels.

3. Discussion

Poor feeding with abdominal distension is a clinical manifestation of congenital hypothyroidism; however, the severity and long duration of symptoms in our newborn, despite biochemical normalization of thyroid hormone levels, are uncommon [3, 5, 6]. Few cases are reported in the literature. Vidwans et al. and Smolkin et al. reported neonates with very similar clinical features of emesis, abdominal distension, and decreased intestinal peristalsis [5, 6]. While these infants had severe primary hypothyroidism, they responded quickly

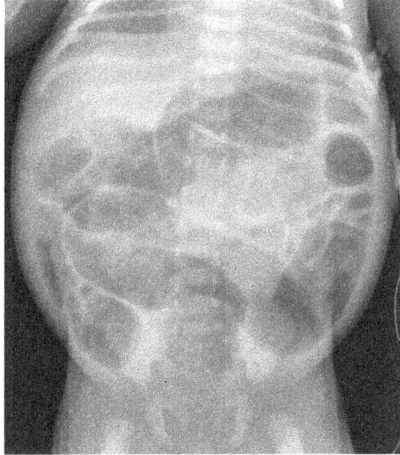

FIGURE 2: A representative abdominal radiograph obtained on HD 11 revealed gaseous distention consistent with an adynamic ileus without evidence of bowel obstruction. A paucity of air in the rectum is again seen.

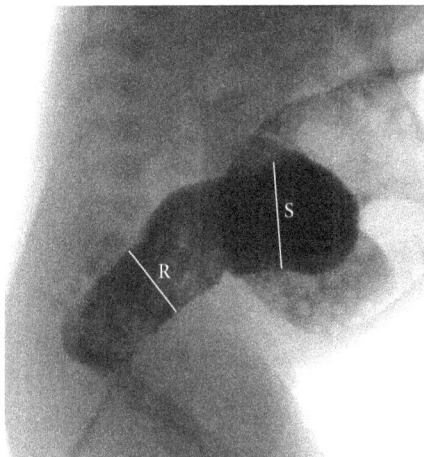

FIGURE 3: Lateral image obtained from the contrast enema demonstrated a mildly narrowed distal rectum (R) compared to a slightly larger caliber sigmoid colon (S). These results demonstrated a diminished rectosigmoid index although there was no apparent transition zone.

to thyroid hormone replacement and were able to tolerate full feeds allowing for discharge home within 4 and 9 days of starting thyroid hormone replacement, respectively. In a more recent case report, Sellappan et al. described a pseudoobstruction syndrome in two premature newborns that have similar responses to thyroid hormone supplementation as well [7]. In our infant, feeds were not well tolerated until 2 weeks after treatment was begun, despite rapid normalization of thyroid hormone levels. It is, however, possible that the later initiation of treatment in our case accounted for the severity and persistence of ileus.

It is unclear what other factors contributed to the delay in resolution of the gastrointestinal symptoms of hypothyroidism in our infant despite normal serum thyroid hormone levels. Based on ultrasound findings of a eutopic thyroid and

increased uptake after administration of I^{123}, hypothyroidism in our infant was likely secondary to dyshormonogenesis. In general, hypothyroidism in athyreosis is more severe than in dyshormonogenesis. However, it is interesting that, despite a eutopic thyroid gland, our patient had severe clinical and biochemical evidence of hypothyroidism. Abdominal distention and ileus are thought to be secondary to decreased intestinal motility, the same mechanism underlying constipation as a symptom of hypothyroidism in children and adults. Perhaps in our patient, improvement in intestinal motility required a longer recovery process related to resetting the pacemaker cells of Cajal or neuromuscular motility system in the intestine [8, 9]. In addition, although there was no thyroid dysfunction or autoimmune disease reported in the mother of our infant, an undetected thyroid disorder could have decreased thyroid hormone levels in the fetus or maternal autoantibodies could have additionally inhibited fetal thyroid function [10].

We thus report a neonate with severe congenital hypothyroidism complicated by recalcitrant ileus and abdominal distention with a prolonged recovery phase despite normalization of thyroid function soon after initiation of treatment. Through this case, we wish to raise awareness of possible uncommon clinical manifestations of congenital hypothyroidism among pediatricians, neonatologists, and endocrinologists to better enable timely and appropriate management perhaps avoiding what may be unnecessary and expensive investigations.

Abbreviations

CH: Congenital hypothyroidism
FT_4: Free thyroxine
HD: Hospital day
NBS: Newborn screening
TSH: Thyroid stimulating hormone.

Conflict of Interests

The authors have no conflict of interests to disclose.

Authors' Contribution

Drs. Caroline Chua and Shilpa Gurnurkar contributed equally to this paper. Both authors conceptualized, drafted, reviewed, and revised the initial paper and approved the final paper as submitted. In addition, both authors are accountable for all aspects of the work and ensure that questions related to the accuracy and integrity of any part of the work will be investigated until resolved. Dr. Yahdira Rodriguez-Prado shared in conceptualizing and drafting the paper. She reviewed and revised the paper and approved the final paper as submitted. In addition, she will be accountable for all aspects of the work and will ensure that questions related to its accuracy and integrity will be investigated until resolved. Dr. Victoria Niklas conceptualized the basis for the paper and supervised its formation contributing to the scholarly content. She critically reviewed and revised all drafts of the paper and approved the final paper as submitted. In addition, she will be accountable for all aspects of the work and ensure that questions related to its accuracy and integrity will be investigated until resolved.

References

[1] K. B. Harris and K. A. Pass, "Increase in congenital hypothyroidism in New York State and in the United States," *Molecular Genetics and Metabolism*, vol. 91, no. 3, pp. 268–277, 2007.

[2] M. V. Rastogi and S. H. LaFranchi, "Congenital hypothyroidism," *Orphanet Journal of Rare Diseases*, vol. 5, no. 1, article 17, 2010.

[3] D. W. Smith, A. M. Klein, J. R. Henderson, and N. C. Myrianthopoulos, "Congenital hypothyroidism—signs and symptoms in the newborn period," *The Journal of Pediatrics*, vol. 87, no. 6, part 1, pp. 958–962, 1975.

[4] M. Virtanen, "Manifestations of congenital hypothyroidism during the 1st week of life," *European Journal of Pediatrics*, vol. 147, no. 3, pp. 270–274, 1988.

[5] A. S. Vidwans, S. Ratzan, and M. R. Sanders, "An unusual presentation of congenital hypothyroidism: a report of two cases," *Journal of Pediatric Gastroenterology and Nutrition*, vol. 31, no. 2, pp. 198–200, 2000.

[6] T. Smolkin, I. Ulanovsky, S. Blazer, and I. R. Makhoul, "Rare presentations of congenital hypothyroidism," *The Israel Medical Association Journal*, vol. 13, no. 12, pp. 779–780, 2011.

[7] B. Sellappan, M. Chakraborty, and S. Cherian, "Congenital hypothyroidism presenting as pseudo-obstruction in preterm infants," *BMJ Case Reports*, 2014.

[8] R. M. Mostafa, Y. M. Moustafa, and H. Hamdy, "Interstitial cells of Cajal, the Maestro in health and disease," *World Journal of Gastroenterology*, vol. 16, no. 26, pp. 3239–3248, 2010.

[9] L. M. Negreanu, P. Assor, B. Mateescu, and C. Cirstoiu, "Interstitial cells of Cajal in the gut—a gastroenterologist's point of view," *World Journal of Gastroenterology*, vol. 14, no. 41, pp. 6285–6288, 2008.

[10] R. Scarpa, R. Alaggio, L. Norberto et al., "Tryptophan hydroxylase autoantibodies as markers of a distinct autoimmune gastrointestinal component of autoimmune polyendocrine syndrome type 1," *Journal of Clinical Endocrinology and Metabolism*, vol. 98, no. 2, pp. 704–712, 2013.

26

Hyperinsulinemic Hypoglycaemia in a Turner Syndrome with Ring (X)

Michela Cappella,[1] **Vanna Graziani,**[1] **Antonella Pragliola,**[2] **Alberto Sensi,**[2] **Khalid Hussain,**[3] **Claudia Muratori,**[1] **and Federico Marchetti**[1]

[1]*Department of Paediatrics, Santa Maria delle Croci Hospital, 48121 Ravenna, Italy*
[2]*Department of Clinical Pathology, Medical Genetics Unit, Pievesestina, 47522 Cesena, Italy*
[3]*London Centre for Pediatric Endocrinology and Metabolism, Great Hormond Street Hospital for Children NHS Trust and the Institute of Child Health, London WC1N 3JH, UK*

Correspondence should be addressed to Federico Marchetti; federico.marchetti@ausl.ra.it

Academic Editor: Ozgur Cogulu

Hyperinsulinemic hypoglycaemia (HH) is a group of clinically, genetically, and morphologically heterogeneous disorders characterized by dysregulation of insulin secretion by pancreatic beta cells. HH can either be congenital genetic hyperinsulinism or associated with metabolic disorder and syndromic condition. Early identification and meticulous management of these patients is vital to prevent neurological insult. There are only three reported cases of HH associated with a mosaic, r(X) Turner syndrome. We report the four cases of an infant with a mosaic r(X) Turner genotype and HH responsive to diazoxide therapy.

1. Introduction

Hyperinsulinaemic hypoglycaemia (HH) is an important cause of hypoglycaemia in childhood based on an unregulated insulin secretion by β cells [1]. Early identification and meticulous management of these patients is vital to prevent neurological insult. We report a case of a child with a mosaic genotype of Turner's syndrome in association with otherwise unexplained persistent HH. This association suggests that HH may be another atypical feature of mosaic Turner's syndrome.

2. Case Report

We report a case of a girl, born preterm at 32 weeks of gestation by caesarean section due to intrauterine growth retardation and alteration of fetal blood flow. Her birth weight was 1455 g (10th–25th centile), length was 40 cm (10th–25th centile), and head circumference was 27 cm (10th). The pregnancy was uneventful and her mother was healthy and nondiabetic. Her family history was unremarkable.

Prenatal ultrasound scans were negative, without any evidence of heart disease. Soon after birth a diagnosis of aortic stenosis with bicuspid aortic valve was made and, at the age of three weeks, she underwent aortic valvuloplasty. Neonatal metabolic screening was normal. No episodes of neonatal hypoglycaemia were documented. After discharge she had no serious illnesses or hospitalization, the cardiologic follow-up was carried out without complications, and she had been growing and developing normally.

At 11 months of age, during her first feed in the morning, she presented an episode of generalized tonic-clonic seizures and staring that lasted five minutes. The episode was not associated with fever or any sign of infection. By the time she arrived at our emergency department, she was a little drowsy, but she could be awakened easily.

Because of her previous history of congenital cardiac defect, we immediately performed an echocardiogram and an electrocardiogram although they did not show any cardiovascular acute disease. Respiratory, abdominal, and neurologic examinations were normal. A complete blood count, C-reactive protein, and electrolyte panel were normal but hypoglycaemia with a blood glucose concentration of 1.8 mmol/l

TABLE 1: Results of the metabolites and hormones measured at the time of hypoglycemia in our child.

Hormone/metabolite	Value	Reference
Plasma glucose (mmol/L)	1.8	3.5–5.5
Serum insulin (mU/L)	7.4	<2
Serum cortisol (mmol/L)	280	<500
Serum growth hormone (mIU/L)	21	>20
Free fatty acids (mmol/L)	0.3	Raised (>0.5)
Total ketone bodies (mmol/L)	0.04 (suppressed)	Raised (>0.6)
Plasma lactate (mmol/L)	1.8	<2
Serum ammonia (μmol/L)	61	<80

(range 3.3–5.5 mmol/l) has been found. Transaminases and creatine phosphokinase were normal. Acid-base balance and lactate showed no abnormality. Her thyroid function test and cortisol, adrenocorticotropic, and growth hormone were normal. Urine analysis was without ketonuria. The levels of organic acids, amino acids in plasma, acylcarnitines, and free carnitine were normal. Electroencephalogram (EEG) and video-EEG as well did not show any abnormalities. No hepatomegaly or pancreatic alteration resulted from abdominal ultrasound. Brain magnetic resonance imaging showed only a delay in myelination but no major abnormalities.

Hypoglycaemia resolved with continuous infusion of glucoelectrolytic solution, but soon after suspension, her random blood glucose controls showed hypoglycaemic episodes especially in the early morning hours, with blood glucose levels around 1.6–2.5 mmol/l (range 3.3–5.5 mmol/l). At the lower glucose value she presented hypoglycaemic symptoms (pallor, sweating, and motor delay) but not seizures. At this time elevated insulin (7.4 mU/L; range < 2 mU/L) was found accompanied by mild hypoketonemia and hypofattyacidaemic hypoglycaemia (0.3 mmol/l) (Table 1).

Then she was commenced on glucose infusion of 10% dextrose (8 mg/kg/min) and hypoglycaemia was corrected. In addition, a positive glycemic response to glucagon has been proven. Overall, the biochemical pictures were consistent with HH.

The serum ammonia concentration was normal and no mutation was found in the ABCC8, KCNJ11 GCK, HADH, UCP2, and HNF4A genes.

On physical examination she presented very mild dysmorphic elements: prominent forehead, plagiocephaly, long palpebral fissures, mild synophrys, thin upper lip, mildly short neck, and irregular palmar creases. Her growth parameters were normal (between 25th and 50th centile in weight and length). She showed a very mild motor delay.

Cytogenetic analysis revealed 2 cell lines: 89% showed a single normal X chromosome and a small ring chromosome, 46 X, r(X); 11% had just a single normal X chromosome, 45 X. No 46 XX cells were found out of 100 examined. Fluorescent in situ hybridization (FISH) studies showed that the X inactivation locus (XIST) was present on the ring X. Cytogenetic findings are associated with Turner syndrome (TS).

After four days glucose infusion was progressively stopped and at the same time an introduction of maltodextrin into her food and drink has been started. She still had intermittent low blood glucose levels. Based on the algorithm for hyperinsulinism's treatment she was treated with diazoxide and responded well at dose of 8 mg/kg/day, with stabilized blood glucose levels and a longer fasting tolerance.

At the time of writing, the proband is 26 months old and is able to fast for 12 hours without developing hypoglycaemia on a low dose of diazoxide (4 mg/kg/day).

3. Discussion

HH can either be due to congenital hyperinsulinism caused by genetic defects (CHI) in key genes regulating insulin secretion or secondary to certain perinatal risk factors (birth asphyxia, intrauterine growth retardation, and maternal diabetes mellitus) or associated with metabolic conditions (congenital disorders of glycosylation, β-oxidation defects). In adults an insulinoma accounts for most cases of HH [1].

Our patient presented at 11 months of age with seizure as the first clinical manifestation of persistent hypoglycaemia and reduced fasting tolerance with no ketonuria. Our work-up to differential diagnosis showed hyperinsulinism (high insulin plasma level, hypoketonaemia, hypofattyacidaemia at lower glucose level, high glucose requirement to maintain normoglycaemia, and positive glycaemic response to glucagon) [1]. The differential diagnosis of β-oxidation defects could be excluded because of the normal plasmatic acylcarnitine.

Nowadays the mutations in nine genes are currently known to cause HH. The most common (about 40–70% of cases) and severe types are due to ABCC8 and KCJN11 (encoding SUR-1 and Kir 6.2, resp.) in which inactivating mutations in these genes encoding the two subunits of the β cell ATP-sensitive potassium channel cause the hyperinsulinism. The effect of these mutations on channel expression and function determines the clinical phenotype, particularly the response to diazoxide [2, 3]. No more common typical mutations in diazoxide-responsive CHI genes were identified. So the response to diazoxide in our patient may suggest that her hyperinsulinaemia is originated from other mechanisms besides disorder of K-ATP channel. The serum ammonia was normal so we ruled out the hyperinsulinism-hyperammonaemia syndrome, the second common form of CHI (caused by mutation in the GLUD1 gene) [2, 3].

Syndromic forms of persistent hyperinsulinism have been recognized in association with trisomy 13, Beckwith-Wiedemann syndrome, congenital disorders of glycosylation, Perlman syndrome, and Soto's syndrome and in some as yet undiagnosed syndromes [1]. The mechanisms of HH in these syndromes are largely unclear [1].

Our patient had the TS. She showed mild dysmorphic elements, her growth parameters were between the 25th and the 50th percentile in weight and length, and just congenital heart disease was suggestive for TS [4].

In the literature another three cases of TS with HH have been described [5–7]. The first case [5] was an infant, who, after newborn hypoglycemia, was studied at 4, 8, and 10 months for hypoglycemic convulsions and with a subsequent leucine loading test compatible with hyperinsulinism. Her complex karyotype showed a monosomic 45 X cell line and two cell lines with an X chromosome derived ring that was duplicated and dicentric in the less frequent cell line: 46 X,+mar[19]/45 X[8]/46 X,+mar2[31].ish r(X)(DXZI+)[81]/dic r(X) (DXZ1++)[2].

A second reported case [6] was a 4-months-old girl with complex mosaic karyotype with four different cell lines: mos 46 X, r(X)/47 X, r(X) + der(X)/46 X,der(X)/45 X. XIST gene was present on the ring, but not on the der(X). This case was admitted with staring episodes and generalized tonic-clonic seizures associated with low blood glucose levels. She showed the typical findings for hyperinsulinism.

The third case [7] was a 13-month-old girl with mosaic TS and mild "Kabuki-like" phenotype as defined by the authors. The karyotype showed a mosaicism with three cell lines: 46 X,r(X)/47 r(X), dup r(X)/45 X. XIST was not investigated, but G banding was considered indicative for XIST presence. She was admitted two times to the hospital with spells; persistent hypoglycemic episodes were associated with a hyperinsulinism.

Unlike our patient, these cases showed their first hypoglycemic episodes during the first days of life and then became symptomatic again at the age of 4 [5, 7] and 9 months [6]. Between these points, any subclinical hypoglycemic episodes remained possibly undetected. Two cases were well responsive to diazoxide and this treatment stabilized blood glucose levels and a longer fasting tolerance. The mechanism leading to HH in mosaic TS is largely not clear [5–7]. The reduced insulin secretion in young, nonobese females with a normal insulin sensitivity implies that beta cell dysfunction or insufficiency is a primary feature of the Turner metabolic syndrome [8].

Moreover it is known that X monosomy increases the risk of glucose intolerance and subsequent diabetes mellitus [9]. However, according to Gravholt et al. [10] in TS there is just "an insignificant tendency towards hypoglycemia": in her large survey on 594 TS she found just 2 cases (0.57 expected, relative risk 3.51, IC: 0.43–12.69). Moreover, our search in PubMed looking for "hypoglycemia and Turner Syndrome" just retrieved the three mosaic cases already cited, all with a ring X chromosome [5–7], a chromosomal abnormality that is found just in 16% of TS karyotypes [11].

So, although large epidemiological data about r(X) and hypoglycemia are lacking, an association between r(X) in TS and HH seems likely.

Our patient presents a mosaic karyotype with a preponderant 46 X,r(X) cell line, showing a tiny ring of the chromosome X (XIST positive) replacing a normal X, and a minor component (11%) with X monosomy (45 X). The presence of the XIST gene on the ring chromosome is correlated with its inactivation while the absence of XIST region prevents the abnormal X chromosome from inactivation, leading to a functional disomy of regions of chromosome X associated with a more severe phenotype with mental retardation and facial features resembling those of the monogenic Kabuki syndrome (in particular the suggestive eversion of the lateral

part of the lower lid was noted) [12–14]. The correlation of this severe phenotype and XIST absence is not absolute [13].

Ring chromosomes often show some instability and cause a "dynamic mosaicism," consisting of mitotic rearrangements (mainly due to the consequences of sister chromatid exchanges in a ring chromosome) that lead to tissues chromosomal heterogeneity [15]. In previously reported cases [5–7] this instability was evident in blood, while in our case it was not; nonetheless instability could be relevant in tissues different from the tested lymphocytes.

Instability generates rearranged chromosomes with duplications and deletions and could also involve XIST or its expression in some tissues.

The pathogenetic mechanism by which the ring X might cause HH is unknown and just speculative hypotheses can be proposed [5–7]. Haploinsufficiency of genes involved in the insulin pathway [6] due to deletion in the ring chromosome seems unlikely, because under this hypothesis homogenous 45 X karyotype should be at least equally predisposing to HH.

Another hypothesis [7] is based on the expression of genes located on the ring, accounting for the functional disomy of part of chromosome X with a mechanism like that proposed for the tiny r(X) for the severe phenotype with mental retardation [16]. This mechanism could be considered also for HH, although XIST seems to be present in all the three cases reported and also in the present case.

A third hypothesis that we put out takes into account the selective mechanism that generally brings to skewed X inactivation: when in a female an X chromosome is structurally abnormal lyonization proceeds randomly, but cells inactivating the normal X are subjected to selective elimination and the great majority of them stop and are eliminated from the cell pool [15]. It is conceivable that in some tissue skewing could be incomplete leaving some unbalanced cells with pathogenetic consequences; moreover the selective apoptotic mechanism involved in cell selection during embryonic stages might interfere with development causing specific pathologies.

4. Conclusions

The recognition of hypoglycaemia in children with TS is important in order to prevent further brain damage caused by hypoglycaemic episodes and seizures. Untreated, or inappropriately treated, these children may suffer from hypoglycaemic brain damage in addition to their mental retardation.

Although the mechanism leading to hyperinsulinism in this condition is still unknown, the present report is the fourth case of a female with TS with ring chromosome X associated with congenital hyperinsulinism. However, the interpretation of the effect of cells with different karyotypes is difficult without karyotyping the pancreatic β cells. Further studies are required to understand whether the mosaic over- or underexpression of unidentified X chromosome gene(s) in the pancreatic cells leads to hyperinsulinaemic hypoglycaemia. Even if the relationship between the presence r(X) and the HH complication in TS has to be proved, it could not only be a casual association.

Abbreviations

CHI: Congenital hyperinsulinism caused by
         genetic defects
EEG: Electroencephalogram
HH: Hyperinsulinemic hypoglycaemia
TS: Turner syndrome.

Conflict of Interests

The authors declare that they have no conflict of interests.

Authors' Contribution

Michela Cappella and Claudia Muratori performed study design, data collection, data interpretation, paper preparation, and literature review, contributed to the diagnosis, and provided clinical assistance. Vanna Graziani performed data collection and data interpretation, contributed to the diagnosis, and provided clinical assistance. Antonella Pragliola and Alberto Sensi performed the cytogenetic and clinical genetic evaluation and participated in writing the paper. Khalid Hussain performed the molecular genetic investigation and participated in writing the paper. Federico Marchetti performed study design, data collection, data interpretation, and paper preparation. All authors approved the final version of the paper.

References

[1] Z. Mohamed, V. B. Arya, and K. Hussain, "Hyperinsulinaemic hypoglycaemia: genetic mechanisms, diagnosis and management," *Journal of Clinical Research in Pediatric Endocrinology*, vol. 4, no. 4, pp. 169–181, 2012.

[2] R. R. Kapoor, S. E. Flanagan, V. B. Arya, J. P. Shield, S. Ellard, and K. Hussain, "Clinical and molecular characterisation of 300 patients with congenital hyperinsulinism," *European Journal of Endocrinology*, vol. 168, no. 4, pp. 557–564, 2013.

[3] K. Lord and D. D. de León, "Monogenic hyperinsulinemic hypoglycemia: current insights into the pathogenesis and management," *International Journal of Pediatric Endocrinology*, vol. 2013, no. 1, article 3, 2013.

[4] L. A. Matura, V. B. Ho, D. R. Rosing, and C. A. Bondy, "Aortic dilatation and dissection in Turner syndrome," *Circulation*, vol. 116, no. 15, pp. 1663–1670, 2007.

[5] Z. Kizaki, K. Matsuo, M. Yoshida et al., "A case of severe hypoglycemia during infancy turned out to be Turner syndrome with ringed X," *Clinical Pediatric Endocrinology*, vol. 12, pp. 69–74, 2003.

[6] H. Alkhayyat, H. B. T. Christesen, J. Steer, H. Stewart, K. Brusgaard, and K. Hussain, "Mosaic turner syndrome and hyperinsulinaemic hypoglycaemia," *Journal of Pediatric Endocrinology and Metabolism*, vol. 19, no. 12, pp. 1451–1457, 2006.

[7] V. Pietzner, J. F. W. Weigel, D. Wand, A. Merkenschlager, and M. K. Bernhard, "Low-level hyperinsulinism with hypoglycemic spells in an infant with mosaic Turner syndrome and mild Kabuki-like phenotype: a case report and review of the literature," *Journal of Pediatric Endocrinology and Metabolism*, vol. 27, no. 1-2, pp. 165–170, 2014.

[8] V. K. Bakalov, M. M. Cooley, M. J. Quon et al., "Impaired insulin secretion in the Turner metabolic syndrome," *Journal of Clinical Endocrinology and Metabolism*, vol. 89, no. 7, pp. 3516–3520, 2004.

[9] V. K. Bakalov, C. Cheng, J. Zhou, and C. A. Bondy, "X-chromosome gene dosage and the risk of diabetes in Turner syndrome," *Journal of Clinical Endocrinology and Metabolism*, vol. 94, no. 9, pp. 3289–3296, 2009.

[10] C. H. Gravholt, S. Juul, R. W. Naeraa, and J. Hansen, "Morbidity in Turner syndrome," *Journal of Clinical Epidemiology*, vol. 51, no. 2, pp. 147–158, 1998.

[11] P. Jacobs, P. Dalton, R. James et al., "Turner syndrome: a cytogenetic and molecular study," *Annals of Human Genetics*, vol. 61, part 6, pp. 471–483, 1997.

[12] M. J. McGinniss, D. H. Brown, L. W. Burke, J. T. Mascarello, and M. C. Jones, "Ring chromosome X in a child with manifestations of Kabuki syndrome," *The American Journal of Medical Genetics*, vol. 70, no. 1, pp. 37–42, 1997.

[13] P. Stankiewicz, H. Thiele, I. Giannakudis et al., "Kabuki syndrome-like features associated with a small ring chromosome X and XIST gene expression," *The American Journal of Medical Genetics*, vol. 102, no. 3, pp. 286–292, 2001.

[14] L. Rodríguez, D. Diego-Alvarez, I. Lorda-Sanchez et al., "A small and active ring X chromosome in a female with features of Kabuki syndrome," *The American Journal of Medical Genetics Part A*, vol. 146, no. 21, pp. 2816–2821, 2008.

[15] R. J. McKinley Gardner, G. R. Sutherland, and L. G. Shaffer, "Autosomal ring chromosomes," in *Chromosome Abnormalities and Genetic Counseling*, R. J. McKinley Gardner, G. R. Sutherland, and L. G. Shaffer, Eds., pp. 201–211, Oxford University Press, 2012.

[16] B. R. Migeon, M. Ausems, J. Giltay et al., "Severe phenotypes associated with inactive ring X chromosomes," *The American Journal of Medical Genetics*, vol. 93, no. 1, pp. 52–57, 2000.

27

Molar Tooth Sign with Deranged Liver Function Tests: An Indian Case with COACH Syndrome

Rama Krishna Sanjeev,[1] Seema Kapoor,[2] Manisha Goyal,[3] Rajiv Kapur,[4] and Joseph Gerard Gleeson[5,6,7]

[1]Department of Pediatrics, ACMS, India
[2]Division of Genetics, Lok Nayak & Maulana Azad Medical College, New Delhi, India
[3]Department of Paediatrics, Maulana Azad Medical College, New Delhi, India
[4]Department of Radiology, ACMS, New Delhi, India
[5]Neurogenetics Laboratory, Department of Neurosciences and Paediatrics, USA
[6]Rady Children's Hospital, USA
[7]Howard Hughes Medical Institute, CA, USA

Correspondence should be addressed to Rama Krishna Sanjeev; rksanjeev88@yahoo.com

Academic Editor: Ozgur Cogulu

We report the first genetically proven case of COACH syndrome from the Indian subcontinent in a 6-year-old girl who presented with typical features of Joubert syndrome along with hepatic involvement. Mutation analysis revealed compound heterozygous missense mutation in the known gene *TMEM67* (also called MKS3).

1. Introduction

COACH syndrome (cerebellar vermis hypo/aplasia, oligophrenia, congenital ataxia, coloboma, and hepatic fibrosis; OMIM# 216360) is a rare autosomal recessive multisystemic disorder first proposed by Verloes and Lambotte [1]. Joubert syndrome (JS) is characterized by the molar tooth sign (MTS), hypotonia, developmental delay, ataxia, irregular breathing pattern, and abnormal eye movements. COACH syndrome is considered by some to be a subtype of Joubert syndrome [2–4]. Mutations in the *TMEM67* gene are responsible for the majority of COACH syndrome, with minor contributions from CC2D2A and RPGRIP1L [5]. Our patient had compound heterozygous mutation in the *TMEM67* gene.

2. Case Summary

A 6-year-old girl presented with global developmental delay, large head, and ataxic gait. The proband was the only child born to nonconsanguineous couple at term after LSCS with birth weight of 3.5 kg. Her motor developmental milestones and speech were grossly delayed.

On examination, her weight was 18.2 kg (50th centile), height 107 cm (50th centile), and head circumference 53 cm (75th–95th centile). Facial features revealed large head, frontal bossing, and hypertelorism with squint. There was pectus excavatum, bilateral clinodactyly, and hepatomegaly (liver span: 10 cm). Neurologically, there was ataxic gait with generalized hypotonia. Eye evaluation showed squint in the right eye (30-degree exotropia) with normal fundus.

Investigations showed normal metabolic parameters except elevated liver enzymes (SGPT = 261 U/L; SGOT = 110 U/L) with normal bilirubin (0.68 mg). MRI brain revealed "molar tooth appearance" (Figure 1(a)) and "Batwing appearance" (Figure 1(b)).

In view of MRI findings with deranged liver function test, COACH syndrome was suspected. Mutation analysis showed the patient to have a compound heterozygous missense

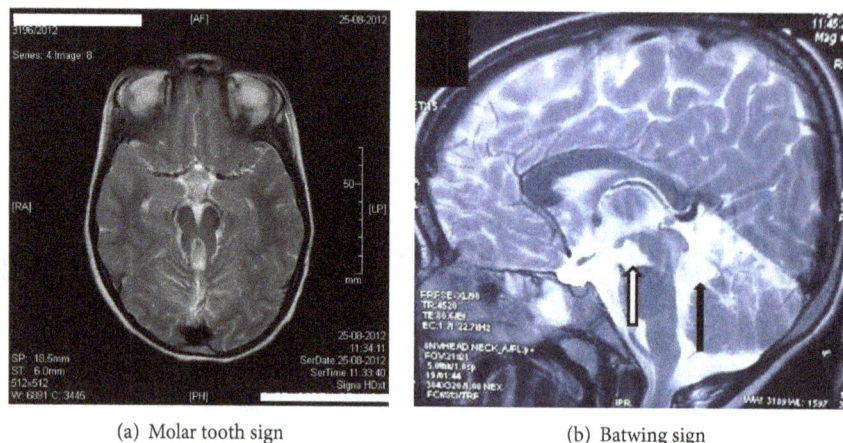

(a) Molar tooth sign

(b) Batwing sign

FIGURE 1: (a) shows thinning of the isthmus with hypoplastic superior cerebellar peduncles forming typical "molar tooth appearance." (b) Hypoplasia of vermis with resultant "batwing appearance" in the fourth ventricle.

mutation at position c.1413-1G>A and c.434T>G in the gene *TMEM67* with father and mother being carriers for c.1413-1G>A and c.434T>G, respectively.

3. Discussion

Joubert syndrome (JS) is a rare genetic disorder affecting the cerebellum characterised by the absence or underdevelopment of cerebellum and malformed brain stem. Diagnosis is based on neurologic signs of hypotonia, ataxia, developmental delay, and oculomotor apraxia along with the "molar tooth sign" (MTS) on MRI, which is the neuroradiologic hallmark of the condition. Disorders that share the MTS have been termed Joubert syndrome (JS). JS comes under the ciliopathies, which are a group of disorders with genetic mutations encoding defective proteins which result in abnormal formation or function of cilia [6].

Cilia are classified into motile and immotile (primary). All the causative JS genes identified to date encode proteins that are localized to the base or axoneme of the cilium [6]. Combinations of additional features such as polydactyly, ocular coloboma, retinal dystrophy, renal disease, hepatic fibrosis, encephalocele, and other brain malformations are classified as Joubert Syndrome Related Disorder (JSRD) [3]. To date, 22 genes, which account for only half of Joubert syndrome cases, have been identified, all encoding for proteins of the primary cilium [6].

Motile cilia when defective cause primary ciliary dyskinesias, which comprise a heterogenous group of disorders characterised by bronchiectasis, left right asymmetry, and infertility [7]. Immotile or primary cilia are present in many differentiated cells of mammalian body like the kidney cells or neurons. All immotile (primary) cilia can now be viewed as sensory cellular antennae with chemosensory, osmosensory, and phototransduction functions [7]. While any organ can be affected by ciliopathic dysfunction, the eye, brain, kidney, and liver are primarily affected [7].

COACH syndrome (OMIM 21630) is considered by some to be a subtype of Joubert syndrome with congenital hepatic fibrosis. The key feature of COACH is congenital hepatic fibrosis (CHF), resulting from malformation of the embryonic ductal plate [1]. In our patient, we found compound heterozygous mutation in the known gene *TMEM67*. Brancati et al. [8] identified compound heterozygous mutation in *TMEM67* gene.

In our patient, we found hepatomegaly and raised liver enzymes with typical features of Joubert syndrome in MRI (molar tooth sign and batwing sign) suggesting COACH syndrome. Clinically, the liver disease can vary from raised liver enzymes to features of portal hypertension [5]. Identification of liver disease is critical because some may develop portal hypertension with variceal bleeding. Known ocular features in COACH syndrome are nystagmus, strabismus, amblyopia, ptosis, and pigmentary retinopathy, of which strabismus was present.

Renal manifestations, reported in subjects with JSRD, were not present in our case. Thus, the presence of mutation in *TMEM67* gene in this patient further delineates the genotype-phenotype correlation in COACH syndrome. JSRD patients with known liver involvement should be tested first for *TMEM67* mutations, followed by CC2D2A and RPGRIP1L. Presymptomatic, gene based diagnosis should make it possible to deliver improved care for systemic complications and prenatal identification.

Conflict of Interests

The authors declare that there is no conflict of interests regarding the publication of this paper.

References

[1] A. Verloes and C. Lambotte, "Further delineation of a syndrome of cerebellar vermis hypo/aplasia, oligophrenia, congenital ataxia, coloboma, and hepatic fibrosis," *The American Journal of Medical Genetics*, vol. 32, no. 2, pp. 227–232, 1989.

[2] D. Satran, M. E. M. Pierpont, and W. B. Dobyns, "Cerebello-oculo-renal syndromes including Arima, Senior-Loken and

COACH syndromes: more than just variants of joubert syndrome," *American Journal of Medical Genetics*, vol. 86, no. 5, pp. 459–469, 1999.

[3] J. G. Gleeson, L. C. Keeler, M. A. Parisi et al., "Molar tooth sign of the midbrain-hindbrain junction: occurrence in multiple distinct syndromes," *American Journal of Medical Genetics*, vol. 125, no. 2, pp. 125–134, 2004.

[4] F. Brancati, B. Dallapiccola, and E. M. Valente, "Joubert syndrome and related disorders," *Orphanet Journal of Rare Diseases*, vol. 5, no. 1, article 20, 2010.

[5] D. Doherty, M. A. Parisi, L. S. Finn et al., "Mutations in 3 genes (*MKS3*, *CC2D2A* and *RPGRIP1L*) cause COACH syndrome (Joubert syndrome with congenital hepatic fibrosis)," *Journal of Medical Genetics*, vol. 47, no. 1, pp. 8–21, 2010.

[6] J. E. Lee and J. G. Gleeson, "Cilia in the nervous system: linking cilia function and neurodevelopmental disorders," *Current Opinion in Neurology*, vol. 24, no. 2, pp. 98–105, 2011.

[7] A. M. Waters and P. L. Beales, "Ciliopathies: an expanding disease spectrum," *Pediatric Nephrology*, vol. 26, no. 7, pp. 1039–1056, 2011.

[8] F. Brancati, M. Iannicelli, L. Travaglini et al., "MKS3/TMEM67 mutations are a major cause of COACH Syndrome, a Joubert Syndrome related disorder with liver involvement," *Human Mutation*, vol. 30, no. 2, pp. E432–E442, 2009.

28

Short Stature in Chronic Kidney Disease Treated with Growth Hormone and an Aromatase Inhibitor

Susan R. Mendley,[1,2] Fotios Spyropoulos,[3] and Debra R. Counts[4]

[1]Department of Pediatrics, University of Maryland School of Medicine, Baltimore, MD 21201, USA
[2]Department of Medicine, University of Maryland School of Medicine, Baltimore, MD 21201, USA
[3]Department of Pediatrics, University of Iowa Children's Hospital, Iowa City, IA 52242, USA
[4]Department of Pediatrics, Sinai Hospital, Baltimore, MD 21215, USA

Correspondence should be addressed to Fotios Spyropoulos; fotios-spyropoulos@uiowa.edu

Academic Editor: Ashraf T. Soliman

We describe an alternative strategy for management of severe growth failure in a 14-year-old child who presented with advanced chronic kidney disease close to puberty. The patient was initially treated with growth hormone for a year until kidney transplantation, followed immediately by a year-long course of an aromatase inhibitor, anastrozole, to prevent epiphyseal fusion and prolong the period of linear growth. Outcome was excellent, with successful transplant and anticipated complete correction of height deficit. This strategy may be appropriate for children with chronic kidney disease and short stature who are in puberty.

1. Introduction

Growth failure is a well-recognized complication of chronic kidney disease (CKD) and if left untreated can adversely affect quality of life [1]. In addition to correction of metabolic acidosis, secondary hyperparathyroidism, and vitamin D deficiency, recombinant human growth hormone (GH) is the most effective therapy to improve growth velocity [2]. However, these strategies may be insufficient in older children who come to attention late with advanced CKD and significant short stature. Advancing puberty and resulting epiphyseal closure may limit the time available for linear growth. We present an alternative approach using an aromatase inhibitor, anastrozole, which has been shown to be effective in idiopathic short stature but has not, to our knowledge, been utilized to maximize height potential in growth failure of CKD.

Inhibition of aromatase activity was initially recognized as beneficial in the therapy of estrogen-sensitive breast cancer. The aromatase enzyme complex, which is formed by cytochrome P450 XIX (CYP19) and the nicotinamide-adenine dinucleotide phosphate cytochrome P450 reductase, is differentially expressed in various tissues. Its role is to aromatize the steroid A ring of androgens (androstenedione and testosterone) resulting in the peripheral conversion of androgens to estrogen as well as the conversion of estrogen to catechol estrogen, 2-hydroxyestrogen, and 6α-hydroxyestrogen [3–5]. The importance of this process to regulating longitudinal growth was recognized in 1994-1995 in reports of two men with tall stature and unfused epiphyses who still manifested adult pubertal development. Further insight into the effect of estrogen on skeletal maturation was demonstrated when these patients were treated with estrogen replacement therapy which led to epiphyseal fusion only in patients with aromatase deficiency [6–8]. Therapeutic use of aromatase inhibition to increase predicted adult height has been shown to be effective in idiopathic short stature [9] although its use remains limited and awaits further study [10]. Despite limited data, the circumstances of this case suggested a benefit to the use of anastrozole to delay epiphyseal fusion in order to prolong linear growth.

2. Case Report

A 14-year-old male was evaluated for short stature and no previous medical problems were known. Height was 146 cm (SDS score −2.17) and weight was 34.8 kg (SDS score −2.30).

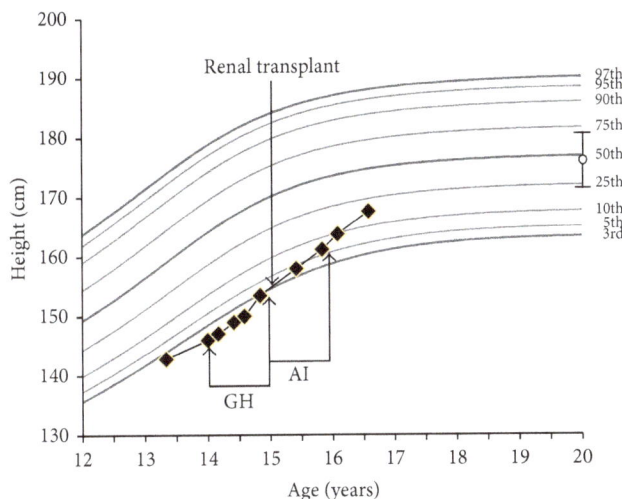

FIGURE 1: Observed growth curve of subject with prediction of final height. GH: interval of growth hormone therapy with growth velocity of 8.5 cm/year; AI: duration of aromatase inhibitor (anastrozole) therapy with growth velocity of 9.8 cm/year. Annualized growth velocity after AI therapy = 5.4 cm/year. Circle with vertical bars denotes predicted adult height by the method of Greulich and Pyle [10].

There was no lower extremity bowing. He was Tanner 1 with bone age 12 6/12 years and predicted adult height was 169 cm (SDS score −1.20) and his midparental height was 174 cm. Both parents reported normal growth pattern with normal timing of puberty. Evaluation revealed serum creatinine of 3.6 mg/dL and serum bicarbonate of 18 mmol/L. Intact parathyroid hormone (PTH) was 188 ng/L. Upon further evaluation, ultrasonographic and radiologic studies demonstrated bilateral hydroureter and hyperechoic kidneys with right grade 5 reflux and left grade 4 reflux, leading to a presumptive diagnosis of longstanding reflux nephropathy.

Initial therapy included sevelamer, sodium citrate, erythropoietin, calcitriol, and GH (0.053 mg/kg/day). There was good control of acidosis and metabolic bone disease with intact PTH maintained between 131 and 177 ng/L. Delayed puberty was treated with a short course of low dose testosterone (50 mg monthly IM for 4 months) in order to improve GH response, which was followed by spontaneous puberty. Annualized growth velocity was 8.5 cm/year (Figure 1), but renal function worsened and the patient was prepared for renal transplantation one year after presentation. At that time, he had Tanner 3 pubic hair and Tanner 2 genitals with a testosterone level of 12.1 nmol/dL and had achieved a height of 155.6 cm (SDS score −1.80). GH was discontinued at the time of transplant because we anticipated early use of glucocorticoids for immunosuppression, which would decrease GH therapy efficacy, and correction of renal function which could make GH therapy unnecessary. Since time for growth became limited by the need for transplant and initial steroid treatment, therapy with an aromatase inhibitor (anastrozole 1 mg daily) was initiated to delay epiphyseal fusion and provide additional time for linear growth. Despite clinician's request, a bone age was not obtained at this time. Transplant immunosuppression included basiliximab induction followed by tacrolimus, mycophenolate mofetil, and glucocorticoids with excellent allograft function. Serum creatinine normalized to 1.0 mg/dL. Prednisone was tapered to 0.1 mg/kg/day by month five and to 0.1 mg/kg every other day by month nine with stable kidney function and no signs of rejection. Ultrasensitive estradiol was <11 pmol/L demonstrating adequate blockade of testosterone conversion. Annualized growth velocity was 9.8 cm/year after transplant (Figure 1) so GH was not restarted. Anastrozole was continued for a total of 12 months and then was stopped when height was 163.8 cm (SDS −1.509), bone age was 14 years, and predicted adult height, by the method of Greulich-Pyle [11], was 177 cm (SDS = 0). Patient has continued to exhibit spontaneous pubertal progression after transplant, and annualized growth velocity off anastrozole and growth hormone therapy was 5.7 cm/yr.

3. Discussion

The age of onset of CKD and the degree of residual renal function are highly correlated with the degree of growth retardation, making early intervention crucial in order to optimize the height outcome and achieve a near normal final height [12]. Current guidelines [13] recommend that acidosis and metabolic bone disease be treated and nutritional deficiencies be corrected and if growth velocity or height SDS score remains abnormal, treatment with recombinant GH should be considered. This was our plan when the patient first presented, but we were concerned that impending puberty would limit our success.

Management of patients who are at pubertal age with significant short stature is challenging. Pubertal hormones lead to advancement of bone age and fusion of the epiphyses, limiting the time available for linear growth. However, there is also an important stimulant effect of testosterone on linear growth which enhances the efficacy of exogenous growth hormone [14, 15] and the combined therapy was initially chosen in our patient to maximize growth velocity as well as promote age-appropriate secondary sexual characteristics. We recognized the possibility that testosterone administration and subsequent pubertal progression might later limit growth duration but were reassured by the availability of anastrozole therapy to delay epiphyseal fusion. While both androgens and estrogens promote epiphyseal growth, estrogens are the major cause of epiphyseal fusion. Aromatase inhibitors have been utilized as adjuvant treatment for boys with disorders of growth of a variety of causes, aiming to extend the duration of linear growth by delaying epiphyseal fusion. Their use increases predicted adult height in boys with GH deficiency, idiopathic short stature, and constitutional delay of growth [9, 16, 17]. This is the first patient reported to our knowledge with growth failure secondary to CKD who has received anastrozole and we wonder whether there is something different about growth in this setting which would make the treatment particularly beneficial. Such a question would require additional study in a larger group of patients and we hope our report is an impetus to this.

An alternative strategy to delay epiphyseal fusion and increase final height might have been to suppress puberty with a gonadotropin (GnRH) analogue. In contrast to GnRH analogues, aromatase inhibitors do not delay the natural progression of secondary sexual characteristics in boys and are less likely to cause adverse psychosocial effects of suppressed puberty. Also, the effectiveness of combined GH and GnRH analogue in patients with short stature is equivocal and a recent consensus statement did not suggest their routine use for short stature [18]. By contrast, there is evidence that aromatase inhibitors increase predicted adult height in adolescent males with a good safety profile [19]. Consistent with its relatively low potency as an inhibitor of cytochrome P450 3A at therapeutic concentrations [20], anastrozole appeared to have no significant effect on tacrolimus levels or renal allograft function in our patient. Since aromatase inhibitors are administered orally rather than by injection, patient acceptance is generally good.

Our patient appears to have completely corrected his large height deficit (using predicted adult height as treatment outcome, shown in Figure 1) with several therapies that were used in combination and in sequence, including correction of metabolic abnormalities, testosterone, 12 months of growth hormone followed by 12 months of anastrozole therapy, and a rapid steroid taper after transplantation. Although the use of anastrozole is a promising measure in this setting we cannot be confident which of the above treatments had the greatest effect. His current treatment with low dose alternate day prednisone and a well-functioning renal allograft appears sufficient to achieve a growth trajectory similar to that which would have occurred in the absence of renal disease. Additional follow-up until near final height will be important to judge the efficacy of these interventions, since predicted height may overestimate true height outcome. In this patient we utilized sequential GH and aromatase inhibitor therapy, but we can foresee a circumstance where combined therapy might be appropriate, depending upon a patient's pubertal status and transplant or dialysis plan. In summary, treatment with GH and an aromatase inhibitor may provide unique benefits in the setting of advanced CKD and should be considered in children who present with significant short stature close to puberty when time for other therapeutic options is limited.

Conflict of Interests

The authors declare that there is no conflict of interests regarding the publication of this paper.

References

[1] A. C. Gerson, A. Wentz, A. G. Abraham et al., "Health-related quality of life of children with mild to moderate chronic kidney disease," Pediatrics, vol. 125, no. 2, pp. e349–e357, 2010.

[2] R. N. Fine, E. Kohaut, D. Brown, J. Kuntze, and K. M. Attie, "Long-term treatment of growth retarded children with chronic renal insufficiency, with recombinant human growth hormone," Kidney International, vol. 49, no. 3, pp. 781–785, 1996.

[3] M. Numazawa, W. Handa, C. Hasegawa, and M. Takahashi, "Structure-activity relationships of 2α-substituted androstenedione analogs as aromatase inhibitors and their aromatization reactions," Journal of Steroid Biochemistry and Molecular Biology, vol. 97, no. 4, pp. 353–359, 2005.

[4] E. Cavalieri, D. Chakravarti, J. Guttenplan et al., "Catechol estrogen quinones as initiators of breast and other human cancers: implications for biomarkers of susceptibility and cancer prevention," Biochimica et Biophysica Acta—Reviews on Cancer, vol. 1766, no. 1, pp. 63–78, 2006.

[5] A. Cavalli, A. Bisi, C. Bertucci et al., "Enantioselective nonsteroidal aromatase inhibitors identified through a multidisciplinary medicinal chemistry approach," Journal of Medicinal Chemistry, vol. 48, no. 23, pp. 7282–7289, 2005.

[6] E. P. Smith, J. Boyd, G. R. Frank et al., "Estrogen resistance caused by a mutation in the estrogen-receptor gene in a man," New England Journal of Medicine, vol. 331, no. 16, pp. 1056–1061, 1994.

[7] A. Morishima, M. M. Grumbach, E. R. Simpson, C. Fisher, and K. Qin, "Aromatase deficiency in male and female siblings caused by a novel mutation and the physiological role of estrogens," Journal of Clinical Endocrinology and Metabolism, vol. 80, no. 12, pp. 3689–3698, 1995.

[8] C. Carani, K. Qin, M. Simoni et al., "Effect of testosterone and estradiol in a man with aromatase deficiency," The New England Journal of Medicine, vol. 337, no. 2, pp. 91–95, 1997.

[9] M. Hero, E. Norjavaara, and L. Dunkel, "Inhibition of estrogen biosynthesis with a potent aromatase inhibitor increases predicted adult height in boys with idiopathic short stature: a randomized controlled trial," Journal of Clinical Endocrinology and Metabolism, vol. 90, no. 12, pp. 6396–6402, 2005.

[10] D. I. Shulman, G. L. Francis, M. R. Palmert, and E. A. Eugster, "Use of aromatase inhibitors in children and adolescents with disorders of growth and adolescent development," Pediatrics, vol. 121, no. 4, pp. e975–e983, 2008.

[11] N. Bayley and S. R. Pinneau, "Tables for predicting adult height from skeletal age: revised for use with the greulich-pyle hand standards," The Journal of Pediatrics, vol. 40, no. 4, pp. 423–441, 1952.

[12] F. Kaskel, "Chronic renal disease: a growing problem," Kidney International, vol. 64, no. 3, pp. 1141–1151, 2003.

[13] "Clinical practice guidelines for nutrition in chronic renal failure. K/DOQI, National Kidney Foundation," American Journal of Kidney Diseases, vol. 35, no. 6, supplement 2, pp. S1–S140, 2000.

[14] N. Mauras, A. Rini, S. Welch, B. Sager, and S. P. Murphy, "Synergistic effects of testosterone and growth hormone on protein metabolism and body composition in prepubertal boys," Metabolism: Clinical and Experimental, vol. 52, no. 8, pp. 964–969, 2003.

[15] D. C. Brown, G. E. Butler, C. J. H. Kelnar, and F. C. W. Wu, "A double blind, placebo controlled study of the effects of low dose testosterone undecanoate on the growth of small for age, prepubertal boys," Archives of Disease in Childhood, vol. 73, no. 2, pp. 131–135, 1995.

[16] S. Salehpour, P. Alipour, M. Razzaghy-Azar et al., "A double-blind, placebo-controlled comparison of letrozole to oxandrolone effects upon growth and puberty of children with constitutional delay of puberty and idiopathic short stature," Hormone Research in Paediatrics, vol. 74, no. 6, pp. 428–435, 2010.

[17] N. Mauras, L. G. De Pijem, H. Y. Hsiang et al., "Anastrozole increases predicted adult height of short adolescent males treated with growth hormone: a randomized, placebo-controlled, multicenter trial for one to three years," *Journal of Clinical Endocrinology and Metabolism*, vol. 93, no. 3, pp. 823–831, 2008.

[18] J.-C. Carel, E. A. Eugster, A. Rogol, L. Ghizzoni, and M. R. Palmert, "Consensus statement on the use of gonadotropin-releasing hormone analogs in children," *Pediatrics*, vol. 123, no. 4, pp. e752–e762, 2009.

[19] N. Mauras, "Strategies for maximizing growth in puberty in children with short stature," *Endocrinology and Metabolism Clinics of North America*, vol. 38, no. 3, pp. 613–624, 2009.

[20] S. W. Grimm and M. C. Dyroff, "Inhibition of human drug metabolizing cytochromes P450 by anastrozole, a potent and selective inhibitor of aromatase," *Drug Metabolism and Disposition*, vol. 25, no. 5, pp. 598–602, 1997.

29

Congenital Portosystemic Shunt: Our Experience

Tiziana Timpanaro,[1] **Stefano Passanisi,**[1] **Alessandra Sauna,**[1] **Claudia Trombatore,**[2] **Monica Pennisi,**[2] **Giuseppe Petrillo,**[2] **Pierluigi Smilari,**[1] **and Filippo Greco**[1]

[1]*Unit of Clinical Pediatrics, Department of Medical and Pediatric Sciences, University of Catania, Via Santa Sofia, 95123 Catania, Italy*

[2]*Radiodiagnostic and Oncological Radiotherapy Unit, University Hospital "Policlinico-Vittorio Emanuele", Via Santa Sofia, 95123 Catania, Italy*

Correspondence should be addressed to Tiziana Timpanaro; timpanarotiziana@yahoo.it

Academic Editor: Josef Sykora

Introduction. Congenital portosystemic venous malformations are rare abnormalities in which the portal blood drains into a systemic vein and which are characterized by extreme clinical variability. *Case Presentations.* The authors present two case reports of a congenital extrahepatic portosystemic shunt (Type II). In the first patient, apparently nonspecific symptoms, such as headache and fatigue, proved to be secondary to hypoglycemic episodes related to the presence of a portosystemic shunt, later confirmed on imaging. During portal vein angiography, endovascular embolization of the portocaval fistula achieved occlusion of the anomalous venous tract. In the second patient, affected by Down's syndrome, the diagnosis of a portosystemic malformation was made by routine ultrasonography, performed to rule out concurrent congenital anomalies. Because of the absence of symptoms, we chose to observe this patient. *Conclusions.* These two case reports demonstrate the clinical heterogeneity of this malformation and the need for a multidisciplinary approach. As part of a proper workup, clinical evaluation must always be followed by radiographic diagnosis.

1. Introduction

Congenital portosystemic shunts are rare vascular abnormalities in which the portal blood drains into a systemic vein. They are the result of embryogenetic alterations or the persistence of the fetal circulation elements, especially those related to the ductus venosus [1]. It is also associated with chromosomal abnormalities, especially Down's syndrome [2].

Anatomically congenital portosystemic venous shunts are classified into extra- and intrahepatic shunts [3]. To date, although these abnormalities are increasingly recognized due to the evolution and development of diagnostic imaging, the total number of cases described in the literature remains low. Of all published cases, 185 and 131 describe an extra- and intrahepatic portosystemic shunt, respectively [4].

Clinical presentation, especially in children, is extremely variable. In some cases, portosystemic malformations may remain asymptomatic, making the diagnosis difficult. In other cases, they may cause metabolic disorders and damage various organs and systems, such as the liver, central nervous system, and respiratory tract.

Imaging plays an important confirmatory role when the diagnosis is suspected and can clearly demonstrate the venous shunt, identify any associated malformations, and suggest the most appropriate management approach.

We present two patients who have been affected by congenital portosystemic shunts. Our two cases demonstrate how the malformation is characterized by heterogeneous clinical variability and can result in different therapeutic implications.

2. Case Report 1

Patient 1 was born from nonconsanguineous parents at the 37th week of gestation by spontaneous vaginal delivery with a birth weight of 2280 g (small for gestational age). At

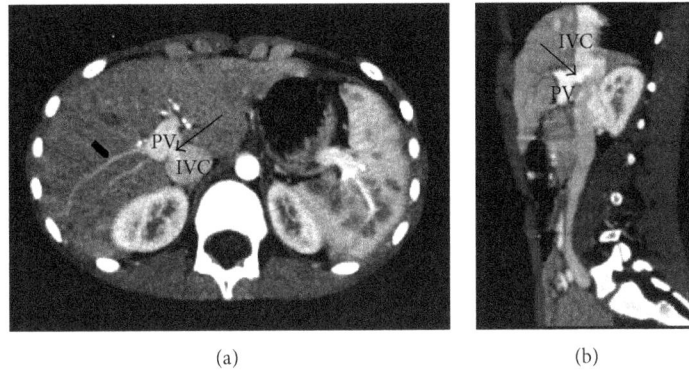

(a) (b)

FIGURE 1: Contrast-enhanced CT images. Axial projection (a); sagittal-oblique projection (b). The arrows in (a) and (b) show a shunt between the posterior wall of the portal vein (PV), just before its intrahepatic hilar division, and the inferior cava vein (ICV); the intrahepatic portal branches appear reduced and filiform (arrowhead in (a)).

birth, he had low glucose levels and received an intravenous 10% glucose infusion with subsequent improvement in the following hours.

Since the age of six, he was regularly followed up by a pediatric neuropsychiatrist for attention hyperactivity disorder, difficulty with concentration, dyscalculia, dyslexia, and a "borderline" IQ.

At the age of 10, due to headache, severe fatigue, and daytime sleepiness he was admitted to our pediatric clinic for further investigation. His height was 149 cm (<90th percentile), his weight was 37.7 kg (25–50th percentile), and his head circumference was 53 cm (75th percentile).

On physical examination, he demonstrated an elongated facies, low-set ears, single palmar creases bilaterally, and hypoplasia of the hypothenar eminence. He also displayed alterations in his osteoarticular system, including arachnodactyly, scapular winging, an ankle valgus deformity, joint laxity, bilateral pes planus, and a hallux valgus deformity.

During the hospitalization, blood tests demonstrated hyperinsulinemia (36 μU/mL; n.v 2.6–24.9) and mild hypoglycemia (49 mg/dL). He underwent oral glucose-tolerance testing, which revealed hyperinsulinemia at 60 minutes (395 μU/mL, associated with a blood glucose value of 42 mg/dL). Testing while fasting was also performed but was stopped at 30 minutes due to hypoglycaemia and general malaise. Suspecting organic disease related to excessive insulin secretion, further diagnostic testing was performed. Ultrasonography (US) showed slight ectasia of the left renal vein coursing cranially and turbulent flow at the inferior vena cava (IVC) through the midline of the aortomesenteric branches. Contrast-enhanced magnetic resonance imaging (MRI) of the abdomen was performed, demonstrating hyperintense hepatic lesions on T1-weighted images and isointense lesions on T2-weighted images (diameters between 9 and 20 mm). No abnormalities of the venous circulation were identified at this point. The patient then underwent contrast enhanced CT (computed tomography) scan, which revealed similar hepatic nodular lesions, characterized by early enhancement with slow washout. These images also showed a close anatomical contiguity between the distal portal vein and the inferior vena cava, along with early uptake

of contrast compatible with a portocaval shunt. An Abernethy malformation (Type II, side-to-side extrahepatic shunt) was confirmed (Figure 1).

In order to correctly classify the shunt, endovascular evaluation of the malformation was performed. The inferior vena cava was catheterized by percutaneous femoral access, and a venogram demonstrated the portocaval shunt. The caliber of the shunt was approximately 10 mm and the balloon occlusion test showed no intraportal pressure peaks. Therefore, embolization of the fistula was performed, achieving occlusion of the anomalous venous tract.

To date, clinical follow-up has been normal and the patient is in good health.

3. Case Report 2

Patient 2 was born from nonconsanguineous parents at the 36th week of gestation by spontaneous vaginal delivery with a birth weight of 1600 g (small for gestational age). The intrapartum diagnosis of Down's syndrome was made by amniocentesis. At the age of two, she underwent surgery for coarctation of the aorta and a patent ductus arteriosus. At the age of nine, she presented at our pediatric clinic for further diagnostic testing, given her underlying disease.

At initial evaluation, she was in good health. Her height was 117.5 cm (<3rd percentile), her weight was 30 kg (>50th percentile), and her head circumference was 45 cm (<3rd percentile). During her hospitalization, laboratory tests were found to be unremarkable. Doppler ultrasonography was performed, revealing a slightly overflowing liver of coarse heterogeneous echotexture, with hypoechoic periportal striae. The pedicle had an irregular morphology with a hyperechoic porta and hypoechoic shadow. There was an apparent communication (10 mm) between the portal vein and inferior vena cava compatible with a portocaval shunt. Color Doppler US showed demodulated, irregular venous flow with no extra- or intrahepatic biliary ductal dilation. An abdominal CT scan was performed to study the splenic-mesentericportal axis. The superior mesenteric and portal vein had an enlarged caliber with slight ectasia of the celiac tripod,

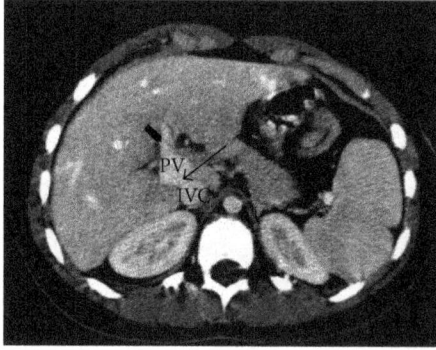

FIGURE 2: Axial contrast-enhanced CT images. The arrow shows the shunt between the portal vein (PV) and the inferior cava vein (ICV); at the hepatic hilum, the PV appears enlarged with only one intrahepatic portal branch (arrowhead).

common hepatic artery, and its branches. The portocaval shunt had only one intrahepatic portal branch, which was of lower caliber (Figure 2). Based on these findings, a diagnosis of Abernethy malformation (Type II, side-to-side shunt) was made. As the shunt was clinically insignificant, we chose to observe the patient. To date, the patient has been followed up with periodic clinical examination and Doppler US; the patient's health has not worsened clinically.

4. Discussion

Congenital portosystemic shunts are classified by their anatomical characteristics into extrahepatic and intrahepatic varieties. Congenital extrahepatic portosystemic shunt (CEPS) was first described by Abernethy in 1793 [5]. In CEPS, the anastomoses are established between the portomesenteric vasculature, before division of the portal vein, and a systemic vein.

In 1994, Morgan and Superina [6] classified CEPS into two types.

(i) Type 1: there is complete diversion of portal blood into the systemic circulation (end-to-side shunt), with absent intrahepatic portal branches.

(ii) Type 2: intrahepatic portal vein is intact, but some of the portal flow is diverted into a systemic vein through a side-to-side shunt.

Congenital intrahepatic shunts, first described by Raskin in 1964, are abnormal intrahepatic connections (diameter > 1 mm) between branches of the portal vein and the hepatic veins or inferior vena cava [7]. Park et al. [8] subdivided them as follows.

(i) Type 1: a single large vessel connecting the right portal vein to the inferior vena cava;

(ii) Type 2: a localized peripheral shunt in which one hepatic segment has one or more communications between peripheral branches of the portal vein and the hepatic veins;

TABLE 1: Clinical manifestations associated with congenital portosystemic shunt [9–15].

Hepatic	Nodular lesions, focal nodular hyperplasia, hepatocellular adenoma, hepatocellular carcinoma, hepatic sarcoma, and newborn cholestasis
Neurological	Behavioral disorders, irritability, dyslexia, lethargy, EEG abnormalities, extrapyramidal signs, and epilepsy
Pulmonary	Dyspnea caused by pulmonary hypertension
Metabolic	Hyperammonemia, hypoglycemia, hyperinsulinaemia, and hypergalactosemia, without evidence of a deficiency of galactokinase or epimerase [1]
Others	IUGR, membranoproliferative glomerulonephritis with proteinuria and IgA stores, coagulation disorders, congestive heart failure, hyperandrogenism, pancreatitis, and autoimmune disorders

(iii) Type 3: an aneurysmal communication between the peripheral portal vein and the hepatic veins;

(iv) Type 4: multiple communications between the portal vein and the hepatic veins, distributed in both lobes.

Congenital portosystemic shunts can cause a broad spectrum of clinical manifestations. The liver, central nervous system, and respiratory tract are usually involved. In a high percentage of cases portosystemic shunt can lead to metabolic dysregulation, while damage to other organs is described in a very small number of cases (Table 1). Table 1 shows the principal clinical manifestations reported in the literature.

Due to the wide variability in clinical presentation, imaging plays an important role to recognize the shunt and related malformations. Color Doppler US demonstrates the presence of the shunt, the type, and the direction of flow of the identified vessels [16]. MR angiography could provide additional information about the hepatic vascular and parenchymal abnormalities. Although using methods that minimize exposure to ionizing radiation is preferable in pediatric patients, this imaging alone is insufficient. Computed tomography angiography is considered the first choice examination [17] because this method displays even small vascular branches compatible with a portocaval shunt. CT also allows imaging of intrahepatic lesions of very small dimensions, as we presented in our first case.

Therapeutic options depend on the type of shunt and its clinical course. If a Type 2 extrahepatic shunt is asymptomatic, as occurs in most children, watchful waiting is indicated and treatment recommended for the first appearance of clinical manifestations inherited to hepatic encephalopathy and liver dysfunction or complications such as pulmonary hypertension. However, these symptoms usually appear in adulthood, especially in those patients with shunts ratio above 60% [18, 19]. Therefore, meticulous clinical and sonographic monitoring must be performed. To date, there are no guidelines on the advisability of earlier treatment only to prevent complications from developing.

Treatment is indicated for patients with clinically significant shunting. Preoperatively, it is necessary to define the shunt anatomically and functionally by invasive endovascular techniques, such as catheter angiography [20]. Shunt occlusion can be performed surgically or with percutaneous endovascular procedures [16]. The aim is to occlude the shunt, while avoiding a rise in portal pressure (secondary portal hypertension). Preoperatively, it is mandatory to complete the anatomical and functional study of the shunt by more invasive techniques, such as catheter angiography [21]. In fact, in some cases, the extremely hypoplastic portal veins distal to the shunt are sometimes difficult to visualize by conventional CT angiography; in these cases, the direct catheterization of the shunt by interventional radiology is essential to study the real vascular anatomy and to distinguish the true Type 1 fistulae (absolute lack of opacification of intrahepatic portal branches) from the Type 2 fistulae with very small portal vein branches [20].

Franchi-Abella et al. [22] proposed a "balloon occlusion test" to estimate the portal pressure trend after temporary closure of the shunt: if the risk for developing portal hypertension would be insignificant, embolization would be performed; otherwise, stepwise treatment, with gradual shunt closure, would be progressively performed to acclimatize the intrahepatic portal system to the new flow, resulting from the spread of hypoplastic intrahepatic portal branches.

In patients with a Type 1 shunt, shunt occlusion is not an option, because it represents the only drainage route for mesenteric and splenic venous blood. In these cases, liver transplantation is the therapeutic approach [23].

5. Conclusion

Due to the wide spectrum of clinical and anatomical features, the diagnosis of portosystemic shunt can occur incidentally. Perhaps the incidence of this rare malformation is underestimated, as the disease often remains undiscovered for several years. Improved knowledge, especially about the clinical aspects, may help to lower the threshold for diagnosis. As we described in the first case, the suspicion may arise at the presence of otherwise unexplained signs and symptoms, such as occasional hypoglycemia. The second case described suggests that, in chromosomal syndromes, such as Down's syndrome, the association with this malformation needs further consideration. Finally, clinical diagnosis must be followed by radiographic evaluation, which is of primary importance to make the diagnosis and to plan management, thus avoiding the most severe consequences of this malformation.

Abbreviations

US: Ultrasonography
IVC: Inferior vena cava
PV: Portal vein
MRI: Magnetic resonance imaging
CT: Computed tomography
CEPS: Congenital extrahepatic portosystemic shunt.

Conflict of Interests

The authors declare there is no conflict of interests regarding the publication of this paper.

Authors' Contribution

Tiziana Timpanaro collected the data and drafted and wrote the paper; Stefano Passanisi helped to draft and write the paper; Alessandra Sauna helped to draft and write the paper; Claudia Trombatore contributed to realize radiological diagnosis with the help of Monica Pennisi and Giuseppe Petrillo; Pierluigi Smilari had been in charge of both the patients and contributed to discussion of the paper; Filippo Greco contributed to discussion and reviewed the paper. The paper has been read and approved by all the authors and each author considers that the paper represents their honest work.

References

[1] M. D. Stringer, "The clinical anatomy of congenital portosystemic venous shunts," *Clinical Anatomy*, vol. 21, no. 2, pp. 147–157, 2008.

[2] N. Golewale, H. J. Paltiel, S. J. Fishman, and A. I. Alomari, "Portal vascular anomalies in Down syndrome: spectrum of clinical presentation and management approach," *Journal of Pediatric Surgery*, vol. 45, no. 8, pp. 1676–1681, 2010.

[3] P. Writters, G. Maleaux, C. George et al., "Congenital veno-venous malformations of the liver: widely variable clinical presentations," *Journal of Gastroenterology and Hepatology*, vol. 23, no. 8, part 2, pp. e390–e394, 2008.

[4] C. Sokollik, R. H. J. Bandsma, J. C. Gana, M. van den Heuvel, and S. C. Ling, "Congenital portosystemic shunt: characterization of a multisystem disease," *Journal of Pediatric Gastroenterology & Nutrition*, vol. 56, no. 6, pp. 675–681, 2013.

[5] J. Abernethy and J. Banks, "Account of two instances of uncommon formation, in the viscera of the human body," *Philosophical Transactions of the Royal Society of London*, vol. 83, pp. 59–66, 1793.

[6] G. Morgan and R. Superina, "Congenital absence of the portal vein: two cases and a proposed classification system for portasystemic vascular anomalies," *Journal of Pediatric Surgery*, vol. 29, no. 9, pp. 1239–1241, 1994.

[7] N. H. Raskin, J. B. Price, and R. A. Fishman, "Portal-systemic encephalopathy due to congenital intrahepatic shunts," *The New England Journal of Medicine*, vol. 270, pp. 225–229, 1964.

[8] J. H. Park, S. H. Cha, J. K. Han, and M. C. Han, "Intrahepatic portosystemic venous shunt," *American Journal of Roentgenology*, vol. 155, no. 3, pp. 527–528, 1990.

[9] C. P. Murray, S. J. Yoo, and P. S. Babyn, "Congenital extrahepatic portosystemic shunts," *Pediatric Radiology*, vol. 33, no. 9, pp. 614–620, 2003.

[10] M. J. Kim, J. S. Ko, J. K. Seo et al., "Clinical features of congenital portosystemic shunt in children," *European Journal of Pediatrics*, vol. 171, no. 2, pp. 395–400, 2012.

[11] A. Watanabe, "Portal-systemic encephalopathy in non-chirrotic patients: classification of clinical types, diagnosis and treatment," *Journal of Gastroenterology and Hepatology*, vol. 15, no. 9, pp. 969–979, 2000.

[12] Y. Eroglu, J. Donaldson, L. G. Sorensen et al., "Improved neurocognitive function after radiologic closure of congenital

portosystemic shunts," *Journal of Pediatric Gastroenterology and Nutrition*, vol. 39, no. 4, pp. 410–417, 2004.

[13] S. Emre, R. Amon, E. Cohen, R. A. Morotti, D. Vaysman, and B. L. Shneider, "Resolution of hepatopulmonary syndrome after auxiliary partial orthotopic liver transplantation in Abernethy malformation. A case report," *Liver Transplantation*, vol. 13, no. 12, pp. 1662–1668, 2007.

[14] J. Duprey, B. Gouin, M. F. Benazet, and J. le Gal, "Glucose intolerance and post-stimulative hypoglycaemia secondary to congenital intra-hepatic porto-caval anastomosis," *Annales de Médecine Interne*, vol. 136, no. 8, pp. 655–658, 1985.

[15] Y. Nishimura, G. Tajima, A. D. Bahagia et al., "Differential diagnosis of neonatal mild hypergalactosaemia detected by mass screening: clinical significance of portal vein imaging," *Journal of Inherited Metabolic Disease*, vol. 27, no. 1, pp. 11–18, 2004.

[16] G. H. Hu, L. G. Shen, J. Yang, J. H. Mei, and Y. F. Zhu, "Insight into congenital absence of the portal vein: is it rare?" *World Journal of Gastroenterology*, vol. 14, no. 39, pp. 5969–5979, 2008.

[17] E. Alonso-Gamarra, M. Parrón, A. Pérez, C. Prieto, L. Hierro, and M. López-Santamaría, "Clinical and radiologic manifestations of congenital extrahepatic portosystemic shunts: a comprehensive review," *Radiographics*, vol. 31, no. 3, pp. 707–722, 2011.

[18] C. Gallego, M. Miralles, C. Marín, P. Muyor, G. González, and E. García-Hidalgo, "Congenital hepatic shunts," *Radiographics*, vol. 24, no. 3, pp. 755–772, 2004.

[19] T. Akahoshi, T. Nishizaki, K. Wakasugi et al., "Portal-systemic encephalopathy due to a congenital extrahepatic portosystemic shunt: three cases and literature review," *Hepato-Gastroenterology*, vol. 47, no. 34, pp. 1113–1116, 2000.

[20] T. B. Lautz, N. Tantemsapya, E. Rowell, and R. A. Superina, "Management and classification of type II congenital portosystemic shunts," *Journal of Pediatric Surgery*, vol. 46, no. 2, pp. 308–314, 2011.

[21] Y. Matsuoka, K. Ohtomo, T. Okubo, J. Nishikawa, T. Mine, and S. Ohno, "Congenital absence of the portal vein," *Gastrointestinal Radiology*, vol. 17, no. 1, pp. 31–33, 1992.

[22] S. Franchi-Abella, S. Branchereau, V. Lambert et al., "Complications of congenital portosystemic shunts in children: therapeutic options and outcomes," *Journal of Pediatric Gastroenterology and Nutrition*, vol. 51, no. 3, pp. 322–330, 2010.

[23] E. S. Woodle, J. R. Thistlethwaite, J. C. Emond et al., "Successful hepatic transplantation in congenital absence of recipient portal vein," *Surgery*, vol. 107, no. 4, pp. 475–479, 1990.

30

Spontaneous Duodenal Perforation as a Complication of Kawasaki Disease

Kambiz Masoumi,[1] **Arash Forouzan,**[1] **Hossein Saidi,**[2] **Hazhir Javaherizadeh,**[3] **Ali Khavanin,**[1] **and Mohammad Bahadoram**[1]

[1]*Department of Emergency Medicine, Imam Khomeini General Hospital, Ahvaz Jundishapur University of Medical Sciences, Ahvaz 6193673166, Iran*
[2]*Department of Emergency Medicine, Hazrate Rasoul Akram Hospital, Iran University of Medical Sciences, Tehran 14455364, Iran*
[3]*Department of Pediatrics, Abouzar Children's Hospital, Ahvaz Jundishapur University of Medical Sciences, Ahvaz 6135715794, Iran*

Correspondence should be addressed to Mohammad Bahadoram; mohammadbahadoram@yahoo.com

Academic Editor: Nan-Chang Chiu

Kawasaki disease is generally known as a systemic vasculitis that often concerns doctors due to its serious cardiac complications; however, other visceral organs may get involved as well. Surgical manifestations of the intestinal tract in Kawasaki disease are rare. In this report, we describe the case of a 2.5-year-old boy with typical Kawasaki disease who presented with GI bleeding and surgical abdomen. The diagnosis of duodenal perforation was confirmed.

1. Introduction

Kawasaki disease (KD) is one of the most common vasculitis of childhood. It is a systemic inflammatory illness that particularly affects medium-sized arteries, especially the coronary arteries. Pathologic studies indicate that multiple organs and tissues are involved but long-term sequelae appear to occur only in the arteries. Possible etiologic factors include immunologic response, infections, and genetic factors [1]. Complications of Kawasaki disease primarily reflect cardiac Sequela, although noncardiac complications also may occur [2]. Vascular changes also can occur in peripheral and visceral arteries. Nonetheless, in rare cases virtually any vascular bed may be affected. Thus, case reports have included KD presenting as a cerebrovascular accident (e.g., acute encephalopathy, stroke, gastrointestinal obstruction, pseudoobstruction, or acute abdominal catastrophe) [3]. GI involvement from KD is not common. However, diarrhea, vomiting, abdominal pain, hepatic dysfunction, and hydrops of the gall bladder (GB) are relatively common, whereas pancreatitis, intestinal obstruction, bowel edema, and acute surgical abdomen are rare. This is a case report regarding acute surgical abdomen (duodenal perforation) due to KD.

2. Case Presentation

A 2.5-year-old boy with fever and erythematous rash on trunk and extremities was brought to the emergency department by his parents. Fever had started about 2 days ago, not relieved by cold compress and acetaminophen. Red eye associated with erythematous lips and oral mucosa appeared a day later. Then, erythematous rash was developed. Regarding his condition, amoxicillin, diphenhydramine, and acetaminophen were prescribed by a general physician in an outpatient clinic. Patient was brought to the emergency department because of unchanging condition in the evening of 3rd day.

On arrival, he seemed very irritated while crying. On examination, we found bilateral nonexudative conjunctivitis, erythematous maculopapular rash on trunk and extremities, oedema, erosion and erythema of lips and oral mucosa, and oedema and erythema of palms and soles. Pharyngitis, cervical, axillary, and inguinal lymphadenopathy were not detected. Heart and lung were normal. Abdomen was soft without tenderness and organomegaly. There was no peripheral cyanosis. Past medical history was negative for allergy. Parents mentioned loss of appetite of their son over the last few days. Patient was admitted with provisional

TABLE 1: Laboratory test results in days 1, 7, 8, and 11.

Test	First day	7th day	8th day	11th day
HB	11 g/dL	6.5 g/dL	9.5 g/dL	11.5 g/dL
Plt	247×10^9/L		293×10^9/L	
WBC	12×10^9 cell/L		8.4×10^9 cell/L	6.9×9 cell/L (PMN: 54%/Eos: 12%/Lymph: 34%)
BS	150 mg/dL			
BUN	17 mg/dL		9 mg/dL	
Creatinine	0.6 mg/dL		0.4 mg/dL	
Sodium	125 meq/L		130 meq/L	
Potasium	4.1 meq/L		3.1 meq/L	
ESR	23 mm/hr		109 mm/hr	11 mm/hr
CRP	+		+++	
UA (Hb)		Trace	Negative	
Reticulocyte count		0.6%		
G6PD level		Deficient		
PT			10.2 sec	
PTT			38 sec	
ALT			51 U/L	
AST			79 U/L	
ANA			Negative	
RF			Negative	
Stool exam			Negative	
Stool culture			Negative	
Urine culture			Negative	
Blood culture			Negative	

diagnosis of Kawasaki disease. The next morning, diagnosis of Kawasaki disease remained unclear. Patient condition was the same as before and he received supportive care. Both results of primary laboratory studies and chest X-ray were normal. On the 5th day of fever, patient's condition remained unchanged. Therefore, based on fulfilled criteria for Kawasaki disease, intravenous immunoglobulin (IVIG) 20 gram/single dose was started (2 gram/kg/single dose over 12 hours, BW: 10 kg) in addition to aspirin 800 mg/day (80 mg/kg/day) in 4 divided doses. Fever and chills occurred following IVIG administration which was controlled by IV fluid therapy and transient discontinuation of IVIG. Then, IVIG was continued more slowly without any problem. Supportive care was continued and patient condition remained unchanged until his mother noted his cola coloured urine (on the 7th day). Immediately, aspirin was discontinued and some lab tests were ordered. Test results are shown in Table 1.

Glucose-6-phosphate dehydrogenase (G6PD) deficiency had been missed. Hydration, serum alkalization, packed cell transfusion (100 cc), and vitamin E were started. Dipyridamole 200 mg/day was started instead of aspirin. The next morning (8th day), other lab tests results came back which were as in Table 1.

At this time, echocardiography was done and normal findings were reported. Melena was reported by mother in the evening. Occult blood testing was obtained whose result was positive. Gastrointestinal bleeding, some specific foods, or medicine were the initial differential diagnosis of positive occult blood test in our case. Clinical manifestations gradually started to eliminate. Fever decreased (38.5). Oral and lips erosions were relieved. Palmar and plantar erythema were declined. Conjunctival congestion was decreased. In the next three days, fever was resolved, restlessness disappeared, appetite increased, and other manifestations were minimal.

Results of some laboratory tests (11th day) are shown in Table 1. On 11th day, regarding fever discontinuation, dipyridamole dose was changed to a 30 mg/day (3 mg/kg/day in 3 divided doses). Unexpectedly the patient vomited in the evening followed by restlessness, fever, and abdominal pain again. Overfeeding, complication of KD, or adverse effects of dipyridamole were suspected for patient symptoms including abdominal pain. Slow feeding and supportive care were recommended but abdominal exam showed tenderness with decreased bowel sound. Then, urgently, abdominal X-ray was ordered which revealed free subdiaphragmatic intraperitoneal air. Patient with diagnosis of acute abdomen underwent emergent laparotomy. Perforated ulcer was seen in anterior portion of descending duodenum. Pathology center reported degeneration and necrosis of the epithelial cells, inflammatory exudates in the tissue layers associated with thrombosis, and hemorrhage of the small submucosal arteries in duodenal specimen. He was discharged of pediatric surgery ward after ten days with good condition. Further investigations showed no cardiac involvement or other complications.

3. Discussion

Kawasaki disease (KD) is a systemic vasculitis, resulting in severe inflammation and necrosis of medium-sized vessels. It involves not only the coronary artery but also the vessels in many other systemic organs. Therefore, KD is a multisystemic disease and unusual symptoms may be part of the systemic illness.

Kawasaki disease is a clinical diagnosis. Although elevated creatinine levels, ESR, and platelets count may also be seen in limited patients [2], in this particular patient we observed CRP+++ by qualitative test and elevated ESR levels that may be because of IVIG infusion in addition to inflammation [4]. Also, hyponatremia (Na, 125 meq/L) means severe inflammation in KD [3], and it may be a clue to the diagnosis of KD [5].

The patient filled all diagnostic criteria of KD except for cervical lymphadenopathy, which is the least common diagnostic criterion [4]. Our patient went under standard treatment for possible diagnosis of typical KD. Following treatment, the patient underwent hemoglobin fall and hematuria on the 7th day. Despite the fact that IVIG therapy and taking aspirin can cause complications such as gastrointestinal bleeding in Kawasaki patients, studies show that their advantages in preventing cardiac complications are far more significant than their possible side effects [2, 6]. There are some causes regarding gross hematuria in KD including aspirin consumption in G6PD deficiency and following hemolysis, renal and urinary complication of KD, and IVIG complication. The risks of aspirin therapy appear to be similar to those reported in other settings, including chemical hepatitis with elevated transaminases, transient hearing loss, and, rarely, Reye's syndrome. However, these risks may be increased in patients with KD. Aspirin-binding studies have suggested that the hypoalbuminemia of children with KD predisposes them to toxic free salicylate levels despite measured (total) values within the therapeutic range [6]. Aspirin in G6PD deficiency in contraindicated and resulted in hemolysis and hematuria. In these cases, other anticoagulants replaced or IVIG only can be administered without use of aspirin. The efficacy of the latter needs further investigation [6]. With the exception of sterile pyuria, urinary abnormalities and renal disease are uncommonly associated with KD. Among the renal complications that have been noted in selected cases are acute interstitial nephritis, mild proteinuria, and acute renal failure. Hemolytic-uremic syndrome, immune complex-mediated glomerulonephritis, and acute interstitial nephritis, for example, have each been reported in a handful of cases [7]. IVIG may cause acute renal injury as well, especially preparations that use sucrose as a stabilizer [6].

Children with KD may present with a wide variety of gastrointestinal manifestations. Gastrointestinal tract involvement is not unusual in KD, and its prevalence is 2.3%. The clinical manifestations include vomiting, diarrhea, abdominal pain, abdominal distension, hepatomegaly, paralytic ileus, and hydrops of gallbladder [7, 8]. Diarrhea associated with vomiting and abdominal pain in 61% and vomiting alone in 44% of Kawasaki cases has been reported [9]. However, surgical manifestations are much less frequent and include small bowel obstruction and strictures, intussusception, ischemic colitis, perforation of duodenum, hemorrhagic enteritis, appendicitis, pancreatitis, bile duct stenosis, and hydrops of gall bladder. A case series from Italy reported 10 children ultimately diagnosed with KD who were treated for acute abdominal catastrophes including gallbladder hydrops and cholestasis, paralytic ileus, appendicular vasculitis, and hemorrhagic duodenitis. Acute surgical abdomen was the clinical presentation of KD in 4.6% of their patients [10]. Surgical abdominal complications of KD have been reported in the literature [3, 8–11].

Despite the studies conducted so far, the cause of early gastrointestinal involvement in some KD patients in not yet known. However, it is interesting to note that a selective expansion of circulating $V\beta2$ T cells has been demonstrated both in the blood and in the jejunal mucosa of patients with KD in the acute phase [12]. The GI mucosa, which may serve as a super antigen presenting organ, because of its large area and the abundance of major histocompatibility complex class II expression by epithelial/macrophages in the GI tract may be the portal of entry to these antigens. Immune system activation during the acute phase of KD is an important factor in pathogenesis of the disease. Selective increase in VB2+ T cells in small intestinal mucosa was found in one series of patients with KD [7, 11, 12]. One study showed various bacterial strains, mainly Gram positive cocci (streptococci and staphylococci), in jejunal biopsies of patients with acute KD compared with controls. This change in small bowel flora was not related to the severity of the GI tract involvement and manifested itself with diarrhea. Because staphylococcus enterotoxin and streptococcus exotoxin might serve as super antigens, the change in the small bowel flora in these patients might play a role in the pathogenesis of the disease [7, 12].

The typical pathology of the small intestine shows degeneration, necrosis, and desquamation of the epithelial cells, as well as inflammatory exudates in the lamina propria and in the muscular layer. Vasculitis and thrombosis of the small submucosal arteries or submucosa hemorrhage are frequently seen [7, 8]. Similar inflammatory changes involving the liver, pancreas, and the lymphoid tissue have also been described [3].

Conflict of Interests

The authors declare that there is no conflict of interests regarding the publication of this paper.

References

[1] R. P. Sundel, "Kawasaki disease," *Rheumatic Disease Clinics of North America*, vol. 41, no. 1, pp. 63–73, 2015.

[2] D. Yim, N. Curtis, M. Cheung, and D. Burgner, "An update on Kawasaki disease II: clinical features, diagnosis, treatment and

outcomes," *Journal of Paediatrics and Child Health*, vol. 49, no. 8, pp. 614–623, 2013.

[3] L. Yaniv, M. Jaffe, and R. Shaoul, "The surgical manifestations of the intestinal tract in Kawasaki disease," *Journal of Pediatric Surgery*, vol. 40, no. 9, pp. E1–E4, 2005.

[4] S. Balasubramanian, M. R. Krishna, K. Dhanalakshmi, S. Amperayani, and A. Ramanan, "Factors associated with delay in diagnosis of kawasaki disease in India," *Indian Pediatrics*, vol. 49, no. 8, pp. 663–665, 2012.

[5] G.-W. Lim, M. Lee, H. S. Kim, Y. M. Hong, and S. Sohn, "Hyponatremia and syndrome of inappropriate antidiuretic hormone secretion in Kawasaki disease," *Korean Circulation Journal*, vol. 40, no. 10, pp. 507–513, 2010.

[6] G. Lee, S. E. Lee, Y. M. Hong, and S. Sohn, "Is high-dose aspirin necessary in the acute phase of Kawasaki disease?" *Korean Circulation Journal*, vol. 43, no. 3, pp. 182–186, 2013.

[7] M. D. Morgan and C. O. S. Savage, "Vasculitis in the gastrointestinal tract," *Best Practice & Research: Clinical Gastroenterology*, vol. 19, no. 2, pp. 215–233, 2005.

[8] F. H. Passam, I. D. Diamantis, G. Perisinaki et al., "Intestinal ischemia as the first manifestation of vasculitis," *Seminars in Arthritis and Rheumatism*, vol. 34, no. 1, pp. 431–441, 2004.

[9] N. R. de M. Alves, C. M. R. de Magalhães, R. de Fátima R. Almeida, R. C. R. dos Santos, L. Gandolfi, and R. Pratesi, "Prospective study of kawasaki disease complications: Review of 115 cases," *Revista da Associacao Medica Brasileira*, vol. 57, no. 3, pp. 295–300, 2011.

[10] F. Zulian, F. Falcini, L. Zancan et al., "Acute surgical abdomen as presenting manifestation of Kawasaki disease," *The Journal of Pediatrics*, vol. 142, no. 6, pp. 731–735, 2003.

[11] G. Casella, B. Bronzino, L. Cutrino, N. Montani, A. Somma, and V. Baldini, "Vasculitis and gastrointestinal involvement," *Minerva Gastroenterologica e Dietologica*, vol. 52, no. 2, pp. 195–214, 2006.

[12] S. Nagata, Y. Yamashiro, Y. Ohtsuka et al., "Heat shock proteins and superantigenic properties of bacteria from the gastrointestinal tract of patients with Kawasaki disease," *Immunology*, vol. 128, no. 4, pp. 511–520, 2009.

31

17-Year-Old Boy with Renal Failure and the Highest Reported Creatinine in Pediatric Literature

Vimal Master Sankar Raj,[1] **Jessica Garcia,**[2] **and Roberto Gordillo**[1]

[1]*Department of Pediatric Nephrology, University of Illinois College of Medicine at Peoria (UICOMP), Peoria, IL 61603, USA*
[2]*Department of Pediatrics, University of Illinois College of Medicine at Peoria (UICOMP), Peoria, IL 61603, USA*

Correspondence should be addressed to Vimal Master Sankar Raj; vraj@uicomp.uic.edu

Academic Editor: Giovanni Montini

The prevalence of chronic kidney disease (CKD) is on the rise and constitutes a major health burden across the world. Clinical presentations in early CKD are usually subtle. Awareness of the risk factors for CKD is important for early diagnosis and treatment to slow the progression of disease. We present a case report of a 17-year-old African American male who presented in a life threatening hypertensive emergency with renal failure and the highest reported serum creatinine in a pediatric patient. A brief discussion on CKD criteria, complications, and potential red flags for screening strategies is provided.

1. Background

Prevalence of chronic kidney disease (CKD) is increasing significantly and it has poor outcomes if not diagnosed and treated early in its course [1]. CKD is a public health issue that affects 9 to 12% of the population in the USA [2, 3]. When management is early and adequate, the rate of progression to kidney failure can be slowed, comorbidities prevented, and the morbidity and mortality of cardiovascular disease associated with CKD decreased. There is lack of information on incidence and prevalence of earlier stages of CKD in children, as most of these patients are asymptomatic [4].

The National Kidney Foundation (NKF) created the Kidney Disease Outcomes Quality Initiative (KDOQI) guidelines and definition of CKD to facilitate the diagnosis and management by primary care physicians. Serum creatinine, a product of muscle metabolism, has been widely used as a marker for glomerular filtration rate (GFR). We describe a clinical case of an adolescent male with the highest serum creatinine reported in a pediatric patient. The primary aim of this case report was to create awareness of chronic kidney disease among general practitioners and to stress that clinical manifestations could be subtle in the early stages of the disease.

2. Case Presentation

A 17-year-old African American male who was previously healthy with the exception of high blood pressure presented to a referring hospital with a 4-day history of coughing, vomiting, headache, facial edema, and lower extremity cramping. One day prior to admission, he also had noticed decreased urine output. At the referring hospital, he was found to be hypertensive with a serum creatinine of 52 mg/dL (4597 μmol/L) and was transferred to our pediatric intensive care unit for further evaluation and treatment.

Patient was born at term gestation and there were no significant health problems. Patient during his routine clinic visits was noted to have high blood pressure by his primary care physician but no further evaluation was done as the blood pressure was attributed to his obesity. Patient did not have any prior surgeries and was not taking any medications. There was no significant history of renal disease, dialysis, or kidney transplant in any of the family members.

On admission, patient was noted to be afebrile, hypertensive with blood pressure of 179/93 mm Hg and heart rate of 88 beats per minute, and tachypneic with respiratory rate in the 40s but saturating at 100% on room air. His anthropometric measurements showed his height to be

180 cm, his weight to be 115 kg, and body mass index to be >99%. Pertinent positives in physical exam include obesity, respiratory distress with nasal flaring, bilateral periorbital edema, and bilateral lower extremity edema. Laboratory results showed the patient to have azotemia with blood urea nitrogen (BUN) of 203 mg/dL and serum creatinine of 52 mg/dL, measured by enzymatic method. He had severe metabolic acidosis with bicarbonate of 10 mmol/L. Patient also had severe electrolyte imbalances including hyponatremia (126 mmol/L), hyperkalemia (6.3 mmol/L), hyperphosphatemia (10.5 mg/dL), hypocalcemia (5.3 mg/dL), and severe anemia with hemoglobin at 5.1 g/dL. Parathyroid hormone levels were elevated at 682 pg/mL (normal 11–80 pg/mL). Urine dipstick showed 3+ protein and 2+ blood and a urine protein to creatinine ratio was elevated at 14 (normal <0.2). Serological workup including complement levels, antinuclear antibodies, antinuclear cytoplasmic antibodies, and antiphospholipid antibodies was negative. Chest X-ray was significant for cardiomegaly and pulmonary edema. Echocardiogram showed severe left ventricular hypertrophy. Renal ultrasound revealed bilateral small, echogenic kidneys (right kidney 7.7 × 5.2 × 4.8 cm; left kidney 8.7 × 4.3 × 4.1 cm) consistent with dysplastic kidneys. Patient emergently underwent hemodialysis for fluid overload and to correct electrolyte imbalance. His anemia and electrolyte imbalances were slowly corrected. He is currently transitioned to peritoneal dialysis awaiting kidney transplant.

3. Discussion

CKD is a heterogeneous group of diseases with altered structure and function of the kidneys with varying manifestation based on underlying etiology. Based on KDIGO guidelines, CKD is classified into various stages using GFR and the degree of albuminuria (Tables 1(a) and 1(b)).

The modified Schwartz formula used to calculate GFR is derived from the CKiD (chronic kidney disease in children) [5] and uses the following formula:

$$\text{eGFR} = K \text{ (height in centimeters)}/\text{Serum creatinine}$$
with the constant K value being 0.413.

GFR varies with age, gender, and body size and increases from infancy to adulthood. Normative data of GFR based on age is presented in Table 2. This needs to be taken into consideration on CKD classification in pediatric population.

4. Epidemiology

Most epidemiological information on adult CKD is available from data on ESRD patients [6]. This represents only the tip of the iceberg and the actual incidence of early stage CKD will be much higher. The exact prevalence of childhood CKD is unknown but it has been estimated at 82 cases per million with ESRD around 15 cases per million based on national registries [7–9]. Though pediatric ESRD contributes only 2% to the total ESRD burden, the mortality rate in adolescents is about 30 to 150% higher compared to the general population [8, 10] indicating the need for specialized

TABLE 1: (a) CKD based on GFR [14]. (b) Persistent albuminuria and risk for CKD [14].

(a)

GFR categories	Description	Range (mL/min/1.73 m^2)
G1	Normal or high	≥90
G2	Mildly decreased	60–89
G3a	Mildly to moderately decreased	45–59
G3b	Moderately to severely decreased	30–44
G4	Severely decreased	15–29
G5	Kidney failure	<15

(b)

Categories	Description	Range
A1	Normally to mildly increased	<30 mg/g
A2	Moderately increased	<3 mg/mmol 30–300 mg/g
A3	Severely increased	3–30 mg/mmol >300 mg/g

Adapted from KDIGO 2012.

TABLE 2: Normal glomerular filtration rate (GFR) in children and adolescents [15].

Age	Mean GFR ± SD (mL/min/1.73 m^2)
1 week (males and females)	41 ± 15
2–8 weeks (males and females)	66 ± 25
>8 weeks (males and females)	96 ± 22
2–12 years (males and females)	133 ± 27
13–21 years (males)	140 ± 30
13–21 years (females)	126 ± 22

Adapted from National Kidney Foundation.

care. The expected remaining life time of children below 14 years of age with ESRD and on dialysis calculated per US renal data system (USRDS) [8] is only 20 years. Hence, the importance of primary prevention with early detection and aggressive intervention cannot be overstated.

5. Etiology

The etiology for ESRD varies with age. Structural anomalies contribute to a large degree to ESRD in younger children, while it is predominantly glomerular diseases in older children. As per NAPRTCS 2011 review data, about 14.2% of all pediatric dialysis patients had ESRD secondary to hypoplastic/dysplastic kidney with obstructive uropathy at 12.6% (Table 3).

6. Screening Strategies for CKD

Screening strategies are aimed at early detection and intervention for CKD so as to slow the progression of disease.

TABLE 3: Pediatric dialysis patient demographics [16].

All dialysis patients	N	%
	7039	100.0
Primary diagnosis		
FSGS	1016	14.4
Hypoplastic/dysplastic kidney	998	14.2
Obstructive uropathy	888	12.6
Reflux nephropathy	244	3.5
SLE nephritis	226	3.2
HUS	216	3.1
Chronic GN	214	3.0
Polycystic disease	201	2.9
Congenital nephrotic syndrome	182	2.6
Prune belly	144	2.0
Medullary cystic disease	140	2.0
Idiopathic crescentic GN	130	1.8
Familial nephritis	130	1.8
MPGN-type I	116	1.6
Pyelonephritis/interstitial nephritis	101	1.4
Cystinosis	99	1.4
Renal infarct	90	1.3
Berger's (IgA) nephritis	86	1.2
Henoch-Schönlein nephritis	67	1.0
MPGN-type II	64	0.9
Wilms' tumor	55	0.8
Wegener's granulomatosis	49	0.7
Drash syndrome	39	0.6
Other systemic immunologic diseases	37	0.5
Oxalosis	32	0.5
Membranous nephropathy	29	0.4
Sickle cell nephropathy	21	0.3
Diabetic GN	10	0.1
Other	887	12.6
Unknown	528	7.5

Adapted from NAPRTCS 2011.

Though routine urine screening for CKD has not been found to be cost effective in the general population and has not been recommended by AAP, it is important to identify and screen children at high risk. Some of the high risk populations at risk for CKD are mentioned below:

(i) Prematurity and being small for gestational age.

(ii) Congenital abnormalities of the kidney and urinary tract.

(iii) H/o poor growth or failure to thrive.

(iv) Family history of kidney diseases and relatives on dialysis or transplant.

(v) Electrolyte or acid-base abnormalities.

(vi) Body mass index (BMI) > 95th percentile.

(vii) Blood pressure greater than the 95% recorded on multiple visits.

(viii) Polyuria or inappropriately dilute urine.

(ix) Gross hematuria.

(x) Dysfunctional voiding, urinary incontinence, or prolonged enuresis.

(xi) H/o recurrent UTI.

A thorough history and physical examination during well child visits could help us in identifying these children with high risk for kidney disease. Once identified, these children should have their urine checked for proteinuria, their renal function analyzed by measuring creatinine, and their blood pressure regularly screened. Children with evidence of kidney damage should be sent to a specialist for further investigation and treatment. For our patient, blood pressure > 95% and the BMI > 95% should have prompted a screening for potential kidney disease.

7. CKD Complications

Cardiovascular disease accounts for most deaths in pediatric CKD similar to adult onset CKD. In contrast to adult CKD patients, where atherosclerosis and coronary vascular disease are much more common, arrhythmias account for the majority of cardiovascular death in children (19.6%) [11]. Traditional risk factors for CVD such as dyslipidemia and hypertension along with nontraditional risk factors such as anemia, disorders of calcium phosphorus metabolism, and increased chronic inflammation are highly prevalent in CKD population. These also contribute significantly to the cardiovascular burden in these children.

Anemia is a common complication in CKD secondary to impaired erythropoiesis. As CKD progresses, so does the prevalence of anemia in these children. Factors such as malnutrition, blood loss, iron deficiency, inadequate dialysis, and uncontrolled secondary hyperparathyroidism should always be kept in mind while managing resistant anemia. KDIGO recommends maintaining hemoglobin levels between 10 and 12 g/dL to reduce need for transfusion. Iron levels should be checked and adequately supplemented in all CKD patients before initiating or increasing dose of erythropoiesis stimulating agents.

Metabolic bone disorder (CKD-MBD) is a major complication in CKD. This occurs secondary to the inability of kidneys to excrete phosphorus and synthesize active vitamin D. Net result is secondary hyperparathyroidism. Disorders in calcium phosphorus balance and secondary hyperparathyroidism play a major role in vascular calcification in CKD and subsequent cardiovascular mortality and morbidity.

Fluid and electrolyte imbalances are especially common in children with CKD secondary to congenital anomalies of the kidneys and urinary tract (CAKUT). In CAKUT impaired urinary concentrating ability could present with polyuria and can present with dehydration. Disorder of sodium, potassium, and acid-base balance is also very common in these children due to impaired tubular handling. As the normal tubular response to ADH is not present, special attention should be paid to the fluid and electrolyte replacement in these children in the setting of dehydration.

Growth failure and neurocognitive delay are important concerns for young children with CKD [12, 13]. Providing adequate calories and protein intake are important in children with CKD as they are more prone to muscle wasting and anorexia. Factors such as systemic inflammation, oral aversion, and alteration in hormonal levels or resistance to action of hormones (follicle stimulating hormone, luteinizing hormone, growth hormone, and thyroid hormone) also contribute to short stature and CKD in children. In infants and toddlers with CKD to maximize nutritional intake a gastrostomy tube is often placed to provide adequate calories and fluids. Optimal nutrition and use of growth hormone replacement are often needed in children with CKD to ensure that they reach their growth potential.

8. Conclusion

Our patient had bilateral dysplastic kidneys and ultimately progressed to ESRD. Though he had potential red flags including obesity and high blood pressure noted on multiple occasions, the thought of kidney disease was not entertained. A screening urine dipstick could have prevented this life threatening admission with hypertensive emergency, severe anemia, and multiple electrolyte imbalances. Earlier detection of kidney disease and control of hypertension and proteinuria could have slowed the progression of disease and also would have allowed the time to plan for his renal replacement therapy in a safe manner. Chronic kidney disease is a growing health burden and awareness of it among primary care physicians is essential in early diagnosis and treatment.

Abbreviations

CKD: Chronic kidney disease
ESRD: End stage renal disease
GFR: Glomerular filtration rate
BUN: Blood urea nitrogen.

Disclosure

The authors have no financial relationships relevant to this paper to disclose.

Conflict of Interests

The authors declare that there is no conflict of interests to disclose.

References

[1] V. Agrawal, A. K. Ghosh, M. A. Barnes, and P. A. McCullough, "Perception of indications for nephrology referral among internal medicine residents: a national online survey," *Clinical Journal of the American Society of Nephrology*, vol. 4, no. 2, pp. 323–328, 2009.

[2] J. Coresh, D. Byrd-Holt, B. C. Astor et al., "Chronic kidney disease awareness, prevalence, and trends among U.S. adults, 1999 to 2000," *Journal of the American Society of Nephrology*, vol. 16, no. 1, pp. 180–188, 2005.

[3] J. Coresh, E. Selvin, L. A. Stevens et al., "Prevalence of chronic kidney disease in the United States," *Journal of the American Medical Association*, vol. 298, no. 17, pp. 2038–2047, 2007.

[4] B. A. Warady and V. Chadha, "Chronic kidney disease in children: the global perspective," *Pediatric Nephrology*, vol. 22, no. 12, pp. 1999–2009, 2007.

[5] L. Copelovitch, B. A. Warady, and S. L. Furth, "Insights from the chronic kidney disease in children (CKiD) study," *Clinical Journal of the American Society of Nephrology*, vol. 6, no. 8, pp. 2047–2053, 2011.

[6] J. Coresh, B. C. Astor, T. Greene, G. Eknoyan, and A. S. Levey, "Prevalence of chronic kidney disease and decreased kidney function in the adult US population: third National Health and Nutrition Examination Survey," *The American Journal of Kidney Diseases*, vol. 41, no. 1, pp. 1–12, 2003.

[7] S. F. Massengill and M. Ferris, "Chronic kidney disease in children and adolescents," *Pediatrics in Review*, vol. 35, no. 1, pp. 16–29, 2014.

[8] U.S. Renal Data System (USRDS), *Annual Data Report: Atlas of End-Stage Renal Disease in the United States*, National Institutes of Health, National Institute of Diabetes and Digestive and Kidney Diseases, Bethesda, Md, USA, 2004.

[9] Clinical Coordinating Center and Data Coordinating Center, *North American Pediatric Renal Transplant Cooperative Study (NAPRTCS)*, Novartis Pharmaceutical, 2005.

[10] S. P. McDonald and J. C. Craig, "Long-term survival of children with end-stage renal disease," *The New England Journal of Medicine*, vol. 350, no. 26, pp. 2654–2662, 2004.

[11] R. Shroff, D. J. Weaver Jr., and M. M. Mitsnefes, "Cardiovascular complications in children with chronic kidney disease," *Nature Reviews Nephrology*, vol. 7, no. 11, pp. 642–649, 2011.

[12] R. H. Mak, W. W. Cheung, J.-Y. Zhan, Q. Shen, and B. J. Foster, "Cachexia and protein-energy wasting in children with chronic kidney disease," *Pediatric Nephrology*, vol. 27, no. 2, pp. 173–181, 2012.

[13] B. J. Foster, L. McCauley, and R. H. Mak, "Nutrition in infants and very young children with chronic kidney disease," *Pediatric Nephrology*, vol. 27, no. 9, pp. 1427–1439, 2012.

[14] KDIGO, "KDIGO 2012 clinical practice guideline for the evaluation and management of chronic kidney disease," *Kidney International Supplements*, vol. 3, no. 1, 2013.

[15] National Kidney Foundation, "K/DOQI clinical practice guidelines for chronic kidney disease: evaluation, classification, and stratification," *The American Journal of Kidney Diseases*, vol. 39, no. 2, supplement 1, pp. S1–S266, 2002.

[16] North American Pediatric Renal Trials and Collaborative Studies (NAPRTCS) 2011 Annual Dialysis Report.

32

Systemic Steroid Treatment for Severe Expanding Pneumococcal Pneumonia

Eran Lavi,[1] David Shoseyov,[1] Natalia Simanovsky,[2] and Rebecca Brooks[1]

[1]*Department of Pediatrics Mount Scopus, Hadassah-Hebrew University Medical Center, P.O. Box 24035, 91240 Jerusalem, Israel*
[2]*Department of Medical Imaging, Hadassah-Hebrew University Medical Center, Mount Scopus, P.O. Box 24035, 91240 Jerusalem, Israel*

Correspondence should be addressed to Eran Lavi; lavi.eran@gmail.com

Academic Editor: Jonathan Muraskas

The treatment of bacterial community-acquired pneumonia (CAP) is based on appropriate antibiotic therapy and supportive care such as intravenous fluids and supplemental oxygen. There is no available data regarding the use of steroids in CAP in children. We present an unusual case of a child with severe respiratory distress, on the brink of mechanical ventilation, due to a rapidly expanding pneumococcal pneumonia. The administration of systemic steroids resulted in a dramatic response with rapid improvement of clinical and radiological abnormalities followed by improvement of laboratory abnormalities. This case report should raise the awareness of the potential benefits of steroids in the treatment of severe pneumonia in children. Prospective randomized trials are needed to confirm the efficacy of steroids in this setting and to determine which patients would benefit most from this.

1. Introduction

Community-acquired pneumonia (CAP) is a significant cause of morbidity and mortality in childhood. Standard treatment for bacterial CAP consists of antibiotic therapy and supportive care, for example, intravenous fluids and supplemental oxygen. The role of systemic corticosteroids in the treatment of bacterial CAP has been reported in adults with conflicting results. We present a case of a child with severe expanding pneumococcal pneumonia that responded to systemic steroids.

2. Case Presentation

A 5-year-old, generally healthy girl, presented to the emergency room with a two-day history of fever, breathing difficulties, and cough. Upon admission she was dyspneic, febrile (38.2°C), and with a heart rate of 160 beats per minute. On auscultation crackles and reduced air entry to the left lung were diagnosed.

Laboratory results showed a normal white blood count with an elevated C reactive protein level (38.6 mg% (N < 0.5 mg%)) and mild respiratory acidosis. Blood cultures taken on admission were positive for *Streptococcus pneumonia* sensitive to Penicillin. The chest X-ray showed an extensive consolidation involving the entire left lung. The patient was admitted to the Pediatric Intensive Care Unit (PICU) where intravenous (IV) Penicillin treatment, IV fluids, and supplemental oxygen were initiated.

Despite the intensive treatment in the PICU, the patient's condition worsened with increased tachypnea and dyspnea requiring escalating amounts of supplemental oxygen. Both physical examination and a repeated chest X-ray showed pleural effusion. A pleural tap was performed and 200 mL of fluid drained. The antigen detection test and pleural fluid culture were positive for *Streptococcus pneumonia*. Despite fluid removal the patient continued to deteriorate. An additional chest X-ray showed severe expanding consolidation with a mediastinal shift to the right (Figure 1(a)). A chest computer tomography scan (CT) confirmed extensive parenchymal consolidation with only minimal pleural effusion.

A single dose of IV methylprednisolone (1 mg/kg) was administered 22 hours after admission to the PICU. Over the following hours the patient's condition improved substantially becoming less dyspneic with improved air entry to her left lung. Oxygen saturations normalized. A repeated

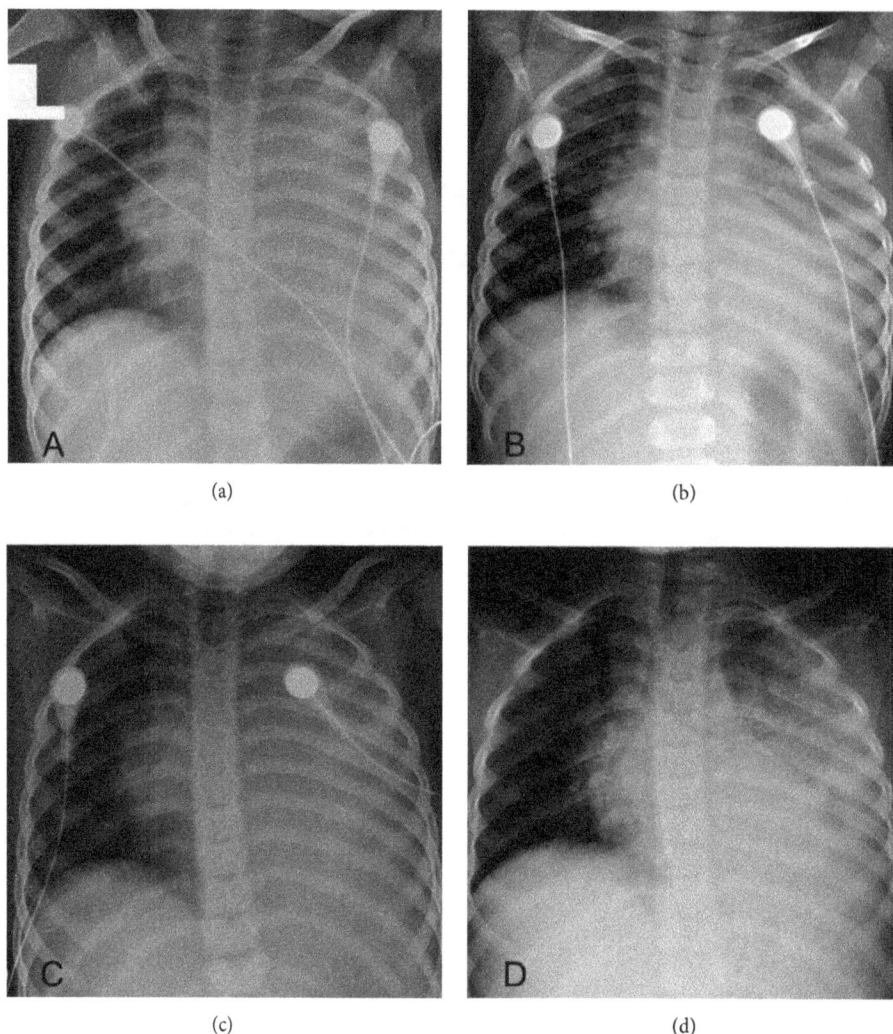

FIGURE 1: A 5-year-old patient with severe expanding pneumococcal pneumonia. (a) Note "white hemithorax" on the left with increased volume causing mediastinal shift to the right. (b) After a single course of left IV methylprednisolone. Significant improvement in the aeration of the left lung with residual consolidation above the diaphragm. (c) A clinical and radiologic deterioration. (d) Improved aeration of the left lung after a second course of IV steroids.

chest X-ray 18 hours after steroid administration showed regression of the lung infiltrate with a normal positioned trachea (Figure 1(b)). However, 24 hours after initial IV steroid treatment she again deteriorated clinically. On the chest X-ray performed 32 hours after steroid treatment a recurrence of the mediastinal shift was detected (Figure 1(c)). A second dose of methylprednisolone was administered to which the patient responded again with the same remarkable response (Figure 1(d)). Steroid treatment was maintained at the dose of 1 mg/kg twice daily for 5 days. The patient continued to improve with no further complications and was discharged home in good condition after a total of 18 days of hospitalization.

It should be emphasized that during the entire period of hospitalization the only additional intervention to the standard treatment consisted of IV steroid therapy. Antibiotics remained unchanged.

3. Discussion

Pneumonia is an acute infection of the lung parenchyma, causing an inflammatory response which changes the balance between pro- and anti-inflammatory cytokines. IL-1β is associated with severity of infection, IL-6 reflects the severity of stress, and TNF-α may be a marker of pneumonia severity [1]. An excessive inflammatory response may lead to severe damage of the pulmonary tissue resulting in respiratory failure and/or septic shock.

Corticosteroids are powerful inhibitors of the inflammatory cascade, suppressing the expression of proinflammatory cytokines and thus potentially preventing an extended inflammatory response.

In infectious diseases the use of corticosteroids is known to reduce complications, such as hearing loss in *Haemophilus influenzae* bacterial meningitis [2], or the need for mechanical ventilation in cases of pneumonia caused by *Pneumocystis jiroveci* in HIV patients [3].

The role of steroids treatment in septic shock and sepsis was examined in several studies and remained controversial without clear evidence of improvement in mortality rate [4]. For this reason steroids are not generally recommended in sepsis management unless adrenal insufficiency is proven.

A small number of studies describe the use of steroids in adult patients with CAP. Meijvis et al. report on a cohort of patients with CAP randomly assigned to receive IV dexamethasone or placebo. Their results showed that length of hospital stay was significantly reduced in the dexamethasone group, whereas no difference was seen in mortality rate between the groups. The study did not include patients in the Intensive Care Unit [5]. Garcia-Vidal et al. showed reduced mortality among patients with CAP who received adjuvant steroid treatment compared with those who received antibiotics alone [6]. In a randomized double-blinded trial performed by Snijders et al., administration of prednisolone (40 mg) for one week did not improve the outcome of patients with CAP. Moreover in this study late failure of treatment was more common among patients treated with prednisolone than those in the placebo group [7].

The role of steroids for the treatment of CAP in the pediatric population has not been extensively studied and is limited mostly to case series. One study has shown clinical improvement after administration of methylprednisolone pulse therapy in 6 children with refractory *Mycoplasma pneumonia* [8].

In a multicenter retrospective study Weiss et al. reported that adjuvant corticosteroid therapy was associated among pediatric patients who received concomitant β-agonist therapy with a shorter hospital length of stay. However, in patients who did not receive β-agonists, systemic corticosteroids were associated with a longer length of stay and greater odds of readmission [9].

The case described here is of a child with severe respiratory distress, on the verge of mechanical ventilation, due to rapidly expanding pneumococcal pneumonia causing a mediastinal shift. The administration of systemic steroids resulted in a dramatic response. It should be emphasized that the patient was not in a septic shock and the deterioration was mainly respiratory. During hospitalization no adverse effects of steroids (hyperglycemia, superadded infection, and bleeding) were noted.

To our knowledge this is the first case report of a significant response to corticosteroids in a pediatric patient with pneumococcal CAP.

In summary, this case report should raise the awareness of the potential benefits of steroids in the treatment of severe pneumonia in children.

As previously shown in a number of studies, steroid treatment in different settings such as sepsis is not beneficial in all cases. The effect of steroids is probably multifactorial and depends on a variety of factors such as genetics, comorbidities, and the severity of the inflammatory response. However, as demonstrated in this case, steroid treatment may significantly reduce mortality in certain cases, yet our findings cannot be generalized to nonbacteremic pneumococcal

pneumonia and prospective randomized trials are needed to determine which patients would benefit most from this treatment in both the adult and pediatric population.

Conflict of Interests

The authors declare that there is no conflict of interests regarding the publication of this paper.

References

[1] A. J. Puren, C. Feldman, N. Savage, P. J. Becker, and C. Smith, "Patterns of cytokine expression in community-acquired pneumonia," *Chest*, vol. 107, no. 5, pp. 1342–1349, 1995.

[2] D. van de Beek, J. de Gans, P. McIntyre, and K. Prasad, "Corticosteroids for acute bacterial meningitis," *Cochrane Database of Systematic Reviews*, no. 1, Article ID CD004405, 2007.

[3] M. Briel, H. C. Bucher, R. Boscacci, and H. Furrer, "Adjunctive corticosteroids for *Pneumocystis jiroveci* pneumonia in patients with HIV-infection," *Cochrane Database of Systematic Reviews*, no. 3, Article ID CD006150, 2006.

[4] G. P. Patel and R. A. Balk, "Systemic steroids in severe sepsis and septic shock," *American Journal of Respiratory and Critical Care Medicine*, vol. 185, no. 2, pp. 133–139, 2012.

[5] S. C. A. Meijvis, H. Hardeman, H. H. F. Remmelts et al., "Dexamethasone and length of hospital stay in patients with community-acquired pneumonia: a randomised, double-blind, placebo-controlled trial," *The Lancet*, vol. 377, no. 9782, pp. 2023–2030, 2011.

[6] C. Garcia-Vidal, E. Calbo, V. Pascual, C. Ferrer, S. Quintana, and J. Garau, "Effects of systemic steroids in patients with severe community-acquired pneumonia," *European Respiratory Journal*, vol. 30, no. 5, pp. 951–956, 2007.

[7] D. Snijders, J. M. A. Daniels, C. S. de Graaff, T. S. van der Werf, and W. G. Boersma, "Efficacy of corticosteroids in community-acquired pneumonia: a randomized double-blinded clinical trial," *The American Journal of Respiratory and Critical Care Medicine*, vol. 181, no. 9, pp. 975–982, 2010.

[8] A. Tamura, K. Matsubara, T. Tanaka, H. Nigami, K. Yura, and T. Fukaya, "Methylprednisolone pulse therapy for refractory Mycoplasma pneumoniae pneumonia in children," *Journal of Infection*, vol. 57, no. 3, pp. 223–228, 2008.

[9] A. K. Weiss, M. Hall, G. E. Lee, M. P. Kronman, S. Sheffler-Collins, and S. S. Shah, "Adjunct corticosteroids in children hospitalized with community-acquired pneumonia," *Pediatrics*, vol. 127, no. 2, pp. e255–e263, 2011.

33

Ameloblastic Fibroma of the Maxilla with Bilateral Presentation: Report of a Rare Case with Review of the Literature

Kranti Kiran Reddy Ealla,[1] **Vijayabaskar Reddy Basavanapalli,**[2]
Surekha Reddy Velidandla,[1] **Sangameshwar Manikya,**[1] **Rajesh Ragulakollu,**[3]
Prasanna M. Danappanavar,[1] **and Vijayasree Vennila**[4]

[1]*Department of Oral and Maxillofacial Pathology, MNR Dental College and Hospital, Sangareddy, Telangana 502294, India*
[2]*Department of Oral and Maxillofacial Surgery, MNR Dental College and Hospital, Sangareddy, Telangana 502294, India*
[3]*Department of Pedodontics and Preventive Dentistry, KLR'S Lenora Institute of Dental Sciences, Rajahmundry,*
 Andhra Pradesh 533294, India
[4]*Department of General Pathology, Kamineni Institute of Medical Sciences, Narketpally, Telangana 508254, India*

Correspondence should be addressed to Kranti Kiran Reddy Ealla; drekkr@yahoo.co.in

Academic Editor: Nina L. Shapiro

Ameloblastic fibroma (AF) is an uncommon benign odontogenic tumour, with both epithelial and mesenchymal neoplastic proliferation. It occurs most frequently in the posterior region of the mandible, while its occurrence in the maxilla is extremely rare. They are usually encountered in children, emphasizing it as an important diagnostic consideration. Herein, we report the first case of a bilateral maxillary ameloblastic fibroma in a 2-year-old female child patient who presented with a chief complaint of swelling in the right mid facial region.

1. Introduction

Ameloblastic fibromas (AFs) are a rare variety of benign odontogenic tumors composed of proliferating odontogenic epithelium embedded in a cellular ectomesenchymal tissue resembling dental papilla [1]. It was first described by Kruse in 1891 and later classified as a separate entity by Thoma and Goldman in 1946 [2, 3]. They are frequently encountered in the posterior mandible with eighty percent cases in the second primary molar or first permanent molar region [4] and 75% associated with an impacted tooth [5]. These tumors are frequently diagnosed between the 1st and 2nd decades of life with 75% of cases being diagnosed before the age of 20 and primarily considered a tumor of childhood and adolescence. Males show a slightly higher prediction than females (M : F = 1.4 : 1) [6].

AFs usually present with a well-defined unilocular or multilocular radiolucencies [7]. Unilocular lesions are predominantly asymptomatic, while the multilocular cases are often associated with jaw swelling [8]. However, most of the cases of AFs are encountered as an incidental finding [9, 10] reiterating their radiographic significance in the differential diagnosis with entities such as dentigerous cyst, ameloblastoma, odontogenic keratocyst, and ameloblastic fibrosarcoma [11, 12].

Microscopically AFs are composed of both the epithelial and connective tissue components; the later appears to recapitulate dental papilla made up of spindled and angular cells with delicate collagen, imparting a myxomatous appearance. The epithelial component is arranged in thin branching cords or small nests with scanty cytoplasm and basophilic nuclei, while stellate reticulum like cells are common in larger nests. Mitoses are not a characteristic feature of ameloblastic fibroma [13]. In contrast to conventional ameloblastoma, the strands of AFs show double or triple layer of cuboidal cells. Numerous mitotic cells or any atypical mitotic figure if noticed suggests a malignant entity such as ameloblastic fibrosarcoma (AFS) in the differential diagnosis [14, 15].

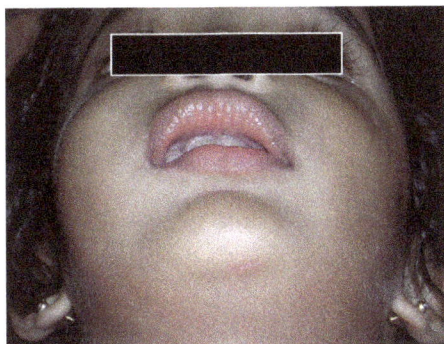

FIGURE 1: Extraoral view showing mild swelling on the right and left mid face.

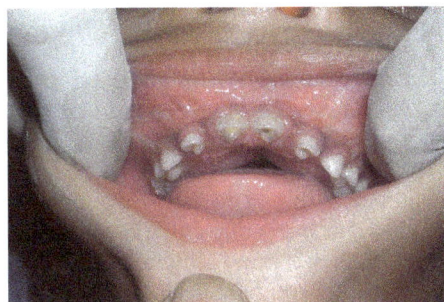

FIGURE 2: Intraoral view showing lobulated, bony hard swelling.

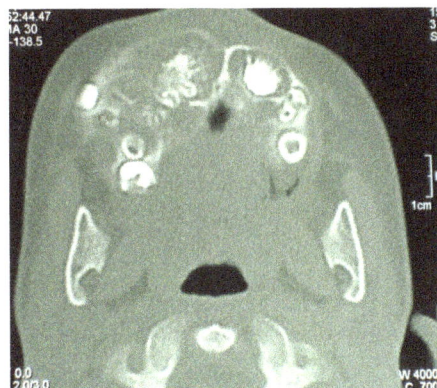

FIGURE 3: CT scan revealing hyperdense mass involving the labial cortex and pterygoid plates.

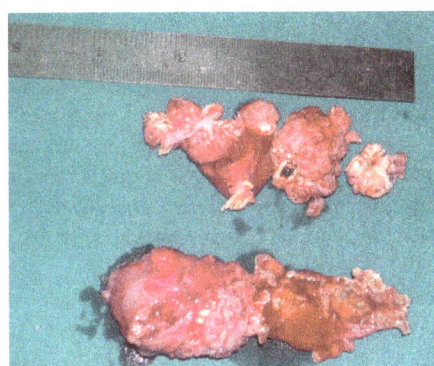

FIGURE 4: Gross picture showing a lobulated and smooth surface.

AFs are usually treated conservatively by enucleation with curettage of the surrounding normal bone, while the aggressive lesions require a radical approach [16]. The present case reports signifies the importance of careful differential diagnosis of intrabony oral lesions with an atypical location.

2. Case Report

A 2-year-old female child patient visited the department of oral and maxillofacial surgery with a complaint of diffuse swelling in the right mid face since one year. The swelling was progressive with gradual increase in size, consequently involving the contralateral side causing a swelling in the left mid facial region after 6 months. Both the swellings exhibited gradual increase in size with evidence of nasal blockage (Figure 1).

On examination, the swellings were diffuse extending on to the zygomatic arch, nontender with no secondary changes. Intraoral examination revealed a nontender, lobulated swelling which was firm to bony hard in consistency (Figure 2). The swelling caused labial and buccal cortical expansion bilaterally and extended up to the pterygoid plates along with palatal bone thickening. The overlying mucosa was intact. The patient's family history revealed that the elder sister, who is currently five years old, had a similar complaint 3 years ago, which was then operated, and a histopathology report of ameloblastic fibroma was rendered. Presently she is free from any recurrence.

Computed tomography with 3D reconstruction was performed which revealed a hyperdense mass involving the labial and buccal cortex and extending up to the pterygoid plates. The palatal bone also showed thickening with irregular surface (Figure 3). Based on the clinical and roentgenographic findings, a presumptive preoperative diagnosis of odontogenic tumor was made. The lesion was excised and curettage of the adjacent maxillary bone was performed under general anesthesia. The surgical specimen was then sent for histopathological analysis. Macroscopically, the specimen measured 3.5 × 1.5 cm in greatest dimension and was firm in consistency with a smooth surface (Figure 4).

Microscopically, the lesion showed proliferation of strands of ameloblastic epithelial cells within a moderately cellular connective tissue stroma that closely simulates the dental papilla. The epithelial islands, nests, and strands were composed of peripheral tall columnar hyperchromatic cells exhibiting reversal of polarity and loosely arranged central cells having angular to spindle shape. The mesenchymal component comprised evenly distributed plump ovoid and stellate cells in a matrix of loose myxoid tissue (Figures 5 and 6).

3. Discussion

Ameloblastic fibroma is a true-mixed neoplasm of odontogenic origin with both epithelial and mesenchymal tissues [4]. These neoplasms are noticed in young patients especially in the first two decades of life [17] and mandible is considered to be the most common site of occurrence than the maxilla by

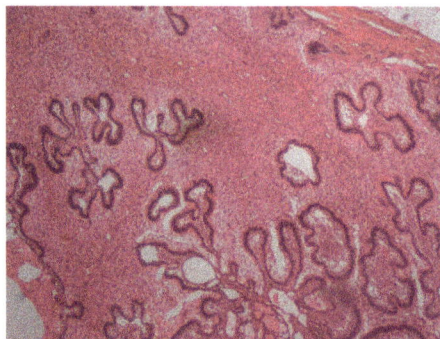

FIGURE 5: Photomicrograph showing ameloblastic islands in a cellular connective tissue stroma.

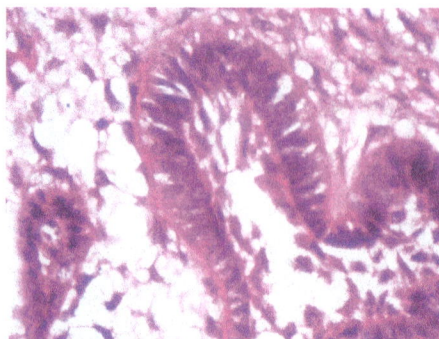

FIGURE 6: Photomicrograph showing tall columnar ameloblasts with reversal of polarity.

a factor 3.1 [18]. Incidence of Maxillary AF is believed to be uncommon by itself; its bilateral presentation is exceedingly rare. To the best of our knowledge, this is the first case presentation of a bilateral maxillary ameloblastic fibroma.

Males are more commonly affected than females, who are usually diagnosed between the first and second decades of life frequently presenting with a painless swelling of the jaw. The present patient was only 2 years old, fitting into the normal spectrum of ameloblastic fibroma, with the youngest age reported in a seven-week-old infant [19].

However, the clinical manifestations of AF are not characteristic and the tumor is frequently observed as an incidental finding in a routine radiographic examination [20]. Normal eruption of the teeth in the affected area is usually altered with more than one-third of cases associated with an impacted tooth [21]. Radiographically they appear unilocular or multilocular with smooth well-demarcated borders [9] which are often misdiagnosed as dentigerous cyst when associated with an impacted tooth. Differential diagnosis of AF must also include entities such as ameloblastoma, odontogenic keratocyst, and ameloblastic fibrosarcoma [12, 13]. Cortical expansion of the affected bone is commonly observed [22] which was noted in the present case elucidating its true neoplastic nature.

Microscopically the epithelial component occupies the mesenchymal stroma in various patterns like thin long strands, cords, nests, or islands. Unlike the strands in ameloblastoma, the strands in AF exhibit double or triple layer of cuboidal cells [23]. The ectomesenchymal component is composed of typical plump fibroblasts with delicate collagen fibrils simulating the dental papilla [24]. The amount of cellularity differs from area to area within the same tumor and between tumors. A narrow cell-free zone bordering the epithelium and juxta-epithelial hyalinization in the connective tissue, which ultrastructurally may represent exuberant basal lamina with or without resemblance to early stage of normal odontogenesis was noted [25, 26].

AFs are classified based on histology as granular cell type, where granular cells predominate in ectomesenchyme, papilliferous with marked proliferation of the epithelium [4], ameloblastoma in association with AF and cystic ameloblastoma [21]. If dentin or enamel were noticed, they are classified as an ameloblastic fibrodentinoma or an ameloblastic

fibroodontoma, respectively. Cahn and Blum proposed the continuum concept by stating that these three mixed tumours were thought to represent various stages of tooth development [27]. There stands a controversy on this spectrum of lesions whether these should be classified as different entities or represent different stages of maturation of the same entity.

The nature of AF still stands enigmatic, as there has been a long debate as to whether ameloblastic fibroma represents a hamartomous growth or is a true benign neoplasm. This controversy further attributes to the difficulties to differentiate between the histology of the neoplastic and the hamartomatous lesions with the histologic features of ameloblastic fibroma [4]. In recent times, it has been proposed that two variants of AF exist, namely, a neoplastic type with no inductive phenomenon and a hamartomatous type revealing inductive capabilities [21]. However, few authors contradicted this view and highlighted the true neoplastic nature by pointing out that AFs are seen in adults (>22 yrs) where odontogenesis is completed and tendency to recur and the recurrent cases do not show further steps of differentiation and potential to turn malignant [24].

AFs show high rate of recurrence with more than 45% turning to malignant ameloblastic fibrosarcoma [24]. In addition to detecting the mitotic figures in the histology, immunohistochemical analysis using ki-67, PCNA, and p53 labelling indices would further aid in delineating AFS from AF [28].

4. Conclusion

A careful treatment planning is necessary considering their recurrence rate and ability to undergo malignant transformation. As it is difficult to differentiate a hamartomatous lesion from a neoplasm based merely on histology, age of the patient should be an important consideration while deciding the treatment plan. Radical therapeutic methods should not be performed in the management of AFs in young patients [29]. Considering the age and high recurrence rate, a long-term follow-up is recommended, particularly in our case where both the siblings were diagnosed with AF necessitating future insight into the genetics.

Conflict of Interests

The authors declare that there is no conflict of interests regarding the publication of this paper.

References

[1] I. R. H. Kramer, J. J. Pindborg, and M. Shear, "The WHO histological typing of odontogenic tumours," *Cancer*, vol. 70, pp. 2988–2994, 1992.

[2] A. Kruse, "Ueber die Entwickelung cystischer Geschwülste im Unterkiefer," *Archiv für Pathologische Anatomie und Physiologie und für Klinische Medicin*, vol. 124, no. 1, pp. 137–148, 1891.

[3] K. H. Thoma and H. M. Goldman, "Odontogenic tumors—a classification based on observations of the epithelial, mesenchymal, and mixed varieties," *The American Journal of Pathology*, vol. 22, no. 3, pp. 433–471, 1946.

[4] P. A. Reichart and H. P. Philipsen, "Ameloblastic fibroma," in *Odontogenic Tumors and Allied Lesions*, p. 121, Quintessence Publishing Co. Ltd., London, UK, 2004.

[5] Y. Takeda, "Ameloblastic fibroma and related lesions: current pathologic concept," *Oral Oncology*, vol. 35, no. 6, pp. 535–540, 1999.

[6] D. M. Cohen and I. Bhattacharyya, "Ameloblastic fibroma, ameloblastic fibro-odontoma, and odontoma," *Oral and Maxillofacial Surgery Clinics of North America*, vol. 16, no. 3, pp. 375–384, 2004.

[7] P. J. Slootweg, "An analysis of the interrelationship of the mixed odontogenic tumors—amelobastic fibroma, ameloblastic fibroodontoma, and the odontomas," *Oral Surgery Oral Medicine and Oral Pathology*, vol. 51, no. 3, pp. 266–276, 1981.

[8] Y. Chen, T. J. Li, Y. Gao, and S. F. Yu, "Ameloblastic fibroma and related lesions: a clinicopathologic study with reference to their nature and interrelationship," *Journal of Oral Pathology and Medicine*, vol. 34, no. 10, pp. 588–595, 2005.

[9] Y. Chen, J.-M. Wang, and T.-J. Li, "Ameloblastic fibroma: a review of published studies with special reference to its nature and biological behavior," *Oral Oncology*, vol. 43, no. 10, pp. 960–969, 2007.

[10] L. Barnes, J. W. Eveson, P. A. Reichart, and P. Sidransky, *Pathology and Genetics of Tumours of the Head and Neck: World Health Organization Classification of Tumours: International Histol Ogical Classification of Tumors*, IARC Press, Lyon, France, 3rd edition, 2005.

[11] R. A. G. Lopez, L. Ortega, M. A. G. Corchon, and A. B. Sandez, "Ameloblastic fibroma of the man dible: report of the two cases," *Medicina Oral*, vol. 8, no. 2, pp. 150–153, 2003.

[12] S. G. Kim and H. S. Jang, "Ameloblastic fibroma: report of a case," *Journal of Oral and Maxillofacial Surgery*, vol. 60, no. 2, pp. 216–218, 2002.

[13] K. Kobayashi, R. Murakami, T. Fujii, and A. Hirano, "Malignant transformation of ameloblastic fibroma to ameloblastic fibrosarcoma: case report and review of the literature," *Journal of Cranio-Maxillofacial Surgery*, vol. 33, no. 5, pp. 352–355, 2005.

[14] C. E. Tomich, "Benign mixed odontogenic tumors," *Seminars in Diagnostic Pathology*, vol. 16, no. 4, pp. 308–316, 1999.

[15] J. A. Regezi, J. J. Sciubba, and R. C. Jordan, *Oral Pathology Clinical Pathologic Correlations*, Elsevier, Amsterdam, The Netherlands, 4th edition, 2003.

[16] R. S. Kulkarni, A. Sarkar, and S. Goyal, "Recurrent ameloblastic fibroma: report of a rare case," *Case Reports in Dentistry*, vol. 2013, Article ID 565721, 4 pages, 2013.

[17] W. G. Shafer, M. K. Hine, and B. M. Levy, "Cysts and tumors of odontogenic origin," in *Shafers Textbook of Oral Pathology*, R. Rajendran and B. Sivapathasundharam, Eds., pp. 402–403, Elsevier, New Delhi, India, 5th edition, 2006.

[18] C. Jindal and R. S. Bhola, "Ameloblastic fibroma in six-year-old male: hamartoma or a true neoplasm," *Journal of Oral and Maxillofacial Pathology*, vol. 15, no. 3, pp. 303–305, 2011.

[19] E. L. Mosby, D. Russell, S. Noren, and B. F. Barker, "Ameloblastic fibroma in a 7-week-old infant: a case report and review of the literature," *Journal of Oral and Maxillofacial Surgery*, vol. 56, no. 3, pp. 368–372, 1998.

[20] D. O. da Costa, A. T. Alves, M. D. Calasans-Maia, R. L. da Cruz, and S. D. Q. C. Lourenço, "Maxillary ameloblastic fibroma: a case report," *Brazilian Dental Journal*, vol. 22, no. 2, pp. 171–174, 2011.

[21] N. J. Mcguinness, T. Faughnan, F. Bennani, and C. E. Connolly, "Ameloblastic fibroma of the anterior maxilla presenting as a complication of tooth eruption: a case report," *Journal of Orthodontics*, vol. 28, no. 2, pp. 115–118, 2001.

[22] B. C. E. Vasconcelos, E. S. S. Andrade, N. S. Rocha, H. H. A. Morais, and R. W. F. Carvalho, "Treatment of large ameloblastic fibroma: a case report," *Journal of Oral Science*, vol. 51, no. 2, pp. 293–296, 2009.

[23] P. A. Reichart and H. P. Philipsen, *Ameloblastic Fibroma. Odontogenic Tumors and Allied Lesions*, Quintessence Publishing Co., Ltd, London, UK, 2004.

[24] B. W. Neville, D. D. Damm, C. M. Allen, and J. E. Bouquot, *Oral and Maxillofacial Pathology*, Elsevier, Amsterdam, The Netherlands, 3rd edition, 2011.

[25] A. G. Farman, A. R. Gould, and E. Merrell, "Epithelium—connective tissue junction in follicular ameloblastoma and ameloblastic fibroma: an ultrastructural analysis," *International Journal of Oral and Maxillofacial Surgery*, vol. 15, no. 2, pp. 176–186, 1986.

[26] C. W. van Wyk and P. C. van der Vyver, "Ameloblastic fibroma with dentinoid formation/immature dentinoma," *Journal of Oral Pathology & Medicine*, vol. 12, no. 1, pp. 37–46, 1983.

[27] L. R. Cahn and T. Blum, "Ameloblastic odontoma: case report critically analyzed," *Journal of Oral Surgery*, vol. 10, pp. 169–170, 1952.

[28] V. F. Bernardes, C. C. Gomes, and R. S. Gomez, "Molecular investigation of ameloblastic fibroma: how far have we gone?" *Head and Neck Oncology*, vol. 4, no. 2, article 45, 2012.

[29] B. L. Nelson and G. S. Folk, "Ameloblastic fibroma," *Head and Neck Pathology*, vol. 3, no. 1, pp. 51–53, 2009.

Invasive Community-Acquired Methicillin-Resistant *Staphylococcus aureus* in a Japanese Girl with Disseminating Multiple Organ Infection: A Case Report and Review of Japanese Pediatric Cases

Ryuta Yonezawa,[1] Tsukasa Kuwana,[2] Kengo Kawamura,[1] and Yasuji Inamo[1]

[1]*Department of Pediatrics and Child Health, Nihon University School of Medicine, 30-1 Oyaguchi-kamimachi, Itabashi-ku, Tokyo 173-8610, Japan*
[2]*Department of Emergency and Critical Care Medicine, Nihon University School of Medicine, 30-1 Oyaguchi-kamimachi, Itabashi-ku, Tokyo 173-8610, Japan*

Correspondence should be addressed to Yasuji Inamo; y-inamo@pb3.so-net.ne.jp

Academic Editor: Maria Moschovi

Pediatric invasive community-acquired methicillin-resistant *Staphylococcus aureus* (CA-MRSA) infection is very serious and occasionally fatal. This infectious disease is still a relatively rare and unfamiliar infectious disease in Japan. We report a positive outcome in a 23-month-old Japanese girl with meningitis, osteomyelitis, fasciitis, necrotizing pneumonia, urinary tract infection, and bacteremia due to CA-MRSA treated with linezolid. PCR testing of the CA-MRSA strain was positive for PVL and staphylococcal enterotoxin b and negative for ACME. SCC *mec* was type IVa. This case underscores the selection of effective combinations of antimicrobial agents for its treatment. We need to be aware of invasive CA-MRSA infection, which rapidly progresses with a serious clinical course, because the incidence of the disease may be increasing in Japan.

1. Introduction

Community-acquired methicillin-resistant *Staphylococcus aureus* (CA-MRSA) has bacteriological and clinical properties different to those of hospital-acquired MRSA. CA-MRSA is classified into staphylococcal cassette chromosome *mec* (SCC *mec*) type IV or type V, which codes a methicillin resistance. The Panton-Valentine leucocidin (PVL) gene of CA-MRSA sometimes occurs, but there is a low occurrence of positivity to this gene in Japan [1]. This infectious disease is very serious and occasionally fatal, regardless of age. However, invasive CA-MRSA infection is still a relatively rare and unfamiliar infectious disease in Japan.

We report the first successfully positive outcome in a 23-month-old Japanese girl with meningitis, osteomyelitis, fasciitis, necrotizing pneumonia, urinary tract infection, and sepsis due to CA-MRSA.

2. Case Presentation

A 23-month-old Japanese girl had presented with a generalized tonic convulsion and pyrexia at a community-based emergency department (ED) 3 days before presentation at our hospital. Her past medical history was unremarkable and she had not recently been hospitalized. On clinical examination at the previous hospital, she had a white cell count of $4900/\mu L$ (stab 17.0%, seg 50.0%, lymph 25.0%, and mono 5.0%) and a C-reactive protein level of 5.88 mg/dL (normal level <0.15 mg/dL). Cerebrospinal fluid (CSF) analysis had been performed with no abnormalities. She was treated with cefotaxime (CTX).

The following morning, MRSA was detected in her blood and urine, and the antimicrobial agent was changed from CTX to vancomycin (VCM) and meropenem (MEPM). However, the CSF was negative. On the third day after admission, she developed swelling in the right femur. Magnetic resonance imaging (MRI) of the right femur revealed necrotizing fasciitis.

She was transferred for further treatment to our hospital at a tertiary emergency department. A computed tomography (CT) scan of the lungs without contrast on admission showed necrotizing pneumonia with multiple nodules and pleural effusion (Figure 1). A CT scan of the brain without contrast was normal. A transthoracic echocardiography did not reveal vegetation or pulmonary embolisms. CSF analysis was performed again and showed a white cell count of 13,603 cells with 914 polymorphonuclear cells/mL, a total protein level of 0.87 g/dL, and a glucose concentration of 50.3 mg/mL (Figure 2). The CSF culture grew MRSA.

LZD and MEPM were started at a dose of 10 mg/kg/day intravenously (IV) every 8 h and 40 mg/kg IV three times daily, respectively. After 3 days of gradual clinical improvement, a gallium-67 citrate scintigraphy and MRI were performed and both showed osteomyelitis of the right femur with necrotizing fasciitis (Figure 3). We continued both antimicrobials until the various infectious lesions had recovered. After 3 weeks of antibiotic therapy, the patient was doing well with significant clinical improvement and no relapse of the infection at 3 months' follow-up. She had no sequelae of invasive CA-MRSA infection or adverse events from the antimicrobials.

Antimicrobial Susceptibility and Genotype Characterization of MRSA Strain. CSF culture grew MRSA. The strain was sensitive to arbekacin, gentamicin, VCM, linezolid (LZD), daptomycin, sulfamethoxazole/trimethoprim, and levofloxacin and resistant to oxacillin, using the broth microdilution method. VCM, LZD, and MEPM MICs were 1.0, 1.0, and 0.25 μg/mL, respectively. Polymerase chain reaction testing of the MRSA strain was positive for Panton-Valentine leucocidin (PVL) and staphylococcal enterotoxin b (*seb*) and negative for arginine catabolic mobile element (ACME). The staphylococcal cassette chromosome (SCC) *mec* type was IVa.

3. Discussion

CA-MRSA has bacteriological and clinical properties different to those of hospital-acquired MRSA (HA-MRSA). HA-MRSA infections are usually defined as MRSA infection in a patient with one of the following risk factors for HA-MRSA: isolation of MRSA ≥2 days after hospitalization; a history of hospitalization, surgery, dialysis, or residence in a long-term care facility within 1 year before the MRSA-culture date; the presence of a permanent indwelling catheter or percutaneous medical procedure at the time of culture; or previous isolation of MRSA [2]. HA-MRSA strains tend to have multidrug resistance and carry SCC *mec* type II or SCC *mec* type III [3]. HA-MRSA strains are typified by a USA100 or USA200 pulsed field gel electrophoresis pattern [4].

CA-MRSA commonly causes skin and soft tissue infections in previously healthy children. CA-MRSA infection is well known in many countries and has become common in the United States, Taiwan, Canada, European countries, and Australia. CA-MRSA is also classified into SCC *mec* type IV

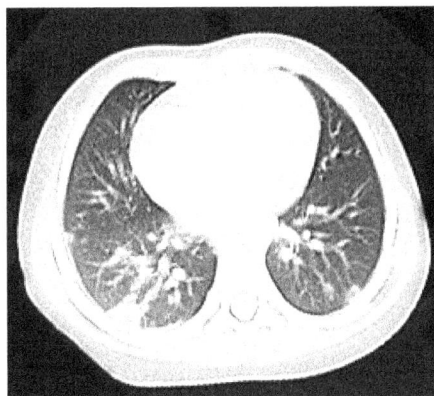

FIGURE 1: Computed tomography scan of the lungs without contrast showing necrotizing pneumonia with multiple nodules and pleural effusion on admission.

or type V, which codes a methicillin resistance. A Japanese nationwide survey showed the incidence of SCC *mec* type IV in positive CA-MRSA as only 2.3% [1]. Japanese ST8 CA-MRSA with SCC *mec* type IVl (ST8 CA-MRSA/J) has emerged in Japan since 2003 and become well adapted to the Japanese community. This strain was negative for PVL and ACME and positive for superantigen (*spa* variants, SaPI), but not enterotoxin gene cluster, egc (*seg*, *sei*, *sem*, *sen*, and *seo*) and enterotoxin u (*seu*). Most strains were resistant to gentamicin [5]. CA-MRSA clones have been genetically reported among countries: ST1-IV (USA400), ST8-IV (USA300), ST30-IV (Southwest Pacific clone also predominant in Japan), ST59 (Taiwan clone), and ST80 (European clone) clones have been predominant.

There are reports of pediatric deaths from Waterhouse-Friderichsen syndrome [6] and pediatric death from CA-MRSA-associated meningitis in the literature [7].

It is important to prevent more severe and disseminated multiple organ involvement because about 20% of invasive CA-MRSA infection remains bacteremic [8].

Despite the PVL, which is known as a strong virulence factor, invasive CA-MRSA infectious disease is severe regardless of PVL positivity or negativity [9, 10] and very serious and occasionally fatal, regardless of age. However, invasive CA-MRSA infection is still a relatively rare and unfamiliar infectious disease in Japan and even in countries that are experienced in CA-MRSA infection [11, 12].

Invasive CA-MRSA infection should be suspected when CA-MRSA is detected from sterile samples such as blood, CSF, and pleural effusion. The disease, which leads to complications such as meningitis, osteomyelitis, fasciitis, necrotizing pneumonia, urinary tract infection, and sepsis, is a critical and serious infection.

Although invasive CA-MRSA infection is still rare worldwide, the infectious disease incidence has gradually increased. The occurrence of pediatric invasive CA-MRSA infectious disease in the United States was 1.1/100,000 persons/year in 2005 and 1.7/100,000 persons/year in 2010 [8]. However, pediatric invasive CA-MRSA infectious disease is rare in Japan and it is difficult to measure its correspondence

		1	2	3	4	5	6	7	8	9	10	21
		Convulsion ↓										
				Pneumonia								
				Meningitis								
		UTI										
		Bacteremia										
		Pyrexia		Fasciitis/osteomyelitis								
		CTX			MEPM							
			VCM		LZD							
				↓ Referral								
Onset day		1	2	3	4	5	6	7	8	9	10	21
WBC and biomarker	WBC	4,900	4,600	7,100	10,100	14,800		14,300	14,300		6,700	
	CRP	5.88	12.62	7.23	4.72	2.63		0.95	0.54		0.94	
	PCT			22.9	11.24	5.66		1.44	0.72		0.12	
CSF	Protein	11.0		87.0				19.0				
	Glucose	94.0		53.0				64.0				
	Cell/3	4		1,363				7				
	M : P	3 : 1		108 : 914				19 : 2				
Urinalysis	Protein	1+	–									
	Blood	2+	–									
	RBCs/hpf	100	–									
	WBCs/hpf	10–19	–									

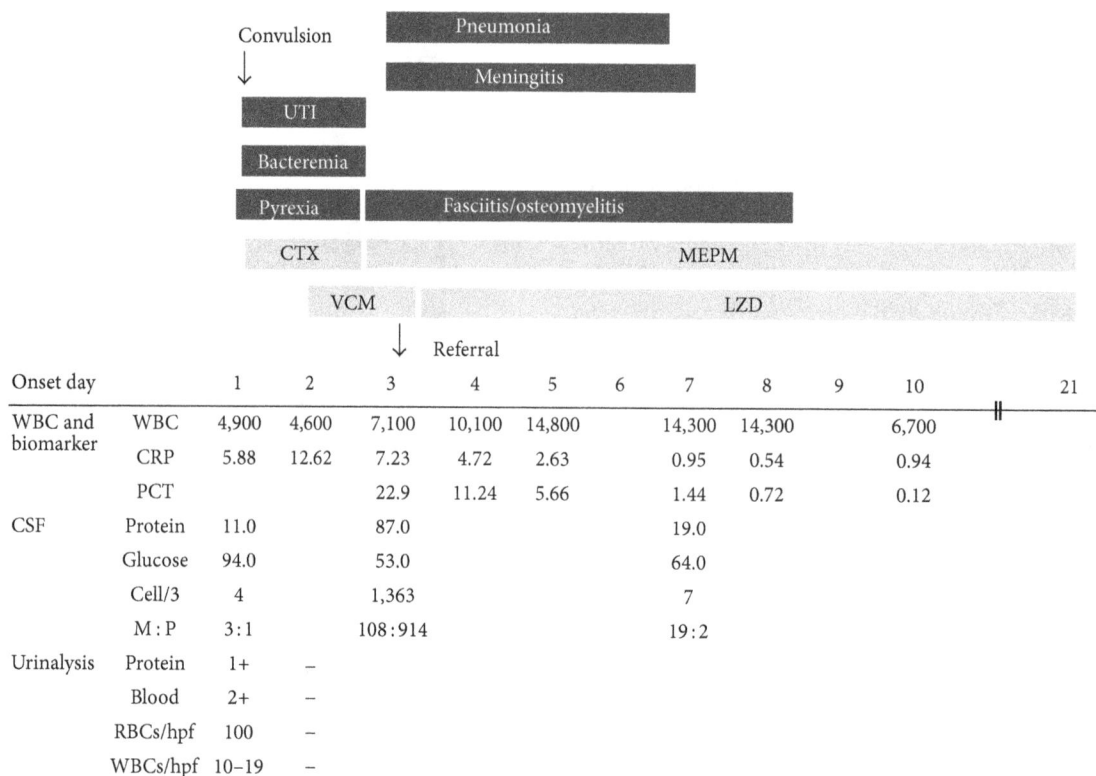

FIGURE 2: Clinical course of a 23-month-old Japanese girl with meningitis, osteomyelitis, fasciitis, necrotizing pneumonia, urinary tract infection, and sepsis due to community-acquired methicillin-resistant *Staphylococcus aureus*. UTI, urinary tract infection; PCT, procalcitonin; VCM, vancomycin (55 mg/kg/day); LZD, linezolid (30 mg/kg/day); CTX, cefotaxime (100 mg/kg/day); MEPM, meropenem (120 mg/kg/day).

to the incidence of CA-MRSA infection. The first pediatric case report of PVL-positive CA-MRSA in Japan was of the death of a 1-year-old patient with severe pneumonia in 2008 [13], the second involved a case report of the death of a 2-year-old patient with severe pneumonia due to PVL-positive CA-MRSA [14], and the third case was the current case involving a positive outcome (Table 1).

The MRSA strain isolated in our study, which was positive for PVL and staphylococcal enterotoxin b (*seb*) and negative for ACME, is a rare molecular characteristic and had not been described before in Japan.

Interestingly, the MRSA strain of the first Japanese case report was positive for PVL and staphylococcal enterotoxin u (*seu*) and enterotoxin gene cluster including seg, sei, sem, sen, and seo genes and negative for ACME [13]. We emphasize that neither our case nor the first case was ST8 CA-MRSA/J. It is possible that this particular isolate has a greater propensity for developing invasive CA-MRSA infection in that it secretes double virulence factors, which are PVL and superantigen.

When infection affects multiple organs in a clinical course, invasive CA-MRSA infection should be considered. Early detection of invasive CA-MRSA in clinical practice is important to prevent a progressively worse outcome. Necrotizing pneumonia, which is caused by invasive CA-MRSA, rapidly develops to respiratory failure with multiple cavities and nodules and pleural effusion in chest X-ray imaging. Invasive CA-MRSA infection is characterized by frequent complications of osteomyelitis and soft tissue infection. When MRSA is detected, we can determine whether it is CA-MRSA according to the circumstances of MRSA detection, for example, from outpatients, detection within 48 hours of admission, no history of MRSA carrier, little antimicrobial response of skin/soft tissue infection, or outbreaks of MRSA in families, nurseries, or sports clubs. The antimicrobial sensitivity of the detected MRSA is different from HA-MRSA and should be rediagnosed as CA-MRSA.

Antibiotics are important to prevent more severe and disseminated multiple organ involvement. Another purpose of antimicrobial therapy is to inhibit production of enterotoxins and PVL, so initial selection of antibiotics can influence the outcome. However, in general, invasive CA-MRSA infection is not familiar to ED physicians. Although early suspicion and/or detection of a rapidly progressive invasive CA-MRSA in a previously healthy child in emergency practice is important, initial empirical therapy for common pediatric infectious diseases in Japan is penicillin or cephalosporin. If a patient suffers from more than one organ infection such as necrotizing pneumonia and fasciitis at their first visit, invasive CA-MRSA is strongly suspected. Empiric therapy such as anti-MRSA antibiotics may be considered [15].

The more severe invasive infections complicated with meningitis have been successfully treated with LZD but not VCM in some case reports [16–20]. Our patient's CSF analysis and CSF culture had no abnormalities at the time of illness

TABLE 1: The review of Japanese pediatric cases with severe CA-MRSA infection.

	Case 1	Case 2	Our case
Age	16-month-old boy	24-month-old boy	23-month-old girl
Reported year	2006	2013	2014
Meningitis	−	−	+
Necrotizing pneumonia	+	+	+
Urinary tract infection	−	−	+
Osteomyelitis	−	−	+
Fasciitis	−	−	+
Bacteremia	+	NA	+
Septic shock	+	+	−
Panton-Valentine leucocidin (PVL)	+	+	+
Cassette chromosome *mec* (SCC *mec*)	IVa	NA	IVa
Staphylococcal enterotoxins	*egc** (+) *seu* (+)	NA	*seb* (+)
Arginine catabolic mobile element (ACME)	Negative	NA	Negative
Initial antimicrobials	SBT/ABPC + CTX	ABPC	CTX
Antimicrobials after MRSA determined	VCM + MEPM	Already dead	VCM/LZD + MEPM
Outcome	Died	Died	Survived

*egc**, enterotoxin gene cluster, including seg, sei, sem, sen, and seo genes.
SBT/ABPC, sulbactam/ampicillin; CTX, cefotaxime; MEPM, meropenem; LZD, linezolid; VCM, vancomycin.

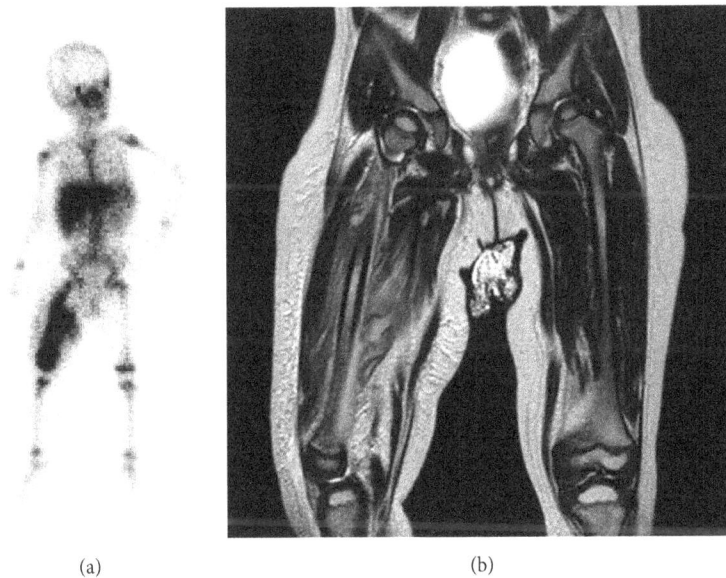

(a)   (b)

FIGURE 3: Gallium-67 citrate scintigraphy showing isolated uptake of the right femur (a) and magnetic resonance imaging scans of the right femur showing osteomyelitis with necrotizing fasciitis (T2-weighted image). There are signal changes in the diaphyseal region of the femurs with circumferential soft tissue involvement (b).

onset despite the presence of convulsions. However, meningitis was detected after 3 days during VCM therapy. Meningitis may have already been developing at the time of the convulsions and was not prevented by VCM. Although there is little consensus for administering LZD [15] and it is used in an off-label manner for meningitis and osteoarticular infections in Japan, ED physicians should consider LZD on VCM failure.

VCM is common for meningitis, but its CSF penetration (CSF to serum ratios) is not particularly high. The percentage of penetration of CSF to serum is 20% in the nonmeningitis phase and 50% in the active meningitis phase [16]. The mainstay of treatment traditionally has been VCM, but there have been a few cases of VCM failure. Data on patients with meningitis treated with LZD therapy are limited, but the LZD percentage penetration of CSF to serum is 70%. There are some cases of complete recovery from meningitis with LZD treatment [21]. Although VCM is the first choice for invasive CA-MRSA infection, LZD may be a better first-line choice for meningitis or in the presence of CNS signs including convulsion and unconsciousness and symptoms of meningitis prior to development of the disease from a viewpoint of CSF penetration.

Although VCM is a first-line antibiotic in pediatric CA-MRSA infection and LZD is second line, there is still no consensus on the management of severe invasive infection. Because there are no published data to generalize recommendation of linezolid use in pediatric meningitis, a clinical study of LZD in CA-MRSA meningitis should be performed to collect prospective data on CA-MRSA meningitis patients and to further determine the efficacy of LZD treatment of CA-MRSA meningitis.

In conclusion, we reported the diagnosis, management, and successful outcome of a female patient with rapidly progressive and severe invasive CA-MRSA infection. The ED physician should be aware of invasive CA-MRSA infection, which follows a life-threatening clinical course, because appropriate antimicrobial treatment is crucial for improving the prognosis.

Abbreviations

MRSA: Methicillin-resistant *Staphylococcus aureus*
CA-MRSA: Community-acquired methicillin-resistant *S. aureus*
CTX: Cefotaxime
PVL: Panton-Valentine leucocidin
ACME: Arginine catabolic mobile element
VCM: Vancomycin
MEPM: Meropenem
LZD: Linezolid.

Conflict of Interests

The authors have no conflict of interests to disclose.

Authors' Contribution

Ryuta Yonezawa (pediatrician) and Tsukasa Kuwana (emergency physician) shared equally in the interpretation of the clinical data and therapy decisions as equal contributors. Kengo Kawamura (pediatrician) treated and planned the management of the patient. Yasuji Inamo conceived the idea and wrote and edited the final paper. All authors read and approved the final paper.

Acknowledgments

The authors gratefully thank Dr. Yuki Uehara (Department of Infection Control Science/General Medicine attached to Juntendo University Faculty of Medicine, Tokyo, Japan) who performed the genotypic characterization of the MRSA strain and Michiko Yagoshi, Ph.D. (Department of Clinical Laboratory, Nihon University School of Medicine, Tokyo, Japan), who performed the microbiological characterization of the MRSA strain. Dr. Kousaku Kinoshita (Department of Emergency and Critical Care Medicine, Nihon University School of Medicine) and Dr. Shori Takahashi (Department of Pediatrics and Child Health, Nihon University School of Medicine) were involved in drafting the paper.

References

[1] K. Yanagihara, N. Araki, S. Watanabe et al., "Antimicrobial susceptibility and molecular characteristics of 857 methicillin-resistant *Staphylococcus aureus* isolates from 16 medical centers in Japan (2008-2009): nationwide survey of community-acquired and nosocomial MRSA," *Diagnostic Microbiology and Infectious Disease*, vol. 72, no. 3, pp. 253–257, 2012.

[2] S. K. Fridkin, J. C. Hageman, M. Morrison et al., "Methicillin-resistant Staphylococcus aureus disease in three communities," *The New England Journal of Medicine*, vol. 352, no. 14, pp. 1436–1505, 2005.

[3] S. Deresinski, "Methicillin-resistant *Staphylococcus aureus*: an evolutionary, epidemiologic, and therapeutic odyssey," *Clinical Infectious Diseases*, vol. 40, no. 4, pp. 562–573, 2005.

[4] L. K. McDougal, C. D. Steward, G. E. Killgore, J. M. Chaitram, S. K. McAllister, and F. C. Tenover, "Pulsed-field gel electrophoresis typing of oxacillin-resistant *Staphylococcus aureus* isolates from the United States: establishing a national database," *Journal of Clinical Microbiology*, vol. 41, no. 11, pp. 5113–5120, 2003.

[5] Y. Iwao, R. Ishii, Y. Tomita et al., "The emerging ST8 methicillin-resistant *Staphylococcus aureus* clone in the community in Japan: associated infections, genetic diversity, and comparative genomics," *Journal of Infection and Chemotherapy*, vol. 18, no. 2, pp. 228–240, 2012.

[6] P. V. Adem, C. P. Montgomery, A. N. Husain et al., "Staphylococcus aureus sepsis and the Waterhouse-Friderichsen syndrome in children," *The New England Journal of Medicine*, vol. 353, no. 12, pp. 1245–1251, 2005.

[7] CDC, "Four pediatric deaths from community-acquired methicillin-resistant *Staphylococcus aureus*—Minnesota and North Dakota, 1997–1999," *Morbidity and Mortality Weekly Report*, vol. 48, no. 32, pp. 707–710, 1999.

[8] M. Iwamoto, Y. Mu, R. Lynfield et al., "Trends in invasive methicillin-resistant *Staphylococcus aureus* infections," *Pediatrics*, vol. 132, no. 4, pp. e817–e824, 2013.

[9] Y. Qiao, X. Ning, Q. Chen et al., "Clinical and molecular characteristics of invasive community-acquired *Staphylococcus aureus* infections in *Chinese children*," *BMC Infectious Diseases*, vol. 14, article 582, 2014.

[10] M. Otto, "A MRSA-terious enemy among us: end of the PVL controversy?" *Nature Medicine*, vol. 17, no. 2, pp. 169–170, 2011.

[11] J. Chen, Y. Luo, S. Zhang et al., "Community-acquired necrotizing pneumonia caused by methicillin-resistant *Staphylococcus aureus* producing Panton-Valentine leukocidin in a Chinese teenager: case report and literature review," *International Journal of Infectious Diseases*, vol. 26, pp. e17–e21, 2014.

[12] C. Nourse, M. Starr, and W. Munckhof, "Community-acquired methicillin-resistant *Staphylococcus aureus* causes severe disseminated infection and deep venous thrombosis in children: literature review and recommendations for management," *Journal of Paediatrics and Child Health*, vol. 43, no. 10, pp. 656–661, 2007.

[13] T. Ito, M. Iijima, T. Fukushima et al., "Pediatric pneumonia death caused by community-acquired methicillin-resistant

Staphylococcus aureus, Japan," *Emerging Infectious Diseases*, vol. 14, no. 8, pp. 1312–1314, 2008.

[14] T. S. T. Takano, R. Tanaka, T. Ohishi, Y. Dantsuji, and H. Hanaki, "A case in PVL possitive MRSA fatal pneumonia with septic shock," *Kansensyogaku Zasshi*, vol. 87, no. 1, p. 172, 2013.

[15] C. Liu, A. Bayer, S. E. Cosgrove et al., "Clinical practice guidelines by the infectious diseases society of America for the treatment of methicillin-resistant *Staphylococcus aureus* infections in adults and children," *Clinical Infectious Diseases*, vol. 52, no. 3, pp. e18–e55, 2011.

[16] R. Naesens, M. Ronsyn, P. Druwé, O. Denis, M. Ieven, and A. Jeurissen, "Central nervous system invasion by community-acquired meticillin-resistant *Staphylococcus aureus*," *Journal of Medical Microbiology*, vol. 58, no. 9, pp. 1247–1251, 2009.

[17] C. Gouveia, A. Gavino, O. Bouchami et al., "Community-associated methicillin-resistant *Staphylococcus aureus* lacking PVL, as a cause of severe invasive infection treated with linezolid," *Case Reports in Pediatrics*, vol. 2013, Article ID 727824, 5 pages, 2013.

[18] O. R. Sipahi, S. Bardak, T. Turhan et al., "Linezolid in the treatment of methicillin-resistant staphylococcal post-neurosurgical meningitis: a series of 17 cases," *Scandinavian Journal of Infectious Diseases*, vol. 43, no. 10, pp. 757–764, 2011.

[19] L. P. Gianni Gattuso, D. Tomasoni, F. Ferri, and A. Scalzini, "A case of community-acquired MRSA (CA-MRSA) sepsis complicated by meningoencephalitis and cerebral abscess, successfully treated with linezolid," *Le Infezioni in Medicina*, vol. 4, no. 4, pp. 244–248, 2009.

[20] R. G. Spini, V. Ferraris, M. P. Glasman, G. Orofino, A. Casanovas, and G. Debaisi, "Methicillin resistant *Staphylococcus aureus* community acquired meningitis. A case report," *Archivos Argentinos de Pediatría*, vol. 112, no. 6, pp. e266–e268, 2014.

[21] A. T. Kessler and A. P. Kourtis, "Treatment of meningitis caused by methicillin-resistant *Staphylococcus aureus* with linezolid," *Infection*, vol. 35, no. 4, pp. 271–274, 2007.

35

Clinical and Imaging Features of a Congenital Midline Cervical Cleft in a Neonate: A Rare Anomaly

Rachelle Goldfisher,[1] **Pritish Bawa,**[1] **Zachary Ibrahim,**[2] **and John Amodio**[1]

[1]*Department of Radiology, SUNY Downstate Medical Center, 450 Clarkson Avenue, Brooklyn, NY 11203, USA*
[2]*Department of Pediatrics, SUNY Downstate Medical Center, 450 Clarkson Avenue, Brooklyn, NY 11203, USA*

Correspondence should be addressed to John Amodio; john.amodio@downstate.edu

Academic Editor: Nan-Chang Chiu

Congenital midline cervical cleft (CMCC) is a rare congenital anomaly. CMCC and its complications and treatment have been well described in ENT, dermatology, and pediatric surgery literature. However, to our knowledge, the imaging work-up has not been reported in the literature thus far. We present a case of CMCC in a neonate with description of clinical presentation and imaging features.

1. Introduction

Congenital midline cervical cleft was first described in 1848 by Luschka [1]; however, it was not fully described until Ombredanne in 1946 [2] explained in his textbook of pediatric surgery. CMCC is uncommon and its diagnosis is usually made on clinical examination. Occasionally, however, CMCC may be confused with a thyroglossal duct or branchial anomaly. The treatment of congenital midline cervical cleft is surgery. To avoid complications of longstanding congenital midline clefts such as limitation of extension of neck or impairment of mandibular growth, early intervention is recommended [3].

Imaging may be requested to differentiate CMCC from these lesions or to determine any coexisting lesions [4]. Magnetic resonance imaging (MRI) is the best modality to determine the extent of the tract, associated ENT anomalies and for presurgical planning.

We present a case of CMCC in a neonate with description of clinical presentation and imaging features.

2. Case Presentation

A full term male neonate was born at 38 weeks of gestation with birth weight of 3465 grams. The infant's mother was a 20-year-old African American female with a history of obesity and pregnancy induced hypertension. Otherwise there was no history of tobacco, drug, or alcohol abuse and all the routine prenatal laboratory tests were normal.

At birth, the child was examined and noted to have a linear craniocaudal pink track in the anterior neck with a skin tag arising from its superior aspect (Figure 1). No discharge was present from the track. A fibrous subcutaneous cord could be palpated beneath the track.

Because of the presence of a cervical cleft an MRI was requested to evaluate the cleft and to look for its internal extension and associated anomalies in the neck.

MRI with contrast was performed which demonstrated a defect in the cutaneous/subcutaneous soft tissues in the midline anterior neck, anterior to the strap muscles. The defect measured 2 cm in craniocaudal dimension and 0.5 cm in its width. It demonstrated low T1 and T2 signal and extended from the level of hyoid bone caudally to the level of manubrium (Figures 2, 3, and 4). No enhancement was seen in postgadolinium images. No extension to the sternum or connection with the deeper soft tissues was identified. The thyroid was normal in location, size, and enhancement. No cyst was identified in relation to thyroid or thyroglossal duct.

3. Discussion

Congenital midline cervical cleft (CMCC) is a rare congenital anomaly, which is thought to be due to failure of fusion of

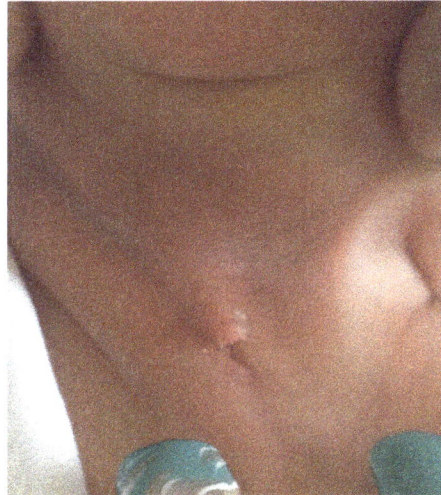

FIGURE 1: Linear craniocaudal pink track in the anterior neck with a skin tag arising from its superior aspect.

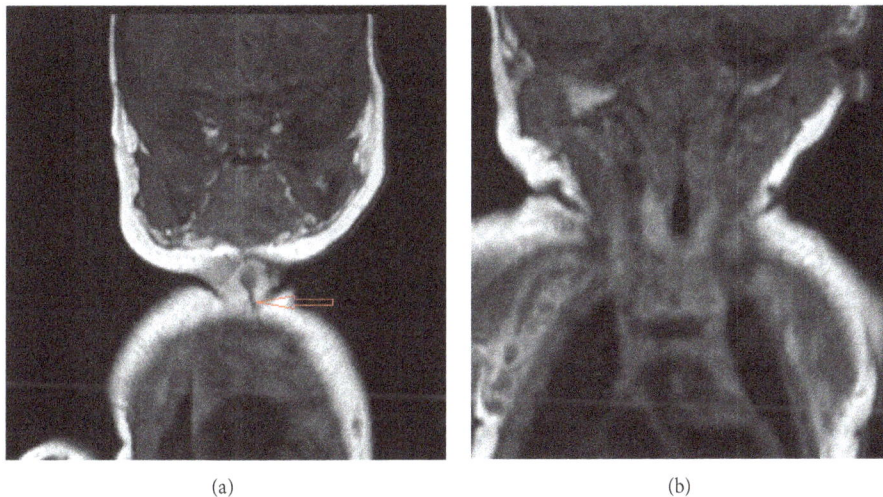

(a)   (b)

FIGURE 2: (a) Coronal T1 weighted MR image of neck demonstrates low T1 signal vertical midline cleft in cutaneous/subcutaneous region (open red arrow). (b) Coronal T1 image demonstrates normal right and left lobes of the thyroid.

the first and second branchial arches during embryogenesis [4]. Less than 100 cases have been reported in the English literature. Most of the cases are reported to be sporadic in Caucasian females with female to male ratio of 2 : 1 [3]. The cleft is located in midline of the anterior neck anywhere between the mandible and the sternum. It may present as a midline defect of the anterior neck skin with a skin projection or sinus or as a subcutaneous fibrous cord. Although not a finding in our patient, at birth, the area often has a discharge [5] and is covered by thin often desquamating epithelium. Over the next few months the epithelium toughens and dries up. Histologically, the lesion consists of skeletal muscle, a fibrous cord, and exocrine tissues [6].

An incidence of 1-2% of congenital cervical malformations has been described in various case series; these include absence of thyroid, ectopic thyroid or thyroglossal duct cyst, ectopic bronchogenic cyst, branchial cyst, midline hemangioma, midline abdominal web, ectopia cordis, clefts

of the lip, chin, tongue, mandible, or sternum, absence of hyoid bone or thyroid cartilage, and rarely congenital cardiac anomalies [6]. Our case had none of the other associations. Ultrasound is sometimes used as a first line imaging modality for other cervical anomalies. However, the full extent of the cervical tract and possible associated anomalies is best demonstrated with MRI. MRI is also useful for presurgical planning.

As the child grows or if there is inadequate repair, the fibrous cord becomes more conspicuous and can lead to contractures of the neck, torticollis, or limited extension [6]. Due to traction on the mandible, a bony prominence of the mandible can be palpated and exostosis of mandible or sternum can be seen on radiographs and/or MRI. Thus an early diagnosis is critical to avoid these complications.

Antibiotics may be required to treat infections or abscesses of congenital midline cervical clefts. Treatment is usually surgical excision and closure of the defect. Although

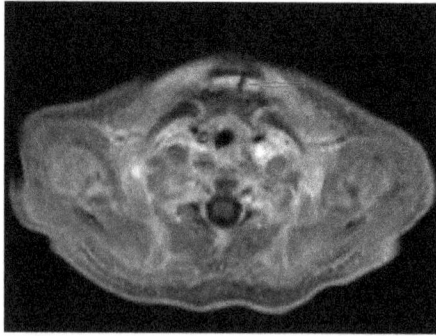

FIGURE 3: Postgadolinium fat saturated T1 axial MR image of the neck shows midline low T1 signal blind ending cleft in the skin/subcutaneous fat (red open arrow).

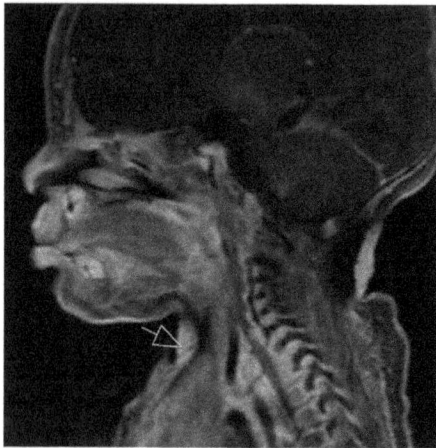

FIGURE 4: Sagittal T1, postgadolinium image shows small cervical tract (arrow) which terminates within the soft tissues and with no extension into deeper structures of the neck.

exact time and technique of surgery are variable in different reports, most of the authors advocate earliest possible intervention for best results. Z-plasty incisions are recommended especially in cases of delayed presentation in order to prevent the development of scar and subsequent cicatrices contractures [6]. Primary anastomosis has been used with some success in patients with small clefts [7].

In summary, a congenital cervical cleft is a rare anomaly. A small number of these are associated with other midline anomalies of the head and neck and the chest. MRI is a useful modality for demonstrating the extent of the cleft, determining if there are any other associated anomalies, and it may be useful for presurgical planning for repair.

Conflict of Interests

The authors declare that there is no conflict of interests regarding the publication of this paper.

References

[1] H. von Luschka, "Ueber fistula colli congenita," *Archiv für Physiologische Heilkunde*, vol. 7, pp. 24–27, 1848.

[2] L. Ombredanne, *Precis Clinique et Operatoire de Chirurgie Infantile*, Masson, Paris, France, 5th edition, 1949.

[3] S. Hirokawa, H. Uotani, H. Okami, K. Tsukada, T. Futatani, and I. Hashimoto, "A case of congenital midline cervical cleft with congenital heart disease," *Journal of Pediatric Surgery*, vol. 38, no. 7, pp. 1099–1101, 2003.

[4] J. P. Eastlack, R. M. Howard, and I. J. Frieden, "Congenital midline cervical cleft: case report and review of the English language literature," *Pediatric Dermatology*, vol. 17, no. 2, pp. 118–122, 2000.

[5] F. H. J. Van der Staak, M. Pruszczynski, R. S. V. M. Severijnen, C. A. Van de Kaa, and C. Festen, "The midline cervical cleft," *Journal of Pediatric Surgery*, vol. 26, no. 12, pp. 1391–1393, 1991.

[6] T. J. Gargan, M. McKinnon, and J. B. Mulliken, "Midline cervical cleft," *Plastic and Reconstructive Surgery*, vol. 76, no. 2, pp. 225–229, 1985.

[7] C. W. McInnes, A. D. Benson, C. G. Verchere, J. P. Ludemann, and J. S. Arneja, "Management of congenital midline cervical cleft," *Journal of Craniofacial Surgery*, vol. 23, no. 1, pp. e36–e38, 2012.

36

45,X/47,XXX Mosaicism and Short Stature

Erica Everest,[1,2] **Laurie A. Tsilianidis,**[1] **Anzar Haider,**[1] **Douglas G. Rogers,**[1] **Nouhad Raissouni,**[1] **and Bahareh Schweiger**[1]

[1]*Cleveland Clinic, 9500 Euclid Avenue, Cleveland, OH 44195, USA*
[2]*Case Western Reserve University School of Medicine, 10900 Euclid Avenue, Cleveland, OH 44106, USA*

Correspondence should be addressed to Erica Everest; ericaeverest@gmail.com

Academic Editor: Ozgur Cogulu

We describe the case of a ten-year-old girl with short stature and 45,X/47,XXX genotype. She also suffered from vesicoureteric reflux and kidney dysfunction prior to having surgery on her ureters. Otherwise, she does not have any of the characteristics of Turner nor Triple X syndrome. It has been shown that this mosaic condition as well as other varieties creates a milder phenotype than typical Turner syndrome, which is what we mostly see in our patient. However, this patient is a special case, because she is exceptionally short. Overall, one cannot predict the resultant phenotype in these mosaic conditions. This creates difficulty in counseling parents whose children or fetuses have these karyotypes.

1. Introduction

Turner syndrome (TS) is a condition characterized by short stature (nearly all girls are <5 feet tall), sexual underdevelopment, a webbed neck, and cubitus valgus (forearm angled away from the body), resulting from a 45,X cell line [1, 2]. Further features may include edema of the hands and feet, characteristic facies, high palate, and short fourth metacarpals [3, 4]. Additionally, renal abnormalities, such as horseshoe kidney, can cause serious health problems [5]. Most concerning are the cardiac abnormalities, such as dilated aortic root, which occur in half of the patients [6]. Women with TS are unlikely to conceive spontaneously, but if they do they are at a high risk of losing the pregnancy or having a baby with congenital anomalies or sex chromosome abnormalities [7]. TS occurs in 1 in 2000 female births [8].

Triple X syndrome is the most common female chromosomal abnormality, occurring in approximately 1 in 1,000 female births, and a review by Tartaglia et al. reveals the subsequent features of the condition [9]. Its most common characteristics are tall stature (>75th percentile), epicanthal folds, clinodactyly, and hypotonia. Possible additional problems can be seizures, renal and genitourinary abnormalities, and premature ovarian failure. The onset of puberty, sexual development, and fertility are usually normal. Also,

more common than in the general population are delays and psychological issues, motor and speech delays, learning disabilities, attention deficits, and mood disorders. There is considerable variation in the phenotype with this disorder. This is reflected by the fact that only 10% of cases are diagnosed clinically.

Mosaic forms of TS tend to have improved prognoses and milder phenotypes. The improved growth and ovarian function of 45,X/46,XX patients over 45,X patients have been well established, and the rarer karyotype 45,X/47,XXX (about 2% of those with TS) also results in more mildly affected girls [10]. The study from Glasgow, Scotland, evaluated the seven 45,X/47,XXX girls registered in the Scottish Turner Syndrome database. Three of the seven subjects did not require growth hormone to achieve a satisfactory height, in comparison to the 45,X and 45,X/46,Xi(X)(q10) matched subjects, all 21 of whom required growth hormone. Additionally, all the 45,X/47,XXX subjects underwent spontaneous puberty, and all five of those older than twelve had spontaneous menarche with regular menstrual cycles. Only 2 of the 14 girls in the 45,X comparison group had spontaneous puberty, and none achieved menarche without the use of estrogen. This is consistent with previous findings [11, 12]. Also, none of the 45,X/47,XXX girls had cardiac or renal abnormalities, though two had middle ear issues. This is in contrast to the 13 of 21 matched subjects with abnormalities to the heart, renal system, or both and is in contrast to the 15 of 21 girls with middle ear issues. The study also had a geneticist, who was blinded to the genotype of the subjects, evaluate for dysmorphic features. 45,X/47,XXX subjects had the most mild expression. Lastly, none of the 45,X/47,XXX subjects had special education needs, in contrast to four in the comparison group. It appears that the haploinsufficiency from the single X chromosome in 45,X is mitigated by the overtranscription of the X chromosome that results from having a 47,XXX cell line [10].

We report a case of a ten-year-old girl with short stature and a history of renal and urinary tract issues. She is a 45,X/47,XXX mosaic. Overall, she represents a mild phenotype, in the fact that she is experiencing few of the Turner stigmata. However, she has significant short stature, and this has not been previously well reported.

2. Case Presentation

A ten-year-three-month-old female presented to the Pediatric Endocrinology Clinic for assessment of short stature. At a height of 4 feet and weight of 51 pounds, she is at the 0.54 and 0.86 percentiles for the CDC 2–20-year stature-for-age and weight-for-age data, respectively. Her parents are of typical height; her mother is $5'5''$ (and had menarche at age 12), and her father is $5'11''$. Her past medical history includes vesicoureteric reflux, urinary tract infections, and decreased kidney function. She was treated with Bactrim from 10 weeks to 3 years for vesicoureteric reflux. She had surgery on her ureters in 2008. She has Tanner stage 1 pubic hair and breasts, normal genitalia, and no axillary hair. She has had body odor and acne for a few years. Neither the review of systems nor the physical examination revealed anything out of the ordinary. She is a fifth grader, who is performing well in school.

Laboratory data showed a normal complete blood count and comprehensive metabolic panel. TSH was 2.260 μU/mL (0.400–5.500 μU/mL) and free T4 was 1.3 ng/dL (0.7–1.8 ng/dL). Transglutaminase antibody (tTG) was 1 unit (normal <20 units). Insulin-like growth factor I was 243 ng/mL (76–478 ng/mL). Bone age was read and interpreted as 8 years 10 months according to the standards of Greulich and Pyle [13], which is considered a normal bone age.

Given the normal thyroid function levels, hypothyroidism is not the cause of her growth failure. Celiac disease is also an unlikely cause of her growth failure, because she did not report abdominal symptoms and her tTG was normal. Normal IGF-1 makes growth hormone (GH) deficiency less likely, because GH stimulates IGF-1 production, but does not necessarily exclude it. Despite the patient not having any of the other stigmata of TS, we ordered a karyotype, because sometimes poor growth is the only presenting symptom.

A chromosome analysis was performed. Thirty metaphase cells were examined from synchronized and unsynchronized PHA-stimulated peripheral blood cultures. Three cells had 45 chromosomes with a single X chromosome (45,X). This chromosome complement is associated with TS. Twenty-seven cells had 47 chromosomes with three X chromosomes (47,XXX). No karyotypically normal cells were identified in the specimen. These two cell lines were presumed to have arisen by a nondisjunctional event at a very early stage of fetal development.

3. Discussion

While 45,X/47,XXX girls have milder phenotypes, as discussed previously, the outcome for any individual is unpredictable. In the case of our patient, we saw urinary system malformations and short stature, but no cardiac, middle ear, pubertal, or learning issues. We are seeing the early stages of spontaneous puberty, and she will probably experience spontaneous menarche shortly [10].

Our patient has a 1 : 9 ratio of 45,X : 47,XXX karyotypes in the cells examined from her peripheral blood smear. However, this does not necessarily reflect the distribution of cells throughout the organ systems of her body. Moreover, most patients assessed for Turner syndrome have only been karyotyped from one tissue, so we do not know which lines dominate in which organs [2]. Researchers at USC Medical Center reported the case of a patient with short stature whose buccal smear showed 45,X/46,XX/47,XXX in a 67/123/10 ratio, whose peripheral leukocyte culture showed 45,X/47,XXX in a 1/1 ratio, and whose skin fibroblast culture showed 45,X/47,XXX in a 5/19 ratio [14]. They confirmed a previous assertion that the proportions of chromosomally different cell lines have little value for phenotype prediction, because the chromosome makeup is so varied depending on the sample tissue [15]. However, they presumed that the 47,XXX line was dominant because of the minor Turner syndrome stigmata. Yet, the 45,X line determined her height.

In contrast to the notion that the ratios do not have predictive value, Akbas et al. present the theory that patients with the 45,X/47,XXX karyotype demonstrate the phenotypes in proportion to their degree of mosaicism [16]. They present the case of a patient with a 35%/65% 45,X/47,XXX ratio. She has short stature and a horseshoe kidney, but what they otherwise describe as a mild phenotype. They compared their patient to a case of a woman with a 90%/10% 45,X/47,XXX ratio and a severe phenotype. She had streak gonads, amenorrhea, thyroiditis, short stature, and learning difficulties [17]. Therefore, the cell ratio may be predictive when it comes to the overall assessment of mild phenotype versus severe phenotype. However, height is not affected proportionally, as demonstrated from this case and others reported [2]. Given that 47,XXX girls present with increased height, if 90% of our patient's sampled cells were 47,XXX, we would not expect her to be at the 0.54 percentile for height.

Overall, making predictions regarding what the future has in store for these mosaic girls is nebulous. For prenatal diagnosis, parents of 45,X/47,XXX girls should be counseled for the possibility of full Turner symptoms but with optimism for a better outcome. Intellectual impairment is reduced compared to 45,X Turner syndrome, which is an important concern for parents who may be considering selective termination [2]. Future fertility also cannot be guaranteed but can be successful in most 45,X/47,XXX women [18].

4. Conclusion

Phenotypes of 45,X/47,XXX mosaic girls are unpredictable. Cell counts that provide a ratio of 45,X cells to 47,XXX cells should not be considered to have predictive value, because they vary by tissue. Fortunately phenotypes tend to be milder, but the height may be quite short in a way that is out of proportion to the relative mildness of the remainder of the phenotype. Fortunately short stature can be corrected with growth hormone, so families should be aware that this is a possible requirement for their girls. More research will need to be done in this area to assess impact of growth hormone on 45,X/47,XXX mosaic female with short stature as this has not been well studied.

Conflict of Interests

The authors declare that there is no conflict of interests regarding the publication of this paper.

References

[1] H. H. Turner, "A syndrome of infantilism, congenital webbed neck, and cubitus valgus," *Endocrinology*, vol. 23, no. 5, pp. 566–568, 1938.

[2] V. P. Sybert, "Phenotypic effects of mosaicism for a 47,XXX cell line in Turner syndrome," *Journal of Medical Genetics*, vol. 39, no. 3, pp. 217–221, 2002.

[3] D. J. Wolff, D. L. van Dyke, and C. M. Powell, "Laboratory guideline for turner syndrome," *Genetics in Medicine*, vol. 12, no. 1, pp. 52–55, 2010.

[4] V. P. Sybert and E. McCauley, "Turner's syndrome," *The New England Journal of Medicine*, vol. 351, no. 12, pp. 1227–1270, 2004.

[5] B. Lippe, M. E. Geffner, R. B. Dietrich, M. I. Boechat, and H. Kangarloo, "Renal malformations in patients with Turner syndrome: imaging in 141 patients," *Pediatrics*, vol. 82, no. 6, pp. 852–856, 1988.

[6] A. E. Lin, B. M. Lippe, M. E. Geffner et al., "Aortic dilation, dissection, and rupture in patients with turner syndrome," *The Journal of Pediatrics*, vol. 109, no. 5, pp. 820–826, 1986.

[7] Q. Zhong and L. C. Layman, "Genetic considerations in the patient with Turner syndrome—45,X with or without mosaicism," *Fertility and Sterility*, vol. 98, no. 4, pp. 775–779, 2012.

[8] J. Nielsen and M. Wohlert, "Chromosome abnormalities found among 34910 newborn children: results from a 13-year incidence study in Arhus, Denmark," *Human Genetics*, vol. 87, no. 1, pp. 81–83, 1991.

[9] N. R. Tartaglia, S. Howell, A. Sutherland, R. Wilson, and L. Wilson, "A review of trisomy X (47,XXX)," *Orphanet Journal of Rare Diseases*, vol. 5, no. 1, article 8, 2010.

[10] J. Blair, J. Tolmie, A. S. Hollman, and M. D. C. Donaldson, "Phenotype, ovarian function, and growth in patients with 45,X/47,XXX Turner mosaicism: Implications for prenatal counseling and estrogen therapy at puberty," *Journal of Pediatrics*, vol. 139, no. 5, pp. 724–728, 2001.

[11] A. M. Pasquino, F. Passeri, I. Pucarelli, M. Segni, and G. Municchi, "Spontaneous pubertal development in Turner's Syndrome," *Journal of Clinical Endocrinology and Metabolism*, vol. 82, no. 6, pp. 1810–1813, 1997.

[12] G. Massa, M. Vanderschueren-Lodeweyckx, and P. Malvaux, "Phenotypic effects of mosaicism for a 47,XXX cell line in Turner syndrome," *European Journal of Pediatrics*, vol. 149, no. 4, pp. 246–250, 1990.

[13] W. W. Greulich and S. I. Pyle, *Radiographic Atlas of Skeletal Development of Hand Wrist*, vol. 2, Stanford University Press, Stanford, Calif, USA, 1971.

[14] S. D. Frasier and M. G. Wilson, "Growth pattern in 45,X/47,XXX mosaicism," *The Journal of Pediatrics*, vol. 81, no. 1, pp. 187–188, 1972.

[15] L. Y. F. Hsu and K. Hirschhorn, "Unusual Turner mosaicism (45,X/47,XXX; 45,X/46,XXqi;45,X/46,XXr): detection through deceleration from normal linear growth or secondary amenorrhea," *The Journal of Pediatrics*, vol. 79, no. 2, pp. 276–281, 1971.

[16] E. Akbas, Z. M. Altintas, S. K. Celik et al., "Rare types of turner syndrome: clinical presentation and cytogenetics in five cases," *Laboratory Medicine*, vol. 43, no. 5, pp. 197–204, 2012.

[17] L. Tauchmanovà, R. Rossi, M. Pulcrano, L. Tarantino, C. Baldi, and G. Lombardi, "Turner's syndrome mosaicism 45X/47XXX: an interesting natural history," *Journal of Endocrinological Investigation*, vol. 24, no. 10, pp. 811–815, 2001.

[18] L. Tarani, S. Lampariello, G. Raguso et al., "Pregnancy in patients with Turner's syndrome: six new cases and review of literature," *Gynecological Endocrinology*, vol. 12, no. 2, pp. 83–87, 1998.

37

Subcutaneous Fat Necrosis of the Newborn: A Case Report of a Term Infant Presenting with Malaise and Fever at Age of 9 Weeks

Ayuk Adaeze Chikaodinaka[1] and Anikene Chukwuemeka Jude[2]

[1]Department of Pediatrics, University of Nigeria Teaching Hospital, PMB 01129, Enugu, Nigeria
[2]University of Nigeria Teaching Hospital, PMB 01129, Enugu, Nigeria

Correspondence should be addressed to Ayuk Adaeze Chikaodinaka; adaraymond@yahoo.com

Academic Editor: Tarak Srivastava

Background. Subcutaneous fat necrosis (SFN) is a rare, temporary, self-limited pathology affecting adipose tissue of full-term or postmature neonates. It is a rare entity especially in Nigeria and usually occurs in the first weeks following a complicated delivery. Because it is not very common, diagnosis is easily missed. It may resolve spontaneously without sequelae but patients need to be followed up because of development of late complications especially hypercalcemia. We report a case of SFN of the newborn noted within one week of birth and highlight the need for proper prompt diagnosis and the need for follow-up to assess possible complications.

1. Background

Subcutaneous fat necrosis (SFN) is a rare, temporary, self-limited pathology affecting adipose tissue of full-term or postmature neonates [1, 2]. It is a rare entity and usually occurs in the first weeks following a complicated delivery [3]. Where the diagnosis is not considered and patient not followed up, complications may arise and patient may be mismanaged. Even though spontaneous resolution without sequelae is the norm, patients should be followed up for development of late complications of SFN, especially hypercalcemia. Symptoms of complications can also be missed because the initial correct diagnosis was not made. We report a case of SFN of the newborn noted within one week of birth and highlight the need for proper prompt diagnosis and the need for follow-up to assess possible complications.

2. Case Presentation

Our patient is a male infant who was born term and presented to the emergency room of our hospital when he was 9 weeks old. His complaints were recurrent fever since discharge from our newborn special care unit at 1 week of birth. He also had developed recurrent vomiting that was usually postprandial with associated significant weight loss. Birth history revealed that he was macrosomic with a birthweight of 4.5 kg. He was born via caesarian section due to cephalopelvic disproportion. Other important perinatal histories were that of meconium-stained liquor, perinatal asphyxia (APGAR 4, 5, 7), and neonatal seizures on 1st day of life. During the initial newborn admission at about 4th day of life, mother noted that the patient had extensive purplish, nontender, firm subcutaneous nodules of uncertain diagnosis. The nodules were localized to the buccal fat region where they were first noted and then later spread to involve the neck, arms, forearms, thighs, and calves (Figures 1, 2, and 3). After discharge he visited several health facilities seeking help for this skin pathology including dermatology consult. During this period he was noted to be having recurrent fever and vomiting. He received several antibiotics before presenting to the emergency ward with the same complaints. At the time of presentation, most of the body swellings had regressed in

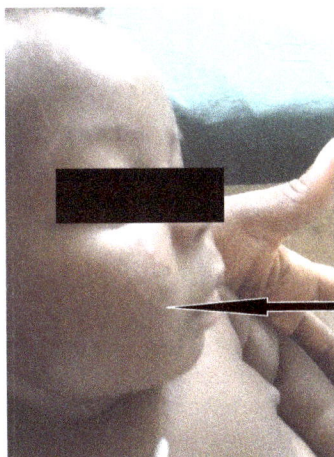

FIGURE 1: Firm nodular erythematous subcutaneous mass on the face noted on 4th day of life at the newborn nursery.

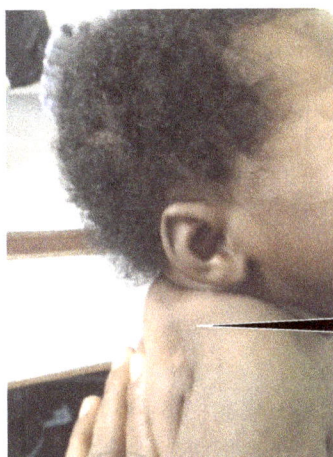

FIGURE 2: Subcutaneous erythematous nodules at nape of the neck noted in first week of life.

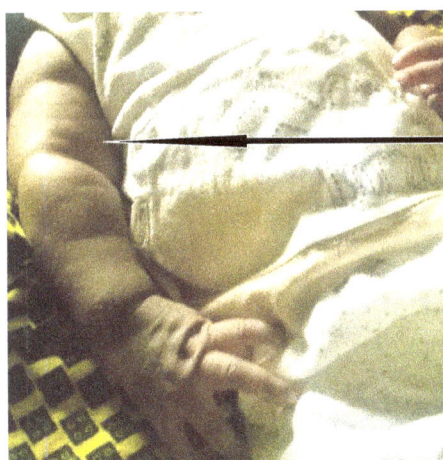

FIGURE 3: Slightly erythematous nodules noted subcutaneously within first week of life involving different parts of the body including the arms and forearms. Thus arms appear larger than they should be due to edema.

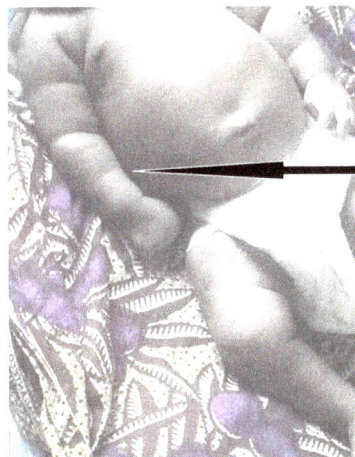

FIGURE 4: General regression in nodules and limb sizes noted at 9th week of life during emergency admission.

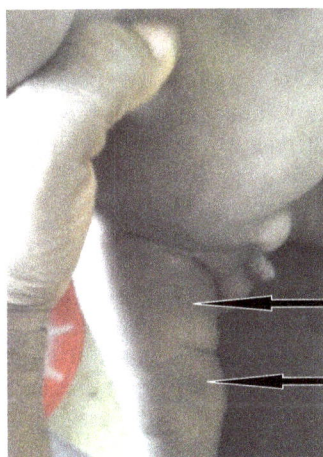

FIGURE 5: Residual hyperpigmented patch on the right thigh with small discrete swellings on the skin over anterior surface of the thighs noted at presentation to the emergency department.

size. The general appearance of the limbs with subcutaneous nodules was now at this admission less massive compared to the first week of life (Figure 4). Further examination revealed an axillary temperature of 38.1°C, slightly depressed anterior fontanelle but normal skin turgor. He still had residual facial nodular swelling that was flat, firm, attached to overlying skin, reddish, and measured about 4 cm in its widest diameter. Some of the child's initial nodules that were noted in the first week of life had substantially regressed and were now only noted as areas of hyperpigmentation as was seen on the skin of the right thigh measuring about 1 cm by 2 cm (Figure 5). His weight loss was evidenced by loose skin folds (arm and thigh) and a weight drop from previously documented 6.1 kg to current weight of 5.3 kg. A complete blood count showed a haemoglobin level of 10.2 g/dL, total WBC 18,300 (neutrophil 48%, lymphocytes 47%, monocytes 2%, and eosinophils 3%). The total platelet count was 534,000 and he had an elevated total ionized calcium level (iCa) of 1.72 mmol (1.12–1.32).

A dipstick urinalysis showed nitrite +, leucocyte ++ which suggested a possible urinary tract infection. A follow-up urine culture was not done as child had been on several antibiotics up to the time of this admission. The routine kidney function results were within normal limits. Immediately following admission into emergency room, dehydration was corrected and parenteral broad spectrum antibiotics commenced. On the 4th day of admission on obtaining the initial calcium result, steps to manage the hypercalcemia were taken. Formula feeding was initially stopped while continuing breast feeding; he was commenced on intravenous fluid hydration therapy of 10% dextrose in 0.45% saline combined with diuretic therapy for 48 hours. The iCa level repeated thereafter was 1.65 mmol and after 2 weeks had dropped further to 1.25 mmol. Skin lesions continued to regress and he continued to do well clinically. With the normalization of calcium levels and the good clinical progress further calcium assays were not continued. He was being followed up in our outpatient clinic at the time of this report.

3. Discussion

Subcutaneous fat necrosis of the newborn (SFN) is a rare form of panniculitis, an inflammation of the subcutaneous and adipose tissue [1]. It typically affects newborns. It is also known as adiponecrosis subcutanea [2]. It is a very rare disorder with no gender predilection [3]. It usually occurs in the first several weeks of life as was seen in our index patient. The exact aetiopathogenesis is unknown but postulations have been made as to the possible causes. A common theory is that stress such as that occuring from birth asphyxia in the newborn with immature fat cells induces inflammation, solidification, and necrosis. This leads to the formation of granulomatous infiltrates [3]. Histology of these granuloma have shown increased expression of 1-alpha hydroxylase known to activate vitamin D3 [4, 5]. The increased activity of vitamin D3 causes increased release of calcium. This could account for the hypercalcemia usually seen in SFN [3].

Another speculation for hypercalcemia is as observed in other conditions that have granulomatous lesions such as sarcoidosis [6]; the presence of granulomatous skin lesions is thought to be a source of extrarenal production of 1,25-OH vitamin D (calcitriol). The calcitriol causes increased intestinal calcium absorption and hence the resultant hypercalcemia [7]. In SFN unregulated production of 1,25-dihydroxyvitamin D by the granulomatous cells of fat necrosis could also result in hypercalcemia as reported by some authors [5, 8]. Furthermore, the combination of hypercalcemia, normal serum concentration of 25-hydroxyvitamin D, elevated 1,25-dihydroxyvitamin D, and a suppressed parathyroid hormone would indicate an abnormal 1,25-dihydroxyvitamin D production with possible increased intestinal absorption of calcium [8]. Unfortunately due to limited finances the 1,25-dihydroxyvitamin D and parathyroid hormone were not assayed and these would have shed further light on the possible sources of hypercalcemia in our index patient.

Susceptible children who may have to undergo body cooling for the management of perinatal asphyxia could also develop subcutaneous necrosis of fat and adipose tissue [4]. Our patient was exposed to stress from birth asphyxia even though he did not receive body cooling therapy. SFN typically occurs in a full-term newborn as was our index patient. The skin lesions usually appear from about day four after delivery [9] and have been associated with certain predisposing factors such as obstetric trauma, meconium aspiration, asphyxia, hypothermia, or peripheral hypoxemia [3]. Many of these factors were present as antecedent clinical history in our patient and may have predisposed our patient to SFN. There has also been a putative report of macrosomia. Mahé et al. [9], in a systematic review of risk factors, clinical manifestations, complications, and outcome in 16 affected children over a 6-year period, reported macrosomia in about half of the children studied. Our patient was also macrosomic with a birthweight of 4.5 kg.

The typical skin lesions appear as erythematous to purplish, firm subcutaneous nodules [10] and are usually asymptomatic. They may appear on the cheeks, buttocks, back, thighs, or upper arms and may be focal or extensive. Sometimes they may be tender during the acute phase [11], as was seen in 4 of the children reviewed by Mahé et al. [9]. Lesions were first noted in the buccal fat region in our patient before spreading to involve other parts of the body.

Among symptoms our patient presented with was persistent fever. Shumer et al. [12] noted fever in 57% of the cases they studied. They postulated this to be due to elevated levels of prostaglandin E2 found in some of the SFN patients with hypercalcemia as well as elaborations of interleukin-1 from the granulomas of SFN [12]. Our patient had elevated calcium levels and this may be the plausible cause of his recurrent fever.

We could also attribute the fever to the possible urinary tract infection as comorbidity which patient had. It may also be part of the symptom complex of SFN. Occurrence of hypercalciuria secondary to hypercalcemia especially in patients diagnosed with rheumatic disease and having a renal comorbidity may lead to sterile leukocyturia [13]. This could mimic a urinary tract infection [13]. In established leukocyturia, however, WBC count is usually more than 15 WBC per hpf [14]. The possibility of UTI as a comorbidity was considered in this patient who had lower WBC of between 5 and 10 WBC per hpf and nitrites in urine. The urinary calcium excretion rate was however not done to further confirm the presence of calcium in urine but the patient had normal kidney function. Elevated levels of serum calcium have been noted as a rare complication of SFN and usually occur with disease regression [15, 16]. Symptoms of hypercalcemia include lethargy, vomiting, poor feeding with attendant weight loss, polyuria, and fever [17]. Severe elevations will lead to nephrocalcinosis with progressive reduction in renal function [17]. Screening for hypercalcemia in children with a possible diagnosis of SFN is therefore important to reduce likelihood of morbidity from hypercalcemia [3]. This requires a high index of suspicion on the part of the attending physician to think early of the diagnosis and know when best to assay for calcium levels. Hypercalcemia occurs as the skin lesions begin to regress and this may coincide with the time when our patient developed fever. The symptom of recurrent vomiting in our patient may also have been part of the symptom complex of hypercalcemia. He also had seizures on day one of life. This may be more attributable as a sequel of birth asphyxia rather than high calcium levels as hypercalcemia is uncommon at that stage of SFN.

The presence of hypercalcemia may also be asymptomatic. Shumer et al. [12] also noted in their study population that 43% of patients with severe hypercalcemia (≥3 mmol/L) were asymptomatic [12].

Apart from clinical diagnosis, SFN can be further confirmed by histopathology following a tissue biopsy, which is an invasive procedure. When the carefully collected biopsy is subjected to histopathology, the following are diagnostic: radially arranged clefts of crystalline triglyceride within fat cells, granulomatous cellular infiltrate composed of lymphocytes which confirms fat necrosis, and presence of histiocytes, multinucleated giant cells, and fibroblasts [11]. Our patient did not get the benefit of histopathology due to the invasive nature of tissue biopsy.

SFN usually runs a self-limiting course [3]. When our patient presented to the emergency room, most of the skin lesion had already regressed. However this also coincides with the period of possible complications of hypercalcemia as was seen in our patient. This could be easily missed if the diagnosis of SFN is not considered. Treatment should aim at preventing and managing the complications of hypercalcemia when present. Hypercalcemia has been successfully managed by a combination of diet modification, fluids, and drugs. Diet modification will include low calcium formula [12]. A combination of saline fluid hydration with calcium wasting diuretics is a recognized standard first-line intervention [18]. Corticosteroids and bisphosphonates may be used for further management when adequate reduction in calcium levels is not obtained with the first-line intervention [3]. Samedi et al. [19], in a case report, noted that the use of pamidronates (a bisphosphonate) had a faster onset of action than corticosteroids and thus advocated it as a possible first-line management of SFN with very severe hypercalcemia. Similarly Alos et al. [20] in a case series involving four infants found that after initial trial of hydration and diuretics and there was not much reduction in iCa levels there was documented good outcome with the use of pamidronates. Our patient however did well with diet modification, optimal hydration, and the use of diuretics.

The possible differential diagnoses to be considered alongside SFN include skin infections in the new born such as bacterial cellulitis, erysipelas, CMV infection, sclerema neonatorum, steroid-induced fat necrosis, deep infantile hemangioma, dermohypodermitis, neurofibromatosis, lipogranulomatosis (Farber disease), sarcomas including pediatric rhabdomyosarcoma, and other panniculitides [3, 21]. The patient however had distinctive features that pointed most to the diagnosis of subcutaneous fat necrosis of the newborn.

As part of management of these babies who have SFN with raised calcium levels, it is recommended that at least biweekly follow-up visits are done for up to a period of 6 months [3, 22]. This is to monitor for manifestations of any complications of hypercalcemia and be able to intervene

appropriately. Calcium assay was repeated at 2 weekly intervals in our index patient until normal values were obtained and follow-up medical check-ups were continued at the outpatient clinic.

4. Conclusion

Subcutaneous fat necrosis is a rare finding in our environment and can present with complications such as hypercalcemia. Presenting this case highlights the need for a high index of suspicion for the medical personnel, to aid early diagnosis and appropriate intervention. If correct diagnosis is made and child is properly followed up, the possible complications arising from hypercalcemia can be prevented or properly managed. Follow-up following resolution of skin lesions is also emphasized. This will help in reducing morbidity or mortality from SFN in the newborn.

Abbreviations

SFN: Subcutaneous fat necrosis.

Consent

Written informed consent was obtained from the parents of the patient for publication of this case report and any accompanying images.

Conflict of Interests

The authors declare that they have no conflict of interests.

Authors' Contribution

Ayuk Adaeze Chikaodinaka and Anikene Chukwuemeka Jude were involved in the review of this patient and the write-up of this case. Ayuk Adaeze Chikaodinaka, Anikene Chukwuemeka Jude participated in the final review of this paper.

References

[1] J. T. Tran and A. P. Sheth, "Complications of subcutaneous fat necrosis of the newborn: a case report and review of the literature," *Pediatric Dermatology*, vol. 20, no. 3, pp. 257–261, 2003.

[2] A. Schwartz, *Cold Panicullitis*, Medscape, 2015, http://emedicine.medscape.com/article/1082003.

[3] S. Grewal, "Subcutaneous fat necrosis of the newborn," *Medscape*, 2014, http://emedicine.medscape.com/article/1081910.

[4] T. Kuboi, T. Kusaka, K. Okazaki et al., "Subcutaneous fat necrosis after selective head cooling in an infant," *Pediatrics International*, vol. 55, no. 2, pp. e23–e24, 2013.

[5] A. Farooque, C. Moss, D. Zehnder, M. Hewison, and N. J. Shaw, "Expression of 25-hydroxyvitamin D3-1α-hydroxylase in subcutaneous fat necrosis," *British Journal of Dermatology*, vol. 160, no. 2, pp. 423–425, 2009.

[6] O. Aladesanmi, X. W. Jin, and C. Nielsen, "A 56-year-old man with hypercalcemia," *Cleveland Clinic Journal of Medicine*, vol. 72, no. 8, pp. 707–712, 2005.

[7] S. M. Moe, "Disorders involving calcium, phosphorus, and magnesium," *Primary Care—Clinics in Office Practice*, vol. 35, no. 2, pp. 215–237, 2008.

[8] K. Kruse, U. Irle, and R. Uhlig, "Elevated 1,25-dihydroxyvitamin D serum concentrations in infants with subcutaneous fat necrosis," *The Journal of Pediatrics*, vol. 122, no. 3, pp. 460–463, 1993.

[9] E. Mahé, N. Girszyn, S. Hadj-Rabia, C. Bodemer, D. Hamel-Teillac, and Y. De Prost, "Subcutaneous fat necrosis of the newborn: a systematic evaluation of risk factors, clinical manifestations, complications and outcome of 16 children," *British Journal of Dermatology*, vol. 156, no. 4, pp. 709–715, 2007.

[10] M. J. Hicks, M. L. Levy, J. Alexander, and C. M. Flaitz, "Subcutaneous fat necrosis of the newborn and hypercalcemia: case report and review of the literature," *Pediatric Dermatology*, vol. 10, no. 3, pp. 271–276, 1993.

[11] J. Morelli, "Diseases of subcutaneous tissues," in *Nelson's Textbook of Pediatrics*, R. M. Kliegman, R. E. Behrman, H. B. Jenson, and B. F. Stanton, Eds., Saunders Elsevier, Philadelphia, Pa, USA, 18th edition, 2007.

[12] D. E. Shumer, V. Thaker, G. A. Taylor, and A. J. Wassner, "Severe hypercalcaemia due to subcutaneous fat necrosis: presentation, management and complications," *Archives of Disease in Childhood: Fetal and Neonatal Edition*, vol. 99, no. 5, pp. F419–F421, 2014.

[13] H.-J. Anders and V. Vielhauer, "Renal co-morbidity in patients with rheumatic diseases," *Arthritis Research & Therapy*, vol. 13, article 222, 2011.

[14] D. Manski, "Urine analysis: sediment and dipstick examination," in *Online Textbook of Urology*, 2015, http://www.urology-textbook.com/urine-analysis.html.

[15] M. P. C. L. de Gomes, A. M. Porro, M. M. S. S. da Enokihara, and M. C. Floriano, "Subcutaneous fat necrosis of the newborn: clinical manifestations in two cases," *Anais Brasileiros de Dermatologia*, vol. 88, supplement, no. 6, pp. 154–157, 2013.

[16] E. Tuddenham, A. Kumar, and A. Tarn, "Subcutaneous fat necrosis causing neonatal hypercalcaemia," *BMJ Case Reports*, 2015.

[17] D. Doyle and A. DiGeorge, "Hyperparathyroidism," in *Nelson's Textbook of Pediatrics*, R. M. Kliegman, R. E. Biehrman, H. B. Stanton, and B. F. Jenson, Eds., Saunders Elsevier, Philadelphia, Pa, USA, 18th edition, 2007.

[18] S.-H. Hung, W.-Y. Tsai, P.-N. Tsao, H.-C. Chou, and W.-S. Hsieh, "Oral clodronate therapy for hypercalcemia related to extensive subcutaneous fat necrosis in a newborn," *Journal of the Formosan Medical Association*, vol. 102, no. 11, pp. 801–804, 2003.

[19] V. M. Samedi, K. Yusuf, W. Yee, H. Obaid, and E. H. Al Awad, "Neonatal hypercalcemia secondary to subcutaneous fat necrosis successfully treated with pamidronate: a case series and literature review," *AJP Reports*, vol. 4, no. 2, pp. e93–e96, 2014.

[20] N. Alos, D. Eugène, M. Fillion, J. Powell, V. Kokta, and G. Chabot, "Pamidronate: treatment for severe hypercalcemia in neonatal subcutaneous fat necrosis," *Hormone Research*, vol. 65, no. 6, pp. 289–294, 2006.

[21] S. Fenniche, L. Daoud, R. Benmously et al., "Subcutaneous fat necrosis: report of two cases," *Dermatology Online Journal*, vol. 10, no. 2, article 12, 2004.

[22] S. B. Hoath and V. Narendran, "The skin," in *Neonatal-Perinatal Medicine*, A. A. Fanaroff, R. J. Martin, and M. C. Walsh, Eds., p. 1705, Elsevier Mosby, St. Louis, Mo, USA, 9th edition, 2011.

38

Two Mutations in Surfactant Protein C Gene Associated with Neonatal Respiratory Distress

Anna Tarocco,[1] **Elisa Ballardini,**[2] **Maria Raffaella Contiero,**[2] **Giampaolo Garani,**[2] **and Silvia Fanaro**[2]

[1]*Pediatric Section, University Hospital S. Anna, Via Aldo Moro 8, 44124 Ferrara, Italy*
[2]*Neonatal Intensive Care Unit and Neonatology, University Hospital S. Anna, Ferrara, Italy*

Correspondence should be addressed to Anna Tarocco; anna.tarocco@unife.it

Academic Editor: Albert M. Li

Multiple mutations of surfactant genes causing surfactant dysfunction have been described. Surfactant protein C (SP-C) deficiency is associated with variable clinical manifestations ranging from neonatal respiratory distress syndrome to lethal lung disease. We present an extremely low birth weight male infant with an unusual course of respiratory distress syndrome associated with two mutations in the SFTPC gene: C43-7G>A and 12T>A. He required mechanical ventilation for 26 days and was treated with 5 subsequent doses of surfactant with temporary and short-term efficacy. He was discharged at 37 weeks of postconceptional age without any respiratory support. During the first 16 months of life he developed five respiratory infections that did not require hospitalization. *Conclusion.* This mild course in our patient with two mutations is peculiar because the outcome in patients with a single SFTPC mutation is usually poor.

1. Introduction

Genetic disorders of lung surfactant proteins determine abnormal surfactant production and function. Several mutations of surfactant genes responsible for a wide range of phenotypical manifestations, from neonatal respiratory distress to adult chronic lung disease, have been described [1]. Pulmonary surfactant is composed of a lipid mixture and specific proteins. ABCA3 and SP-B are important to absorb surfactant phospholipids into specialized secretory organelles; SP-C and SP-B are required for absorption of the secreted phospholipids into the alveolar surface. SP-C deficiency is a rare autosomal dominant condition associated with interstitial lung disease in children and adults with a variable clinical course [2].

2. Case Report

An extremely low birth weight male infant was born at 27th week of gestational age by emergency Caesarean section for onset of labor. Parents were both of African ethnicity (Senegal), not consanguineous, and without family history of note. At birth he required neonatal resuscitation with positive pressure ventilation and intubation. Apgar score was 2-5-8 at 1, 5, and 10 minutes, respectively. During the first hours of life the infant showed a progressive increase of respiratory distress with increased oxygen requirement (up to 60%). The chest radiograph revealed a diffuse haziness of both lungs as shown in Figure 1. The administration of porcine surfactant (200 mg/kg Curosurf, Chiesi) improved ventilatory parameters and allowed extubation. The infant was maintained with continuous positive airway pressure until day 3 of life without supplemental oxygen. On day 4 the physical examination revealed tachypnea, chest retractions, and episodes of apnea requiring reintubation. Mechanical ventilation was then continued for 26 days. During this period he was treated with five subsequent doses of surfactant (100 mg/kg/dose) with temporary efficacy so that three attempts at extubation failed. Chest radiographs showed bilateral diffuse alveolar opacities due to persistent diffuse pulmonary infiltrates (Figure 2). Abundant white fluid tracheal aspirates (repeatedly reported as negative for bacteria

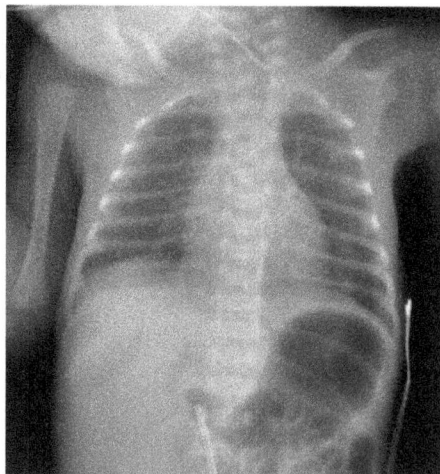

FIGURE 1: Chest radiograph (first day of life) revealing diffuse haziness of both lungs.

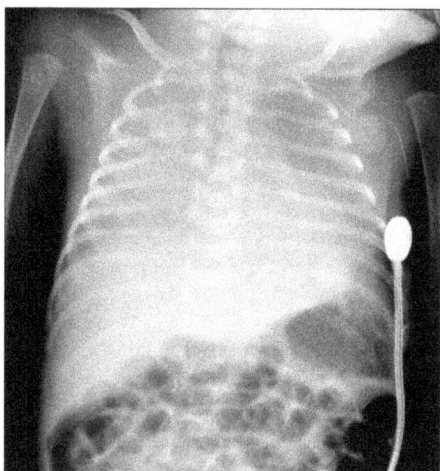

FIGURE 2: Chest radiograph (20 days of life) showing bilateral diffuse alveolar opacities.

and fungi) were documented. The patient was treated with four different antibiotics, fluconazole, and corticosteroids (7-day low-dose treatment with dexamethasone: 0.1 mg/kg/day for 5 days followed by 0.05 mg/kg/day for 2 days) without significant efficacy. On the basis of the clinical response to surfactant, radiographic findings, and white tracheal secretions, surfactant protein deficiency was suspected. Tracheal aspirates and blood for molecular typing for surfactant protein were analyzed: DNA sequencing showed two mutations in the SFTPC gene (C43-7G>A and 12T>A). Parents refused to be examined. The infant was maintained on high flow nasal cannula with oxygen until the 59th day of life. He was discharged at 73 days of life with a weight of 2,700 g without any respiratory support or supplemental oxygen.

During the first 16 months of life the infant developed 5 episodes of bronchiolitis, never requiring hospitalization.

3. Discussion

Surfactant, which is secreted by type II alveolar cells, reduces the surface tension maintaining the stability of the lungs. Multiple mutations of the gene of SP-C have been identified, which cause dysfunction of surfactant metabolism and are associated with interstitial lung disease. Nogee et al. described the first case in 2001 [3]. They reported a female term infant with a heterozygous mutation in SFTPC who developed severe respiratory insufficiency at 6 weeks of age. Thomas et al. in 2002 described a large family with variable phenotypic expressions of interstitial lung disease [4]. Three members had been previously described by Donohue et al. in 1959 [5] and Young in 1966 [6] as having a lethal manifestation of pulmonary fibrosis called "fibrocystic pulmonary dysplasia." Brasch et al. published a case of lethal severe respiratory insufficiency in a 13-month-old baby associated with de novo missense mutation of SFPTC [7]. Tredano et al. published another case of full term baby with early onset of respiratory distress. He progressively developed respiratory distress at 1 month of age, with recurrent bronchitis and dyspnea requiring oxygen supplementation [8]. Soraisham et al. in 2006 reported a case of a term newborn with an unusual presentation and course of lung disease due to single novel mutation in SFTPC gene [9]. Turcu et al. in 2013 described 7 cases of single SP-C gene mutation diagnosed from 3 months of age to 10 years. In two of them symptoms were present at birth; the other children presented later chronic cough, failure to thrive, or oxygen dependency. One of them died at 16 days of life [1]. Recently, Van Hoorn et al. presented a successful weaning from mechanical ventilation in a term newborn with SP-C mutation with severe neonatal respiratory distress treated with methylprednisolone pulse therapy and oral prednisolone [10].

The pathophysiology of this disorder involves intracellular accumulation of a structurally defective SP-C protein. In addition the activity of produced surfactant may be defective [9]. On the basis of the few cases reported, it is evident that clinical manifestations are variable and that the onset ranges from the neonatal period to adulthood. Surfactant protein C deficiency varies from mild temporary tachypnea to lethal respiratory failure due to idiopathic pulmonary fibrosis [11].

At present, no medical therapy for the SFTPC mutation is available. Lung transplantation may be an option in case of severe irreversible respiratory failure. In our report, two mutations of the SFTPC gene were identified. The first one, c43-7G>A, has already been described by Lawson et al. and is associated with idiopathic pulmonary fibrosis [11]. The second, c12T>A, has been reported in dbSNP as a rare variant of the SP-C gene (rs200469074; available at http://www.ncbi.nlm.nih.gov/projects/SNP/). In our patient respiratory distress syndrome resulted from a combination of both prematurity and surfactant abnormality, which accounted for prolonged ventilatory support and for the need of repeated surfactant doses and corticosteroid treatment. At the age of 16 months he is in good clinical condition without any respiratory support and has a normal nutritional status and neurodevelopment. He has developed five respiratory infections that have not required hospitalization. This clinical case highlights the need for molecular and genetic characterization of the surfactant gene especially in preterm patients, when the respiratory distress syndrome has an unusually prolonged course. Our case of two mutations is remarkable since, differently from most cases with even single SFTPC mutations, it was characterized by a particularly mild clinical presentation. There are no reports on the clinical effect of these associated mutations and we may speculate that the c12T>A SP-C gene variant may have no pathogenic effect.

Conflict of Interests

The authors declare no competing financial interests in relation to this work.

References

[1] S. Turcu, E. Ashton, L. Jenkins, A. Gupta, and Q. Mok, "Genetic testing in children with surfactant dysfunction," *Archives of Disease in Childhood*, vol. 98, no. 7, pp. 490–496, 2013.

[2] W. A. Gower and L. M. Nogee, "Surfactant dysfunction," *Paediatric Respiratory Reviews*, vol. 12, no. 4, pp. 223–229, 2011.

[3] L. M. Nogee, A. E. Dunbar, S. E. Wert, F. Askin, A. Hamvas, and J. A. Whitsett, "A mutation in the surfactant protein C gene associated with familial interstitial lung disease," *The New England Journal of Medicine*, vol. 344, no. 8, pp. 573–579, 2001.

[4] A. Q. Thomas, K. Lane, J. Phillips III et al., "Heterozygosity for a surfactant protein C gene mutation associated with usual interstitial pneumonitis and cellular nonspecific interstitial pneumonitis in one kindred," *American Journal of Respiratory and Critical Care Medicine*, vol. 165, no. 9, pp. 1322–1328, 2002.

[5] W. L. Donohue, B. Laski, I. Uchida, and J. D. Munn, "Familial fibrocystic pulmonary dysplasia and its relation to Hamman-Rich syndrome," *Pediatrics*, vol. 24, pp. 786–813, 1959.

[6] W. A. Young, "Familial fibrocystic pulmonary dysplasia: a new case in a known affected family," *Canadian Medical Association Journal*, vol. 94, no. 20, pp. 1059–1061, 1966.

[7] F. E. Brasch, M. Griese, M. Tredano et al., "Interstitial lung disease in a baby with a *de novo* mutation on the SFTPC gene," *European Respiratory Journal*, vol. 24, no. 1, pp. 30–39, 2004.

[8] M. Tredano, M. Griese, F. Brasch et al., "Mutation of SFTPC in infantile pulmonary alveolar proteinosis with or without fibrosing lung disease," *The American Journal of Medical Genetics*, vol. 126, no. 1, pp. 18–26, 2004.

[9] A. S. Soraisham, A. J. Tierney, and H. J. Amin, "Neonatal respiratory failure associated with mutation in the surfactant protein C gene," *Journal of Perinatology*, vol. 26, no. 1, pp. 67–70, 2006.

[10] J. Van Hoorn, A. Brouwers, M. Griese, and B. Kramer, "Successful weaning from mechanical ventilation in a patient with surfactant protein C deficiency presenting with severe neonatal respiratory distress," *BMJ Case Reports*, Article ID 203053, 2014.

[11] W. E. Lawson, S. W. Grant, V. Ambrosini et al., "Genetic mutations in surfactant protein C are a rare cause of sporadic cases of IPF," *Thorax*, vol. 59, no. 11, pp. 977–980, 2004.

39

Isolated Splenic Vein Thrombosis: 8-Year-Old Boy with Massive Upper Gastrointestinal Bleeding and Hypersplenism

Mohammad Ali Kiani,[1] Arash Forouzan,[2] Kambiz Masoumi,[2] Behnaz Mazdaee,[2] Mohammad Bahadoram,[3] Hamid Reza Kianifar,[1] and Hassan Ravari[4]

[1]*Pediatric Gastroenterology Ward, Department of Pediatrics, Mashhad University of Medical Sciences, Mashhad 9177948564, Iran*
[2]*Department of Emergency Medicine, Imam Khomeini General Hospital, Ahvaz Jundishapur University of Medical Sciences, Ahvaz 6193673166, Iran*
[3]*Medical Student Research Committee and Social Determinant of Health Research Center, Ahvaz Jundishapur University of Medical Sciences, Ahvaz 6193673166, Iran*
[4]*Vascular and Endovascular Surgery Research Center, Imam Reza Hospital, Faculty of Medicine, Mashhad University of Medical Sciences, Mashhad 9177948564, Iran*

Correspondence should be addressed to Kambiz Masoumi; emdajums@yahoo.com

Academic Editor: Denis A. Cozzi

We present an 8-year-old boy who was referred to our center with the complaint of upper gastrointestinal bleeding and was diagnosed with hypersplenism and progressive esophageal varices. Performing a computerized tomography (CT) scan, we discovered a suspicious finding in the venography phase in favor of thrombosis in the splenic vein. Once complementary examinations were done and due to recurrent bleeding and band ligation failure, the patient underwent splenectomy. And during the one-year follow-up obvious improvement of the esophageal varices was observed in endoscopy.

1. Introduction

Splenic vein thrombosis (SVT) is known as one of the rare causes of upper gastrointestinal bleeding and is mostly seen in the fifth decade of life and male sex [1, 2]. So far, 37 different etiologies have been reported for SVT [3]. The typical manifestations are bleeding from gastric varices characterized by anemia, hematemesis, melena, or hematochezia seen in 15%–50% of patients. Splenomegaly is observed in all patients with SVT whether it be in physical examination or imaging evaluation or during surgery [3]. Sometimes other symptoms of splenomegaly such as thrombocytopenia or pancytopenia and abdominal pain are also manifestations of the disease [4]. It must be noted that since liver cirrhosis is absent in SVT, these patients do not have chronic liver disease [4]. Being asymptomatic, in most cases, makes the diagnosis of SVT difficult. However reports of SVT have increased in recent years which could be due to advancement

in imaging techniques [5]. Previously, though, most cases of SVT were distinguished in postmortem autopsy but now with the developments such as celiac angiography and splenoportography most cases are readily detectable. Since abdominal CT is used for patients with acute pancreatitis as well as preoperative patients of chronic pancreatitis, SVT is often an incidental finding in the computerized tomography (CT) scan [5]. The diagnosis test of choice for the assessment of SVT is venous-phase celiac angiography [5]. This condition results in increased localized sinistral portal pressure, which is also known as sinistral portal hypertension. The majority of patients with SVT and the resulting sinistral portal hypertension, in contrast to patients with generalized portal hypertension, are asymptomatic and have normal hepatic function. Gastrointestinal bleeding secondary to esophageal or gastric varices may occur in these patients (Figure 1). Most patients with SVT have peripheral arteries other than gastric varices which never go bleeding. As a result asymptomatic

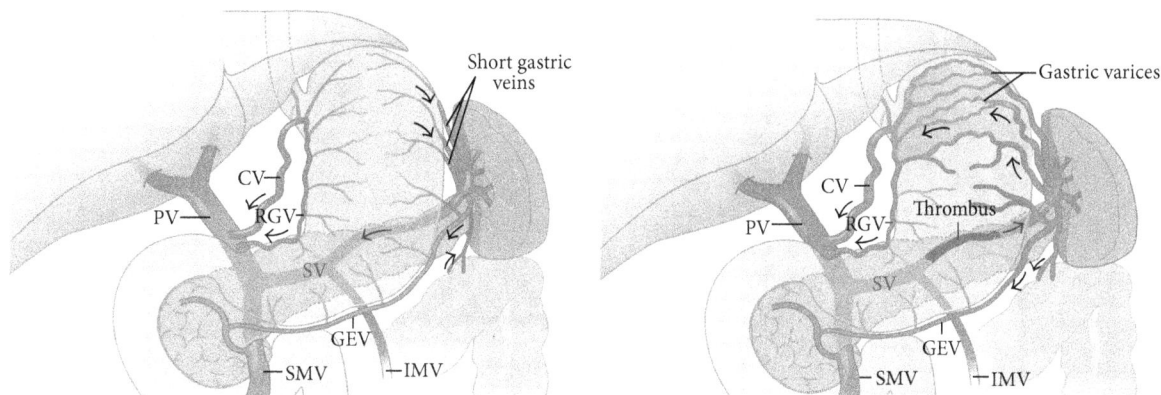

FIGURE 1: The effects of splenic vein thrombosis on normal venous anatomy. Note the gastric varices, dilatation of short gastric, and gastroepiploic (GEV) and coronary (CV) veins. The portal vein (PV), superior mesenteric vein (SMV), and inferior mesenteric vein (IMV) are patent. RGV: right gastric vein; SV: splenic vein [6].

patients without gastric varices should be monitored and do not need treatment for SVT [4]. In other words SVT alone does not need treatment. In symptomatic patients splenectomy is the treatment of choice done by shunting collateral flow [4].

2. Case Report

Patient was an 8-year-old boy referred to our center with massive upper gastrointestinal bleeding. The patient was found to have splenomegaly. He went through multiple evaluations including endoscopy and underwent band ligation for progressive esophageal varices. The patient had no history of neonatal blood exchange and umbilical venous catheters during infancy. No finding suggestive of portal venous thrombosis was observed in Doppler sonography. All the experiments indicated normal hepatic function. Due to recurrent bleeding and signs of hypersplenism and bicytopenia (thrombocytopenia and anemia), CT scan in venography phase was performed, which presented suspicious findings in splenic vein. Patient's CT angiography of the abdomen revealed splenomegaly (Figure 2), dilation and tortuosity of spleen hilum veins and veins lining the esophagus and stomach (Figure 3), and dilation of coronary and left renal veins (Figure 4). Haziness was observed throughout the mesenteric fat of the spleen hilum and splenic vein pathway. However, the size and density of the pancreas were normal. Additionally, lipase and amylase levels were also normal both in initial evaluations and in subsequent follow-ups. Given the portal hypertension symptoms and the history of cytopenia and splenic vein thrombosis, complementary evaluations were made considering PNH. Flow cytometry of peripheral blood was carried out on white blood cells in which CD55 and CD59 were reported as 90% positive. Gallbladder as well as intra- and extrahepatic biliary ducts were seen as normal. Splenorenal shunt was observable through left renal vein and splenogastric shunt was visible because of the tortuosity and dilation of gastric veins and enlargement of coronary vein. Regarding the clinical status of the patient, such as recurrent bleeding and failure to respond to band

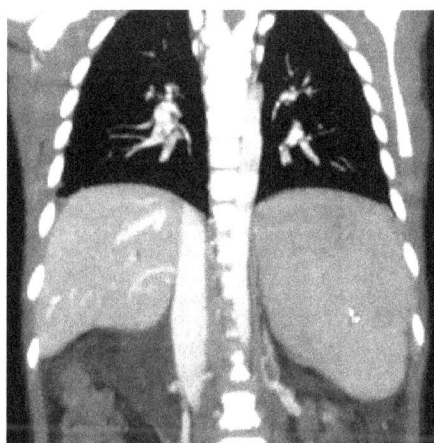

FIGURE 2: Patient's CT angiography of the abdomen revealed splenomegaly.

ligation in the specified time, the patient was scheduled for surgery. He underwent laparotomy under general anesthesia and in sterile conditions. The laparotomy findings were as follows: normal liver in inspection and palpation. There were plenty of omental adhesion bands surrounding the spleen. The spleen was larger than usual. Dilated veins surrounding the spleen and stomach and esophagus were observed. To release adhesions surrounding the spleen, the splenic vessels ligations were cut. Splenectomy was completed. It is worth noting that, due to signs of hypersplenism and the presence of splenic thrombosis, diagnostic assessments were done prior to surgery on MPS including ET and PV. JAK2 mutation was checked and reported as negative. Aspiration and bone marrow biopsy were also performed which reported bone marrow as normocellular and reactive. During the one-year follow-up the patient did not go into relapse and control endoscopies showed improvement of esophageal varices. In the assessments that followed hereditary deficits of pro S, pro C and Antithrombin III were checked for and reported as negative. The normal values are added to Table 1.

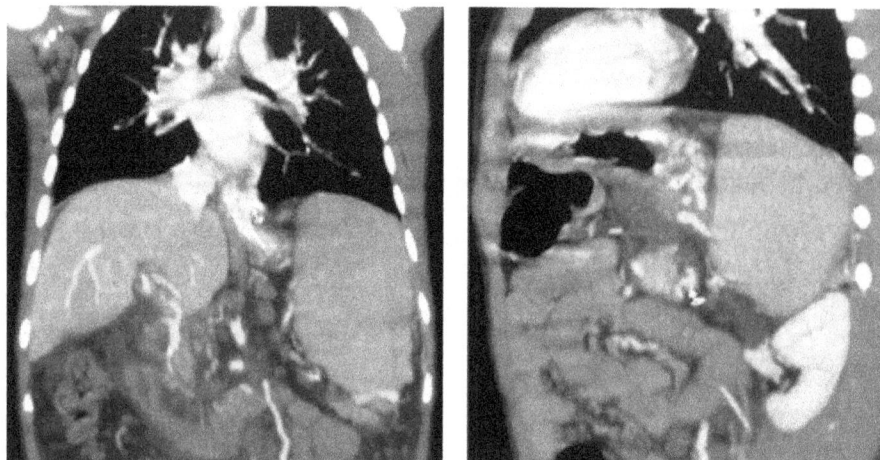

FIGURE 3: Dilation and tortuosity of spleen hilum veins and veins lining the esophagus and stomach.

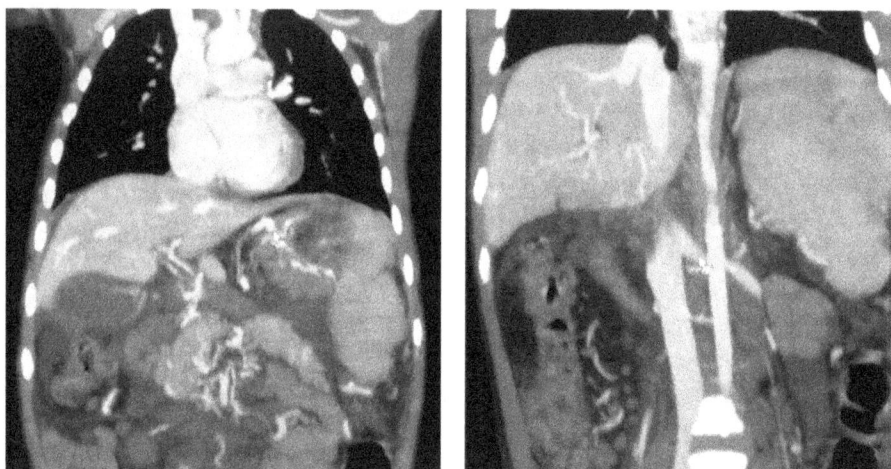

FIGURE 4: Dilation of coronary and left renal veins.

TABLE 1: Laboratory evaluation.

Beta 2 GP1 level	
IgG	4.3 AU/mL (normal: <5)
IgM	3.2 AU/mL (normal: <8)
IgA	2.4 AU/mL (normal: <8)
Anticardiolipin Ab	
IgM	9.63 MPL/mL
Lupus anticoagulant Ab	Absent
Protein C	85.6 (normal: 70%–130%)
Protein S	120.2 (normal: 77%–143%)
Antithrombin III	97% (normal: >75%)
Factor V Leiden	Absent

3. Discussion

Portal hypertension resulting from SVT can lead to massive gastrointestinal bleeding from esophageal or gastric varices or cause hypertensive gastropathy [1]. In 7%–20% of patients SVT is accompanied by acute and chronic pancreatitis, pancreatic pseudocysts, and pancreatic adenocarcinoma [1, 2]. Even after recovery, symptoms of pancreatitis have been reported [1, 4]. The most common cause of SVT is chronic pancreatitis and perivenous inflammation [4]. Although SVT has been reported in more than 45% of patients with chronic pancreatitis, most of SVT patients are asymptomatic [3]. Pancreatitis leading to SVT may be mild and the patients show no clinical sign indicating chronic pancreatitis [3].

Unlike patients with portal vein hypertension, most patients with SVT are asymptomatic and have normal hepatic function [4]. SVT can cause localized hypertension of splenic veins and create collaterals from spleen to the fundus. From that point, blood returns to the main portal system via coronary vein. In such a case, gastric varices are not often associated with esophageal varices except for collaterals at the site of gastroesophageal junction, where bleeding is common. In other cases, despite the formation of large and multiple collaterals, spontaneous bleeding seldom occurs.

Patients with the following characteristics are suspected of having SVT [4]: patients with history of pancreatitis or GI bleeding, patients with splenomegaly without portal vein hypertension, cirrhosis, or hematologic disease, and finally patients with gastric varices alone. There are other reasons for gastric bleeding in patients with chronic pancreatitis which include the following: arterial pseudoaneurysm, pancreatic pseudocysts, hemosuccus pancreaticus, peptic ulcer disease, gastritis, and Mallory-Weiss tears [7].

Therefore, an overall assessment in patients with SVT and gastrointestinal bleeding is necessary as less than half the bleeding is related to gastric varices. SVT in acute or chronic pancreatitis results from factorial perivenous inflammation and includes intrinsic endothelial damage caused by inflammation and extrinsic damage secondary to venous pressure resulting from fibrosis, adjacent pseudocysts, or edema [3]. In any patient with signs of splenic vein thrombosis and the resulting hypersplenism, the underlying cause for hypercoagulation state should be investigated. Hypercoagulable states are inherited or acquired conditions. They are associated with a predisposition to vein thrombosis. These include a wide range of thrombolytic disorders throughout the body such as brain vein thrombosis, extremity deep venous thrombosis, arterial thrombosis (such as stroke, myocardial infarction), and intra-abdominal venous thrombosis. The most prevalent clinical feature resulting from hypercoagulable states is venous thromboembolic disease. Some other resulting disorders include myeloproliferative and hyperhomocysteinemia syndromes and antiphospholipid antibodies (APAs). As mentioned earlier our patient turned negative for MPS but in the subsequent tests blood homocysteine level was checked to be normal. APS panel was checked to show no specific underlying disorder (values are cited in Table 1) [8].

Obstruction of the splenic vein could result from enlarged retroperitoneal lymph nodes and pancreatic or perisplenic nodes [3]. These lymph nodes surround splenic veins and if they get enlarged due to inflammation or malignancy, put pressure on veins and cause obstruction and thrombosis [7]. Despite earlier reports pointing to pancreatic carcinoma as the most common cause of SVT [7, 9] most recent studies conclude that acute or chronic pancreatitis particularly in pancreatic tail is the probable cause of SVT in most patients [1, 9].

Pancreatitis is the initiating cause of thrombosis in 60% of patients; however, diagnosis of SVT in these patients does not always occur during an acute attack [3, 9]. Other causes for SVT include the following: adenopathy of metastatic carcinoma and lymphoma and iatrogenic reasons after operations such as partial gastrectomy and distal splenorenal shunt [1, 2]. Splenectomy is the treatment of choice for SVT [5]. In patients with gastric varices bleeding resulting from SVT, splenectomy must be done as an emergency because gastric varices have a relatively higher potential for massive bleeding than esophageal varices. And also no other treatment is available to put the bleeding under control [7, 10]. The role of prophylactic splenectomy in asymptomatic patients is still controversial. Previous studies showed high rates of variceal hemorrhage in patients with SVT; therefore many authors recommended splenectomy in this group of patients. But recent studies indicate that gastric varices bleeding only occurs in 40% of patients and thus prophylactic splenectomy is not recommended [7]. In this case no underlying disorders such as pancreatic associated etiologies (e.g., traumas, gastric operations, umbilical vein catheterizations, malignancies, retroperitoneal disease, splenic artery aneurysms, myeloproliferative disease, protein S deficiency, protein C deficiency, antithrombin III deficiency, and factor V Leiden mutation) were present and no evidence of antiphospholipid syndrome was seen. This convinced us that this case was interesting enough to be reported as an idiopathic isolated splenic vein thrombosis case.

Conflict of Interests

The authors declare that there is no conflict of interests regarding the publication of this paper.

References

[1] A. Kumar, P. Sharma, and A. Arora, "Review article: portal vein obstruction—epidemiology, pathogenesis, natural history, prognosis and treatment," *Alimentary Pharmacology & Therapeutics*, vol. 41, no. 3, pp. 276–292, 2015.

[2] N. Hidajat, H. Stobbe, V. Griesshaber, R. J. Schroder, and X. Felix, "Portal vein thrombosis: etiology, diagnostic strategy, therapy and management," *Vasa*, vol. 34, no. 2, pp. 81–92, 2005.

[3] S. Köklü, Ş. Çoban, O. Yüksel, and M. Arhan, "Left-sided portal hypertension," *Digestive Diseases and Sciences*, vol. 52, no. 5, pp. 1141–1149, 2007.

[4] N. A. Nadkarni, S. Khanna, and S. S. Vege, "Splanchnic venous thrombosis and pancreatitis," *Pancreas*, vol. 42, no. 6, pp. 924–931, 2013.

[5] B. C. Chen, H. H. Wang, Y. C. Lin, Y. L. Shih, W. K. Chang, and T. Y. Hsieh, "Isolated gastric variceal bleeding caused by splenic lymphoma-associated splenic vein occlusion," *World Journal of Gastroenterology*, vol. 19, no. 40, pp. 6939–6942, 2013.

[6] J. R. Butler, G. J. Eckert, N. J. Zyromski, M. J. Leonardi, K. D. Lillemoe, and T. J. Howard, "Natural history of pancreatitis-induced splenic vein thrombosis: a systematic review and meta-analysis of its incidence and rate of gastrointestinal bleeding," *HPB*, vol. 13, no. 12, pp. 839–845, 2011.

[7] S. M. Weber and L. F. Rikkers, "Splenic vein thrombosis and gastrointestinal bleeding in chronic pancreatitis," *World Journal of Surgery*, vol. 27, no. 11, pp. 1271–1274, 2003.

[8] S. R. Deitcher, E. Caiola, and A. Jaffer, "Demystifying two common genetic predispositions to venous thrombosis," *Cleveland Clinic Journal of Medicine*, vol. 67, no. 11, pp. 825–836, 2000.

[9] S. Koklu, A. Koksal, O. F. Yolcu et al., "Isolated splenic vein thrombosis: an unusual cause and review of the literature," *Canadian Journal of Gastroenterology*, vol. 18, no. 3, pp. 173–174, 2004.

[10] G. Karagiannis, A. Anagnostara, V. Samaras, and S. Mylona, "Isolated splenic vein thrombosis," *Journal Belge de Radiologie—Belgisch Tijdschrift voor Radiologi*, vol. 95, no. 2, article 105, 2012.

40

NIV-Helmet in Severe Hypoxemic Acute Respiratory Failure

Joana Martins, P. Nunes, C. Silvestre, C. Abadesso, H. Loureiro, and H. Almeida

Pediatric Intensive Care Unit, Professor Doutor Fernando Fonseca Hospital, Lisbon, Portugal

Correspondence should be addressed to Joana Martins; joana.jm@gmail.com

Academic Editor: Bibhuti Das

Noninvasive ventilation (NIV) is a method to be applied in acute respiratory failure, given the possibility of avoiding tracheal intubation and conventional ventilation. A previous healthy 5-month-old boy developed low-grade intermittent fever, flu-like symptoms, and dry cough for 3 days. On admission, he showed severe respiratory distress with SpO_2/FiO_2 ratio of 94. Subsequent evaluation identified an RSV infection complicated with an increase of inflammatory parameters (reactive C protein 15 mg/dL). Within the first hour after NIV-helmet CPAP SpO_2/FiO_2 ratio increased to 157. This sustained improvement allowed the continuing of this strategy. After 102 h, he was disconnected from the helmet CPAP device. The NIV use in severe hypoxemic acute respiratory failure should be carefully monitored as the absence of clinical improvement has a predictive value in the need to resume to intubation and mechanical ventilation. We emphasize that SpO_2/FiO_2 ratio is a valuable monitoring instrument. Helmet interface use represents a more comfortable alternative for providing ventilatory support, particularly to small infants, which constitute a sensitive group within pediatric patients.

1. Background

Respiratory Syncytial Virus (RSV) is a major cause of viral respiratory tract infections in infants and children. The course of RSV infection is usually benign, with low mortality rates (estimated 2–5%), even for high-risk patients [1].

Acute respiratory failure (ARF) secondary to RSV infection has its prevalence estimated in 0.8–2.5%. However, this risk is difficult to access, since different groups within the pediatric population show different prevalence of ARF. For instance, 7.3–42% of children with bronchopulmonary dysplasia develop ARF in the context of RSV infection [2].

The mainstay of treatment for patients with severe ARF has been intubation and mechanical ventilation. However, noninvasive ventilation (NIV) can be considered as an alternative, given the possibility of avoiding direct complications of tracheal intubation and conventional ventilation [3, 4]. Nonetheless, it should be closely monitored in order to intubate and ventilate the patient in the presence of complications.

The main goals of using NIV, continuous positive airway pressure (CPAP) or bilevel positive airway pressure (BPAP), in patients with ARF are to improve oxygenation, to unload the respiratory muscles, and to relieve dyspnea, all of which should decrease the intubation rate.

Neuromuscular drive, inspiratory muscle effort, and relief of dyspnea significantly improve with BiPAP, compared to CPAP; however, oxygenation is better correlated with higher CPAP level (10 cm H_2O) [4].

In this case report, we used the SpO_2/FiO_2 ratio as a descriptive measurement of ARF severity.

Oxygen saturation as measured by SpO_2/FIO_2 ratio has been demonstrated to correlate well with the PaO_2/FiO_2 ratio in both adult and pediatric studies, as long as SpO_2 is between 80 and 97%. When SpO_2 is over 97%, the oxyhemoglobin dissociation curve flattens and the SpO_2/FiO_2 ratio reliability is lost [5]. Rice et al. [6] validated this measurement for adults, by demonstrating that, for $SpO_2 \leq 97\%$, PaO_2/FiO_2 ratio of 200 corresponds to SpO_2/FiO_2 ratio of 235.

2. Case Report

A previous healthy 5-month-old boy (10 Kg), with unknown familiar history, presents with low-grade intermittent fever, flu-like symptoms, and dry cough 3 days prior to admission. The symptoms progressively worsened, leading to an

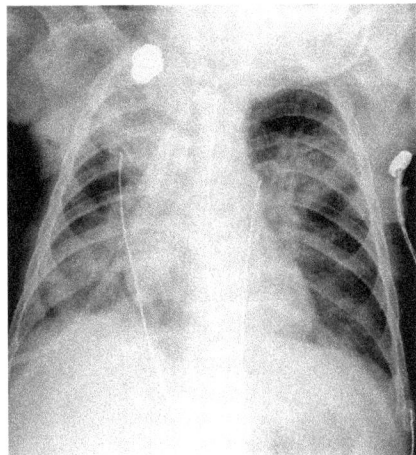

FIGURE 1: Thoracic X-ray on admission.

increased respiratory rate (RR: 80 bpm), respiratory distress (use of accessory respiratory muscles and subcostal and sternal retractions), and tachycardia (150–200 bpm). At pulmonary auscultation, subcrepitant rales were present with no increase of expiratory time.

On PICU admission, he presented SpO_2 of 81% on room air (FiO_2 0.21) which responded poorly to oxygen administration, leading to the use of high oxygen flow mask (Venturi mask) with an initial FiO_2 of 0.6 (SpO_2 increases to the maximum of 91%), quickly ascending to FiO_2 1.0 (SpO_2 of 92–94%: SpO_2/FiO_2 ratio 94).

Laboratory work-up revealed venous pH 7.430, pCO_2 34.8, HCO_3 22.6, and base excess of −1,3, microcytic hypocromic anemia, normal leucocyte count (leucocyte 6000/mm^3, neutrophils 44.2%, and lymphocytes 41.7%), and a reactive protein C of 15 mg/dL. Respiratory secretions rapid immunological test identified RSV infection.

Thoracic X-ray (Figure 1) evaluation identified multiple hypotransparent foci, mainly at the upper right lobe, affecting three quadrants out of four, leading to the presumptive diagnosis of bronchopneumonia.

SpO_2/FiO_2 index was calculated, minimum of 94 (prior to NIV-CPAP implementation).

3. Treatment

The patient was then started on antibiotics, crystalline G penicillin 300 000 UI/Kg/day, and was connected to the helmet CPAP device (Figure 2), with an initial FiO_2 0.6 and PEEP 10 cm H_2O.

Initially, there was a need for sedation boluses with midazolam (0.1 mg/kg q2 administration).

4. Follow-Up

Within the first hour after starting NIV, SpO_2/FiO_2 rose to 156, leading to SpO_2/FiO_2 of 240 by the second hour after connection (Figure 3).

By the same time, prominent improvement was also detected in respiratory rate and signs of respiratory effort (mainly intercostal and subcostal retractions).

In the first 48 h after admission, NIV suspension (need for secretions removal, for instance) caused a rapid oxygenation drop and a subsequent increase of the respiratory effort. Progressively, periods without ventilatory support became larger and more tolerated by the patients.

During the NIV administration period, there was no need for further sedative boluses. The patient was kept quiet using chloral hydrate 1-2 administrations a day, mainly in the first 48 hours of ventilatory support.

After 102 h of ventilatory support, he was definitely disconnected from the helmet CPAP device, keeping O_2 administration through nasal prongs. He was transferred to a general pediatric ward at the 9th day after admission.

5. Discussion

NIV has shown positive effects in adult patients with different types of respiratory failure, being specially safe and effective for patients with hypercapnic ARF due to chronic obstructive pulmonary disease (COPD) exacerbation and hypoxemic ARF due to cardiogenic pulmonary oedema, community-acquired pneumonia, and immunocompromised patients with pulmonary infiltrates [7–9].

In pediatric population, NIV use in ARF patients showed a success rate between 57% and 92% [4], but this rate heterogeneity may be due to different age groups under analysis.

This patient represents a not so prevalent evolution for a RSV respiratory infection in a previously healthy child: within 3 days after the first symptoms, he progressed to hypoxemic ARF.

This patient was submitted to a numerous other tests (cultural analysis of blood and sputum) in order to identify other possible respiratory agents, but no other causes were determined. Nonetheless, the patient was started on antibiotics (intravenous penicillin 300 000 UI/Kg/day) right after admission, as bacterial coinfection was suspected mostly through the reactive protein C determination.

Much thought was dedicated to the possibility of this patient being an ARDS patient; however, according to the Berlin definition [10], he does not fulfill the diagnosis criteria, as the time between the beginning of the symptoms and the ARF was less than a week. Also we did not use PaO_2 measurements to determine the PaO_2/FiO_2 ratio as recommended by this task force.

Essouri et al. [11] determined success rate in pediatric ARF patients under NIV of 73%. However, in the ARDS group, this success reached only 22%.

There are however other factors that can be used to predict NIV failure: lower age, apnea, bacterial coinfection [12], lower weight [13], higher clinical severity score (PRISM score, for instance), smaller respiratory and heart rate decrease within 1 hour after NIV, and increasing need for supplementary oxygen [13].

Mayordomo-Colunga et al. [13] suggested SpO_2/FiO_2 ratio of 193 one hour after NIV as the cut-off value under

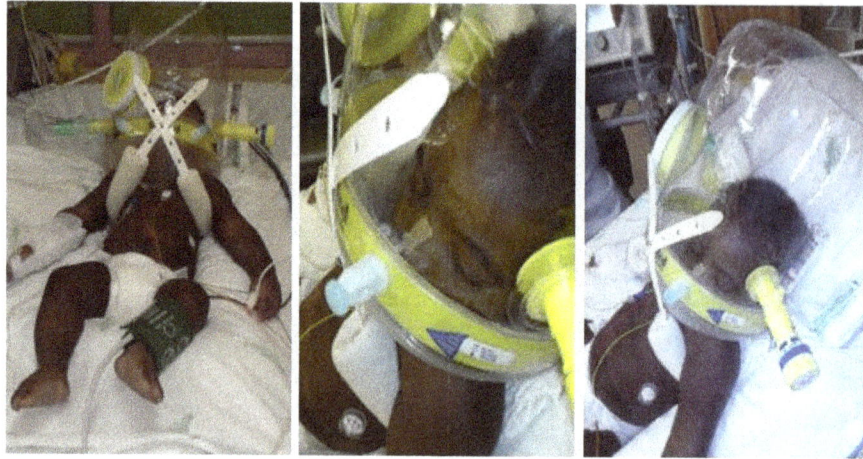

FIGURE 2: Helmet interface use with significant comfort for the patient.

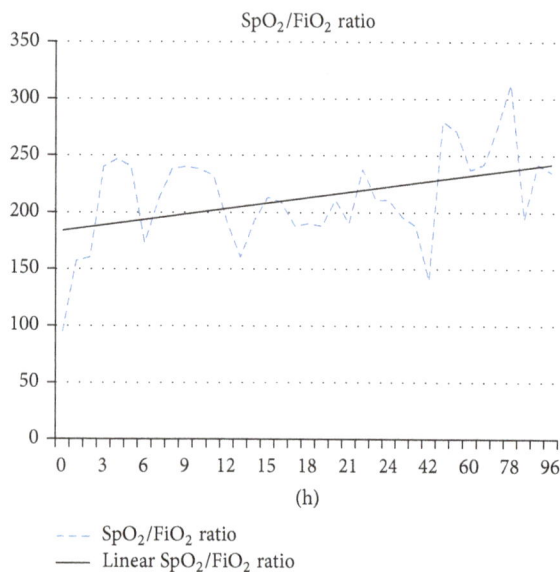

FIGURE 3: SpO$_2$/FiO$_2$ evolution after helmet CPAP connection.

which endotracheal intubation should be considered in any ARF patient. In our case, 1 h after connection, our patient was still under the cut-off value, but the hemodynamic stability, the absence of gasometrical deterioration, a decrease in the FiO$_2$ supplied, and a steady improvement in respiratory effort lead us to continue with NIV strategy under close surveillance.

By the second hour after NIV, the SpO$_2$/FiO$_2$ ratio was above the suggested cut-off value, granting us the support to maintain the chosen treatment. Nonetheless, severe ARF patients under NIV require close attention: Antonelli et al. refer to as much as seventy percent of the NIV failure of adult population being intubated within 48 hours [14]; however, Mayordomo-Colunga et al. showed that, in a pediatric population, the mean time of NIV support prior to failure and intubation was 13 to 16 h [11–13].

The choice between interfaces is mainly determined by the comfort that can be provided to the patient. In the adult population, face mask or helmet use have had the same rate of success (52% versus 49%) [14]. In pediatric patients, it is globally assumed that the different interfaces do not cause differences in the NIV success ratio, but it is only logical to assume that the difficulty in achieving a good ventilatory-child synchrony can be responsible for some of the failure cases. Most authors refer to the difficulty in fighting leakage, finding the appropriate mask size according to each child and preventing skin pressure lesions. Additionally, there is a comprehensible need of sedative use in these patients which can somehow compromise respiratory drive.

Skin pressure lesions are the NIV's more frequent complications: their incidence is estimated in 23% [15], and both facial and nasal interfaces share the same problems.

The helmet interface choice was mainly determined by this child's context: being a heavy and reactive 5 months old infant, we suspected that the adaptation to an oronasal interface would not be easy and would require sedative use.

The helmet adaptation was, nonetheless, simple and fast, with sedative use in boluses needed only in the first day. Two hours after NIV connection, the early response was notorious, with a significant reduction in FiO$_2$ need and RR, but mainly the SpO$_2$/FiO$_2$ ratio increased in a steady way from 156–160 1 h after connection to above 200 <48 h after the connection.

6. Learning Points

(i) NIV use in severe ARF should be closely monitored.

(ii) The first hours after NIV connection are crucial to determine the risk of NIV failure.

(iii) Helmet use represents a more comfortable alternative for providing ventilatory support, particularly to small infants, which constitute a sensitive group within pediatric patients.

Conflict of Interests

The authors declare that there is no conflict of interests regarding the publication of this paper.

References

[1] J. Hammer, A. Numa, and C. J. L. Newth, "Acute respiratory distress syndrome caused by respiratory syncytial virus," *Pediatric Pulmonology*, vol. 23, no. 3, pp. 176–183, 1997.

[2] J. G. de Dios and C. O. Sangrador, "Consensus conference on acute bronchiolitis (I): methodology and recommendations," *Anales de Pediatría*, vol. 72, no. 3, pp. 221.e1–221.e33, 2010.

[3] R. Agarwal, A. N. Aggarwal, and D. Gupta, "Role of noninvasive ventilation in acute lung injury/acute respiratory distress syndrome: a proportion meta-analysis," *Respiratory Care*, vol. 55, no. 12, pp. 1653–1660, 2010.

[4] J. Mayordomo-Colunga, A. Medina, C. Rey et al., "Predictive factors of non invasive ventilation failure in critically ill children: a prospective epidemiological study," *Intensive Care Medicine*, vol. 35, no. 3, pp. 527–536, 2009.

[5] R. G. Khemani, N. J. Thomas, V. Venkatachalam et al., "Comparison of SpO2 to PaO2 based markers of lung disease severity for children with acute lung injury," *Critical Care Medicine*, vol. 40, no. 4, pp. 1309–1316, 2012.

[6] T. W. Rice, A. P. Wheeler, G. R. Bernard et al., "Comparison of the SpO_2/FiO_2 ratio and the PaO_2/FiO_2 ratio in patients with acute lung injury and ARDS," *Chest*, vol. 132, pp. 410–417, 2007.

[7] M. Antonelli, G. Conti, M. L. Moro et al., "Predictors of failure of noninvasive positive pressure ventilation in patients with acute hypoxemic respiratory failure: a multi-center study," *Intensive Care Medicine*, vol. 27, no. 11, pp. 1718–1728, 2001.

[8] M. Antonelli, G. Conti, M. Bufi et al., "Noninvasive ventilation for treatment of acute respiratory failure in patients undergoing solid organ transplantation: a randomized trial," *The Journal of the American Medical Association*, vol. 283, no. 2, pp. 235–241, 2000.

[9] M. Antonelli, G. Conti, M. Rocco et al., "A comparison of noninvasive positive-pressure ventilation and conventional mechanical ventilation in patients with acute respiratory failure," *The New England Journal of Medicine*, vol. 339, no. 7, pp. 429–435, 1998.

[10] The ARDS Definition Task Force, "Acute respiratory distress syndrome: the Berlin definition," *Journal of the American Medical Association*, vol. 307, no. 23, pp. 2526–2533, 2012.

[11] S. Essouri, L. Chevret, P. Durand, V. Haas, B. Fauroux, and D. Devictor, "Noninvasive positive pressure ventilation: five years of experience in a pediatric intensive care unit," *Pediatric Critical Care Medicine*, vol. 7, no. 4, pp. 329–334, 2006.

[12] C. Abadesso, P. Nunes, C. Silvestre, E. Matias, H. Loureiro, and H. Almeida, "Non-invasive ventilation in acute respiratory failure in children," *Pediatric Reports*, vol. 4, no. 2, article e16, 2012.

[13] J. Mayordomo-Colunga, M. Pons, Y. López et al., "Predicting non-invasive ventilation failure in children from the SpO_2/FiO_2 (SF) ratio," *Intensive Care Medicine*, vol. 39, no. 6, pp. 1095–1103, 2013.

[14] M. Antonelli, G. Conti, A. Esquinas et al., "A multiple-center survey on the use in clinical practice of noninvasive ventilation as a first-line intervention for acute respiratory distress syndrome," *Critical Care Medicine*, vol. 35, no. 1, pp. 18–25, 2007.

[15] C. S. James, C. P. J. Hallewell, D. P. L. James, A. Wade, and Q. Q. Mok, "Predicting the success of non-invasive ventilation in preventing intubation and re-intubation in the paediatric intensive care unit," *Intensive Care Medicine*, vol. 37, no. 12, pp. 1994–2001, 2011.

41

Central Hypoventilation: A Case Study of Issues Associated with Travel Medicine and Respiratory Infection

Kam Lun Hon,[1] **Alexander K. C. Leung,**[2] **Albert M. C. Li,**[1] **and Daniel K. K. Ng**[3]

[1]*Department of Paediatrics, The Chinese University of Hong Kong, Prince of Wales Hospital, Shatin, Hong Kong*
[2]*Department of Pediatrics, University of Calgary, Calgary, AB, Canada T2M 0H5*
[3]*Department of Paediatrics, Kwong Wah Hospital, Kowloon, Hong Kong*

Correspondence should be addressed to Kam Lun Hon; ehon@hotmail.com

Academic Editor: Alexander Binder

Aim. We presented the case of a child with central hypoventilation syndrome (CHS) to highlight issues that need to be considered in planning long-haul flight and problems that may arise during the flight. *Case.* The pediatric intensive care unit (PICU) received a child with central hypoventilation syndrome (Ondine's curse) on nocturnal ventilatory support who travelled to Hong Kong on a make-a-wish journey. He was diagnosed with central hypoventilation and had been well managed in Canada. During a long-haul aviation travel, he developed respiratory symptoms and desaturations. The child arrived in Hong Kong and his respiratory symptoms persisted. He was taken to a PICU for management. The child remained well and investigations revealed no pathogen to account for his respiratory infection. He went on with his make-a-wish journey. *Conclusions.* Various issues of travel medicine such as equipment, airline arrangement, in-flight ventilatory support, travel insurance, and respiratory infection are explored and discussed. This case illustrates that long-haul air travel is possible for children with respiratory compromise if anticipatory preparation is timely arranged.

1. Introduction

Travel medicine is the branch of medicine that deals with the prevention and management of health problems of international travelers [1–4]. We presented the case of a child with central hypoventilation syndrome (CHS) to highlight issues that need to be considered in planning long-haul flight and problems that may arise during the flight.

2. Case

In the summer of 2013, the pediatric intensive care unit (PICU) of a hospital in Hong Kong received an 8-year-old boy with central hypoventilation with respiratory infection and decompensation en route to Hong Kong on a make-a-wish campaign. He was diagnosed with central hypoventilation (medullary atrophy) or Ondine's curse and had been well managed in Toronto, Canada. He was ambulatory, only needed home ventilatory support at night via tracheostomy, and inhaled salbutamol puffs on a *prn* basis, and he was on

PEG (percutaneous endoscopic gastrostomy) feeding with puree food. Advanced fitness for air-travel arrangement was well negotiated with the respective commercial airline. However, he developed symptoms of respiratory infections with intermittent fever (up to 39°C), cough, and sputum for 2 days prior to departure. The child was seen at the emergency department of a children's hospital in Toronto and was treated with an oral course of cefuroxime. During the long-haul flight, symptoms of respiratory infections persisted and desaturations (86%) developed. The patient had his own oxygen monitoring and air compressor on board which needed to be increased to 1 L/min. On arrival in Hong Kong, he was taken to the emergency department. His vital signs were as follows: tympanic temperature 38.6°C, heart rate 157/min, and SpO$_2$ 98% on own ventilator with flow 1 L/min. The home ventilator's electric plug was in Canadian style and did not fit the Hong Kong standard socket. Chest radiograph revealed mild right sided haziness. He was admitted to PICU for management. He weighed 23.2 kg and his vital signs were as follows: temperature 36.5°C, heart rate 121/min, respiratory rate 23/min, BP 97/57 mmHg, and SpO$_2$ 97% in room air on arrival at PICU. The child received physiotherapy and the tracheostomy was temporarily connected to the ICU ventilator on SIMV mode with pressure control (PC) and pressure support (PS). Settings were FiO$_2$ 0.25, inspiratory time (Ti) 0.9 seconds, intermittent mandatory ventilation (IMV) rate 20/min, positive end expiratory pressure (PEEP) 5 cm H$_2$O, pressure control 15 cm H$_2$O above PEEP, and PS 13 cm H$_2$O above PEEP. There was no further desaturation, and the settings were gradually reduced to IMV 10/min and FiO$_2$ of 0.21. The child gave a history of drug allergy to Ativan (lorazepam) and gluten sensitivity. Sedation was not needed. He received a course of intravenous amoxicillin/clavulanate (30 mg/kg/dose, 8 hourly). The patient remained playful, talkative, and not in distress. Laboratory data were normal complete blood count with white blood cell count of 16.1 × 10^9/L, neutrophil differential of 77%, and elevated C-reactive protein of 44.1 (normal < 9.9 mg/L). There was no bacterial or respiratory viral isolation in the tracheal aspirate. Blood culture was negative. The patient was discharged from the PICU 2 days later and went on with his make-a-wish journey to Disneyland in Hong Kong prior to returning home.

3. Discussion

Ondine's curse, also called congenital central hypoventilation syndrome (CCHS) or primary alveolar hypoventilation, is a serious form of central nervous system failure, involving an inborn failure of autonomic control of breathing. Patients generally require tracheotomies and lifetime mechanical ventilator support. With advances of home ventilatory support, patients with central hypoventilation are no longer "cursed." They can live a relative normal life at home, as reported by Hon et al., even in the remote countryside setting in one case report [5–7].

Travel medicine is the branch of medicine that deals with the prevention and management of health problems of international travelers [1–4]. The field of travel medicine encompasses a wide variety of disciplines including epidemiology, infectious disease, public health, tropical medicine, high altitude physiology, travel related obstetrics, psychiatry, occupational medicine, military and migration medicine, and environmental health. In our case, potential problems that may arise during travel include cardiopulmonary disease mortality, injury, and accident. Infectious disease accounts for about 2.8–4% of deaths during/from travel [1–4, 8–10]. In terms of morbidity, traveler's diarrhea is the most common problem encountered [9, 10].

In this day and age, international travel is made possible even for patients who need ventilatory support. Prior to a long-haul air travel, parents should negotiate with airline to detail the transport and inflight plans [8, 11, 12]. The following part gives 4 website addresses of checklists for commercial air-travel preparation for ventilated children. In our case of CCHS with specific needs for ventilatory support, the patient, family, and the airline collaborated well. In general, the patient's usual emergency medication such as inhaled salbutamol should be readily accompanying the patient. Additional space is required to station the ventilator, air compressor, and monitor. An international travel insurance policy is mandatory in this age of unexpected and unavoidable disasters [8].

Websites of checklists for commercial air-travel preparation for ventilated children are as follows:

(1) A Special Needs Preflight Checklist: 16 Things You Need to Do before Heading to the Airport (http://www.friendshipcircle.org/blog/2012/01/09/a-special-needs-pre-flight-checklist/).

   (i) Booking your tickets:

      (a) Stopover or direct flight?
      (b) Best time of day to travel.
      (c) Choose airline wisely.
      (d) What seat is best for your child?

   (ii) Medical preparation:

      (a) Travel prescriptions.
      (b) A letter from a doctor.
      (c) Medications and medical records.
      (d) Medical equipment.
      (e) In case of emergency.

   (iii) Preparing your child to fly:

      (a) Read about airports and airplanes.
      (b) Airplane videos.
      (c) Social stories.
      (d) Airport visits.
      (e) Mock flights.

   (iv) Before you head to the airport:

      (a) Call Transportation Security Administration (TSA) in the USA.
      (b) Small bills.
      (c) Check in at home.
      (d) Have a backup plan.
      (e) Take a deep breath and smile.

(2) Medical Guidelines for Airline Passengers, Aerospace Medical Association, Alexandra, VA (May, 2002) (http://www.asma.org/asma/media/asma/Travel-Publications/paxguidelines.pdf).

   (i) General advice:

      (a) Have all medication in carry-on luggage and be sure it is in its original container with the prescription label.
      (b) If you have significant medical problems, carry an abbreviated copy of your medical records.
      (c) Alert airlines in advance of special requirements.
      (d) Wear loose comfortable clothing.
      (e) Allow extra time.
      (f) Consider buying insurance which includes provision for air evacuation home in event of any medical condition.

(3) Travel with a Ventilator: Ventilation Resource Site (http://www.livingwithavent.com/pages.aspx?view=noninv&page=Living/Travel).

    (i) Talk with other ventilator users.

    (ii) Consider power.

    (iii) Include supplies.

    (iv) Check transportation procedures:

        (a) Plan travel well in advance.

        (b) Obtain approval for in-flight ventilation.

        (c) Get to the airport with ample time before departure.

        (d) Protect the ventilator.

        (e) Bring adequate power for the use of the ventilator in flight, or check if the aircraft has outlets for medical use.

        (f) Check oxygen availability during flight.

        (g) Prepare for possible technical problems with the ventilator.

    (v) Know ventilator settings.

(4) Air Travel and Ventilator Users, International Ventilator Users Network, 2003 (http://www.ventusers.org/edu/valnews/val17-3c.html#air).

    This website gives some tips about travelling with a ventilator.

One more issue pertinent to the discussion of travel medicine is advice regarding feasibility of long-haul travel in a patient with acute or intercurrent respiratory infection. Since the days of SARS (severe acute respiratory syndrome) and recently MERS (Middle East respiratory syndrome) and SARI (severe acute respiratory infection), travel transmission of novel respiratory infections has become hot issues [13–15]. Ideally, patients with an acute respiratory infection should not be travelling for the patient's own sake as well as for the sake of other passengers. However, travel may be once-in-a-lifetime opportunity for a young person with chronic illness as was in our case. This may be inhumane to the child if his/her opportunity was removed from him/her due to a non-life threatening chest infection. On the other hand, the risk has to be weighed between a seemingly minor infection which may predispose a major decompensation during long-haul travel in a child with already compromised respiratory health.

No published literature on mortality and morbidity in children travelling with central hypoventilation syndrome or Ondine's curse is available. Critically ill children are transported safely via medical evacuation teams [16, 17]. However, critically ill children cannot be transported via commercial airlines. Our case illustrates that children who are ventilator dependent may travel in commercial airlines if they are stable. The issue of quarantine to prevent international transmission of SARI is a much more complicated issue that is likely to remain a contemporary controversy. This case illustrates the many issues associated with long-haul flight in a pediatric patient with a chronic respiratory disorder. Air travel is possible for children with respiratory compromise if anticipatory preparation is timely arranged.

Conflict of Interests

The authors declare that they have no conflict of interests.

References

[1] M. Cupa, "Air transport, aeronautic médecine, health," *Bulletin de l'Academie Nationale de Medecine*, vol. 193, no. 7, pp. 1619–1631, 2009.

[2] F. Al-Zurba, B. Saab, and U. Musharrafieh, "Medical problems encountered among travelers in Bahrain International Airport clinic," *Journal of Travel Medicine*, vol. 14, no. 1, pp. 37–41, 2007.

[3] O. Eray, M. Kartal, N. Sikka, E. Goksu, O. E. Yigit, and F. Gungor, "Characteristics of tourist patients in an emergency department in a Mediterranean destination," *European Journal of Emergency Medicine*, vol. 15, no. 4, pp. 214–217, 2008.

[4] P. Felkai, "Analysis of prevention in travellers diseases on the basis of latest results in travel medicine," *Orvosi Hetilap*, vol. 149, no. 36, pp. 1707–1712, 2008.

[5] E. K. Hon, M. Wilson, and R. C. Hindle, "The survival story of a child with Ondine's curse in Northland," *New Zealand Medical Journal*, vol. 107, no. 976, pp. 149–150, 1994.

[6] G. Juan, M. Ramon, M. A. Ciscar et al., "Acute respiratory insufficiency as initial manifestation of brain stem lesions," *Archivos de Bronconeumología*, vol. 35, no. 11, pp. 560–563, 1999.

[7] T.-C. Wang, Y.-N. Su, and M.-C. Lai, "PHOX2B mutation in a Taiwanese newborn with congenital central hypoventilation syndrome," *Pediatrics and Neonatology*, vol. 55, no. 1, pp. 68–70, 2014.

[8] R. Cocks and M. Liew, "Commercial aviation in-flight emergencies and the physician," *Emergency Medicine Australasia*, vol. 19, no. 1, pp. 1–8, 2007.

[9] K. Harvey, D. H. Esposito, P. Han et al., "Surveillance for travel-related disease—GeoSentinel Surveillance System, United States, 1997–2011," *Morbidity and Mortality Weekly Report. Surveillance Summaries*, vol. 62, no. 3, pp. 1–15, 2013.

[10] H. Kollaritsch, M. Paulke-Korinek, and U. Wiedermann, "Traveler's diarrhea," *Infectious Disease Clinics of North America*, vol. 26, no. 3, pp. 691–706, 2012.

[11] H. Matthys, "Fit for high altitude: are hypoxic challenge tests useful?" *Multidisciplinary Respiratory Medicine*, vol. 6, no. 1, pp. 38–46, 2011.

[12] A. Basu, "Middle ear pain and trauma during air travel," *BMJ Clinical Evidence*, vol. 2007, article 0501, 2007.

[13] K. L. Hon, "Just like SARS," *Pediatric Pulmonology*, vol. 44, no. 10, pp. 1048–1049, 2009.

[14] K. L. Hon, "Severe respiratory syndromes: travel history matters," *Travel Medicine and Infectious Disease*, vol. 11, no. 5, pp. 285–287, 2013.

[15] P. L. Lim, T. H. Lee, and E. K. Rowe, "Middle east respiratory syndrome coronavirus (MERS CoV): update 2013," *Current Infectious Disease Reports*, vol. 15, no. 4, pp. 295–298, 2013.

[16] K. L. Hon, H. Olsen, B. Totapally, and T.-F. Leung, "Hyperventilation at referring hospitals is common before transport in intubated children with neurological diseases," *Pediatric Emergency Care*, vol. 21, no. 10, pp. 662–666, 2005.

[17] K.-L. E. Hon, H. Olsen, B. Totapally, and T.-F. Leung, "Air versus ground transportation of artificially ventilated neonates: comparative differences in selected cardiopulmonary parameters," *Pediatric Emergency Care*, vol. 22, no. 2, pp. 107–112, 2006.

42

Bladder Wall Telangiectasia in a Patient with Ataxia-Telangiectasia and How to Manage?

Fatma Deniz Aygün, Serdar Nepesov, Haluk Çokuğraş, and Yıldız Camcıoğlu

Department of Pediatric Infectious Diseases, Clinical Immunology and Allergy, Istanbul University, Cerrahpasa Medical Faculty, 34098 Istanbul, Turkey

Correspondence should be addressed to Fatma Deniz Aygün; fdenizaygun@gmail.com

Academic Editor: Mohammad Ehlayel

Ataxia-telangiectasia (A-T) is a rare neurodegenerative, inherited disease causing severe morbidity. Oculocutaneous telangiectasias are almost constant findings among the affected cases as telangiectasia is considered the main clinical finding for diagnosis. Vascular abnormalities in organs have been reported infrequently but bladder wall telangiectasias are extremely rare. We aimed to report recurrent hemorrhage from bladder wall telangiectasia in a 9-year-old boy with A-T who had received intravenous cyclophosphamide for non-Hodgkin's lymphoma. Since A-T patients are known to be more susceptible to chemical agents, we suggested that possibly cyclophosphamide was the drug which induced bladder wall injury in this patient.

1. Introduction

Ataxia-telangiectasia is an immunodeficiency syndrome with a wide spectrum of findings including progressive cerebellar ataxia, oculocutaneous telangiectasia, ionizing radiation hypersensitivity, susceptibility to developing lymphoreticular malignancy, and defects in DNA repair [1]. It is an autosomal recessive inherited disorder caused by mutations in the ATM gene, a serine/threonine kinase located on the long arm of chromosome 11, that activates proteins in cellular response to DNA damage [2]. Approximately 10% of A-T homozygotes develop malignancy, mostly of the lymphoid system, including Hodgkin's lymphoma [1, 3]. Telangiectasia is pathognomonic component of the disease, partially giving the disease its name. Oculocutaneous area is the most commonly affected, vascular involvement in other parts of the body have been reported [4], but bladder wall telangiectasia is extremely rare and reported only in a few patients. This report describes development of bladder wall telangiectasia and hemorrhagic cystitis in a patient with ataxia-telangiectasia who had been treated with cyclophosphamide for NHL.

2. Case Report

A 9-year–old boy was admitted to the Immunology Department due to recurrent pulmonary infections and meningitis. He was the son of nonconsanguineous parents with no known diseases. His developmental stages were delayed. His height and weight measurements were less than 3rd percentile. He had ataxia and ocular telangiectasia, without cutaneous involvement. He did not have any other cerebellar sign. Physical examinations of chest, abdomen, and cardiovascular system were in normal limits. Laboratory analysis including complete blood count and liver and renal function tests were all in normal ranges. Serum immunoglobulin G level was low, 427 mg/dL (normal range 780–1600), IgA was low, 32 mg/dL (normal range 70–400), but IgM was very high, 1330 mg/dL (normal range 40–320). Flow cytometric analysis of T, B, and NK cells revealed normal values. Serum alpha fetoprotein (AFP) was elevated to 196,45 IU/mL (normal range < 5.8 IU/mL) supporting the diagnosis of ataxia-telangiectasia, and cranial MRI revealed cerebellar atrophy. A-T was also subsequently confirmed by identification of c.7788G>A(p.Glu2596Glu) homozygous mutations in both alleles of the ATM gene.

At the age of 9, he developed B-cell NHL in the lower pole of left kidney. He was treated with R-CHOP protocol, including cyclophosphamide (CPA), doxorubicin, vincristine, and prednisolone, which achieved cure. Concomitant Mesna administration and massive hydration were given to prevent bladder damage during the course of treatment.

Six months after the cure, he developed massive, painless hematuria requiring blood transfusion for two times. His blood pressure was normal. In laboratory studies, blood urea nitrogen, creatinine level, and coagulation parameters were all normal; thrombocytopenia was not seen at any time. The polymerase chain reaction (PCR) analysis of urine for adenovirus and polyoma BK virus tests were both negative; urine culture was sterile. The viral serology including cytomegalovirus (CMV), Epstein-Barr virus, and CMV DNA was negative. No calculi or signs of damage at renal parenchyma were seen in ultrasonography. Cystoscopy revealed a blood clot in the bladder with multiple telangiectasias in the bladder wall. A large clot was removed from the bladder following catheter irrigation of the bladder with regular saline solution. Later on, bilateral ureteral stents were placed. We were able to perform PCR assay for polyomavirus JC in his serum during his follow-up and viremia was not demonstrated. During the 6th month of follow-up, he still had telangiectasia in bladder wall but a gradual improvement was observed in the patient's clinical symptoms with the ureteral stents and he did not need further urological treatment.

3. Discussion

Telangiectasia is the hallmark of ataxia-telangiectasia. In most cases, telangiectasias first appear when the child reaches three to five years of age; they are progressive and have symmetric distribution. In our patient, telangiectasia first appeared when he was 4 years old. He was diagnosed to have bladder wall telangiectasias when he was 9 years old.

Telangiectasias of blood vessels are seen primarily on the bulbar conjunctivae and on exposed areas of the skin, typically the pinnae, nose, face, and neck [5]. Vascular anomalies in various organs, like brain, hepatic vein, and intestinal mucosa, have been reported, but bladder wall telangiectasia is very rare.

Significant bleeding from telangiectasia is also very infrequent in AT. There are only few reported cases describing mucosal hemorrhage from cerebral telangiectasia besides the reported infrequent bladder wall hemorrhages before our case [6].

Bladder wall telangiectasia was first described in 2008 with two patients of A-T and lymphoma who also received CPA including chemotherapy [7]. Authors suggested that hematuria could be due to the toxic effect of CPA during lymphoma therapy. They concluded that since A-T is a DNA repair disorder and the ATM gene has an important role in cell cycle arrest in response to cellular stress, it is possible that A-T patients are more sensitive than normal individuals

to CPA induced bladder damage which leads to the development of clinically significant telangiectasias.

In the same year, another patient with A-T who developed massive hematuria due to bladder wall varices was reported from Japan [8]. He was also treated with CPA for autoimmune thrombocytopenia 3 years ago.

Patients with A-T and diagnosis of malignancy are more susceptible to toxic effects of chemotherapy. Despite significant toxicity, CPA remains as a drug of choice in cancer chemotherapy. The exact mechanism causing the induction of cell death is unknown, but Goldstein et al. considered that DNA interstrand cross-links can be responsible for its cytotoxicity. They also showed the apoptotic death induced by mafosfamide, a CPA analogue by contribution of DNA replication and transcription inhibition [9].

Hemorrhagic cystitis is a well-known side effect of CPA caused by exposure of bladder mucosa to acrolein, a urinary toxic metabolite of CPA. The damage of bladder wall induced by acrolein is followed by ulceration, neovascularization, and hemorrhage which leads to hemorrhagic cystitis. As A-T patients are more sensitive to chemical agents, acrolein may accelerate the development of telangiectasia in bladder wall mucosa.

Sandoval and Swift reported hemorrhagic cystitis in 50% of A-T patients receiving 1200 mg/m² or more CPA despite hyperhydration [10], but these patients did not receive Mesna which is known to reduce bladder toxicity of CPA. Concomitant administration of Mesna with CPA is recommended as we did.

It is suggested that some of the patients with A-T who receive CPA therapy may subsequently develop bladder hemorrhage regardless of the single or cumulative dose. So the use of CPA, even at a relative low dose, should be avoided in the treatment of patients with A-T.

The last case of bleeding from bladder wall telangiectasia in A-T patient was reported by Christmann et al. in 2008. The patient was a 10-year-old boy having bladder wall telangiectasia and infection with polyomavirus JC. BK and JC virus are from the Polyomaviridae family and cause hemorrhagic cystitis in immunocompromised patients. But the patient reported in that article had also received CPA for lymphoma like other cases [11]. We investigated our patient for polyomavirus, adenovirus, and cytomegalovirus and therefore excluded these viral causes.

In conclusion, A-T is caused by mutations in the ATM gene, which is involved in the detection of DNA damage, and plays an important role in cell cycle progression. The defect in DNA repair in A-T also explains the sensitivity of patients to chemotherapeutic agents. It is possible that our case developed hemorrhagic cystitis after CPA therapy. Despite our support of massive hydration and Mesna administration, his underlying defective DNA damage was the probable cause of bleeding.

Conflict of Interests

The authors declare that there is no conflict of interests regarding the publication of this paper.

References

[1] R. A. Gatti, S. Becker-Catania, H. H. Chun et al., "The pathogenesis of ataxia-telangiectasia: learning from a Rosetta Stone," *Clinical Reviews in Allergy and Immunology*, vol. 20, no. 1, pp. 87–108, 2001.

[2] R. Kitagawa and M. B. Kastan, "The ATM-dependent DNA damage signaling pathway," *Cold Spring Harbor Symposia on Quantitative Biology*, vol. 70, pp. 99–109, 2005.

[3] F. Gumy-Pause, P. Wacker, and A.-P. Sappino, "ATM gene and lymphoid malignancies," *Leukemia*, vol. 18, no. 2, pp. 238–242, 2004.

[4] M. Kamiya, H. Yamanouchi, T. Yoshida et al., "Ataxia telangiectasia with vascular abnormalities in the brain parenchyma: report of an autopsy case and literature review," *Pathology International*, vol. 51, no. 4, pp. 271–276, 2001.

[5] S. Greenberger, Y. Berkun, B. Ben-Zeev, Y. B. Levi, A. Barziliai, and A. Nissenkorn, "Dermatologic manifestations of ataxia-telangiectasia syndrome," *Journal of the American Academy of Dermatology*, vol. 68, no. 6, pp. 932–936, 2013.

[6] E. Nardelli, E. Fincati, M. Casaril, and A. M. Iannucci, "Multiple cerebral hemorrhages in ataxia-telangiectasia. A case report," *Acta Neurologica*, vol. 7, no. 6, pp. 494–499, 1985.

[7] J. M. Cohen, P. Cuckow, and E. G. Davies, "Bladder wall telangiectasis causing life-threatening haematuria in ataxia-telangiectasia: a new observation," *Acta Paediatrica, International Journal of Paediatrics*, vol. 97, no. 5, pp. 667–669, 2008.

[8] K. Suzuki, K. Tsugawa, E. Oki, T. Morio, E. Ito, and H. Tanaka, "Vesical varices and telangiectasias in a patient with ataxia telasngiectasia," *Pediatric Nephrology*, vol. 23, no. 6, pp. 1005–1008, 2008.

[9] M. Goldstein, W. P. Roos, and B. Kaina, "Apoptotic death induced by the cyclophosphamide analogue mafosfamide in human lymphoblastoid cells: contribution of DNA replication, transcription inhibition and Chk/p53 signaling," *Toxicology and Applied Pharmacology*, vol. 229, no. 1, pp. 20–32, 2008.

[10] C. Sandoval and M. Swift, "Treatment of lymphoid malignancies in patients with ataxia-telangiectasia," *Medical and Pediatric Oncology*, vol. 31, no. 6, pp. 491–497, 1998.

[11] M. Christmann, S. Heitkamp, E. Lambrecht, K. Doerries, R. Schubert, and S. Zielen, "Haemorrhagic cystitis and polyomavirus JC infection in ataxia telangiectasia," *Journal of Pediatric Urology*, vol. 5, no. 4, pp. 324–326, 2009.

43

A Rare Cause of Prepubertal Gynecomastia: Sertoli Cell Tumor

Fatma Dursun,[1] **Şeyma Meliha Su Dur,**[2] **Ceyhan Şahin,**[3] **Heves Kırmızıbekmez,**[1] **Murat Hakan Karabulut,**[4] **and Asım Yörük**[5]

[1]*Ümraniye Training and Research Hospital, Pediatric Endocrinology, 34766 Istanbul, Turkey*
[2]*Ümraniye Training and Research Hospital, Radiology, Istanbul, Turkey*
[3]*Ümraniye Training and Research Hospital, Pediatric Surgery, Istanbul, Turkey*
[4]*Ümraniye Training and Research Hospital, Pathology, Istanbul, Turkey*
[5]*Göztepe Training and Research Hospital, Pediatric Oncology, Istanbul, Turkey*

Correspondence should be addressed to Fatma Dursun; fatmadursun54@yahoo.com

Academic Editor: Anup Mohta

Prepubertal gynecomastia due to testis tumors is a very rare condition. Nearly 5% of the patients with testicular mass present with gynecomastia. Sertoli cell tumors are sporadic in 60% of the reported cases, while the remaining is a component of multiple neoplasia syndromes such as Peutz-Jeghers syndrome and Carney complex. We present a 4-year-old boy with gynecomastia due to Sertoli cell tumor with no evidence of Peutz-Jeghers syndrome or Carney complex.

1. Introduction

Prepubertal gynecomastia is characterized by the presence of palpable unilateral or bilateral breast tissue in boys, without other signs of sexual maturation. Gynecomastia is common in normal males in the neonatal period, at early puberty, and with increasing age [1]. Prepubertal gynecomastia is a rare condition, and there are limited numbers of case reports in the medical literature. Some cases were associated with excessive aromatase activity or estrogen producing adrenal or testis tumors [1].

Sertoli cell tumors (SCTs) account for 2% of prepubertal testicular tumors and very few have occurred in the first decade of life. The most common presenting symptom of a testicular tumor is painless scrotal mass. Gynecomastia can be seen in approximately 5% of patients with testicular mass. Most of the SCTs in prepubertal boys, which are generally bilateral and diffuse, are in the content of Peutz-Jeghers Syndrome (PJS) or Carney complex [2].

2. Case Report

A 4-year-old boy was referred to pediatric endocrinology because of bilateral breast enlargement. There was no history of a chronic disease, medication, or a familial disorder. Height was 114 cm (+1.2 SDS), weight was 20 kg (+0.7 SDS), and physical examination revealed bilateral gynecomastia. Breast development appeared as Tanner Stage-2 (Figure 1), axillary and pubic hair were absent, stretched penile length was 6 × 1.5 cm, and right testis was 2 mL and left testis was 5 mL (Figure 2). Hormone levels were in normal ranges (Table 1); tumor markers were negative while scrotal ultrasonography (USG) exhibited a 8 × 12 mm solid lesion with cystic component in the left testis. The committee on tumoral diseases agreed on the decision to perform a testis-sparing surgery in the light of examination of frozen sections. However the large and cystic mass left no adequate testis tissue to conserve, so a left orchiectomy was performed. Abdomen and thorax Computed Tomography (CT) imaging were normal. Histopathological investigation revealed a SCT which had positive staining with inhibin, vimentin, and calretinin. Gynecomastia regressed at the end of three months following the operation.

3. Discussion

Gynecomastia is common in boys at early puberty, while prepubertal gynecomastia is a rare condition. It is generally

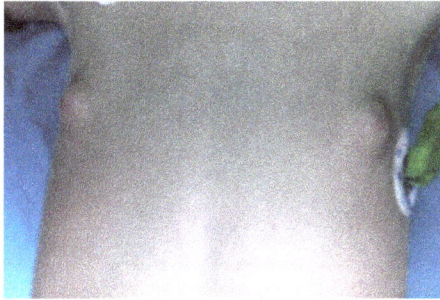

FIGURE 1: Bilateral gynecomastia.

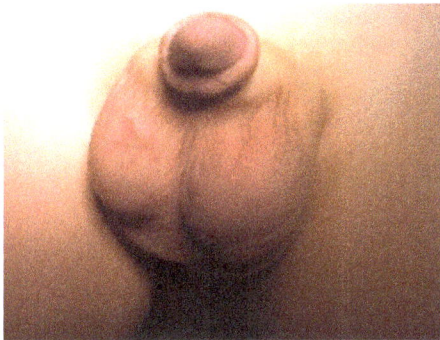

FIGURE 2: Asymmetrical testicles.

TABLE 1: Results of laboratory and imaging studies of the patient.

LH* ($N < 0.05$)	0.05 mIU/mL
FSH* (N: 0.1–3)	0.11 mIU/mL
Total testosterone (N: <0.14)	0.13 ng/mL
TSH* (N: 0.7–6.4)	1.02 mIU/mL
Free T4* (N: 0.8–2.2)	1.17 ng/dL
17OHP* (N: 0.03–0.9)	0.9 ng/mL
Prolactin (N: 2.89–35)	23 ng/mL
Cortisol ($N > 9$)	13.4 mcg/dL
DHEA-S* (N: 5–57)	17.8 mcg/dL
Estradiol ($N < 10$)	<10 pg/mL
SHBG* (N: 11.2–100)	125.3 nmol/L
Bone age	5 years 9 months
Beta-HCG* ($N < 1$)	0.1 mIU/mL
Alpha fetoprotein ($N < 9$)	0.3 ng/mL
Carcinoembryogenic antigen (N: 0–3)	0.9 ng/mL
Scrotal ultrasonography	Right testis: 0.5 mL. 12 × 8 mm solid mass with cystic component in the central area was detected in left testis.
Thorax Computed Tomography	Normal
Abdomen Computed Tomography	Normal

*LH: luteinizing hormone; FSH: follicle stimulating hormone; TSH: thyroid stimulating hormone; Free T4: free tiroksin-4; 17OHP: 17-hydroxy-progesterone; DHEA-S: dehydroepiandrostenedione-sulphate; SHBG: sex-hormone-binding-globulin; Beta-HCG: beta-human chorionic gonadotropin; N: normal range.

considered a pathological sign of a possible endocrinopathy, requiring a detailed history, physical examination, and laboratory work-up [1]. Most of the patients have peripubertal gynecomastia (25%) or drug-induced breast development (20%). The frequencies of some remaining causes have been estimated as follows: cirrhosis (8%), primary hypogonadism (8%), testicular tumors (3%), secondary hypogonadism (2%), hyperthyroidism (1.5%), and renal disease (1%). In other cases, prepubertal gynecomastia has been the endocrine manifestation of rare syndromes, such as PJS [3].

The records of Prepubertal Testicular Tumor Registry include forty-two patients with stromal tumors, of whom only 10 patients had SCT with an overall mean age of 52.5 months at presentation [1, 4]. They are sporadic in 60% of the reported cases, but in the remaining cases they are linked to multiple neoplasia syndromes such as PJS and Carney complex [5, 6]. The neoplastic Sertoli cells overexpress p450 aromatase (CYP19A1), which is normally found in only low concentrations in prepubertal Leydig cells. Aromatase allows for increased conversion of 1.4-androstenedione (the major source of androgens from the adrenal gland in prepubertal males with SCTs) to estrone. As only minimal elevations of estrogens are needed to advance the bone maturation and cause gynecomastia, physicians should take into consideration the sensitivity of the assay used to measure estrogens [6]. We could not measure level of serum estrone. Testosterone is also converted to estradiol, but this is less of an issue in prepubertal boys with SCTs [5]. Although these hormone levels may still remain below the detection limit of standard assays, the sensitivity of the growth plates and breast tissue

to estrogens may lead to growth acceleration, advanced bone age, and gynecomastia in prepubertal boys. Such presentation is similar to that observed in cases of aromatase excess syndrome due to rearrangements in the CYP19A1 gene [7].

There is no specific differential immunoprofile for this tumor. Vimentin, inhibin, and calretinin seem more widely expressed and may help the diagnosis of SCTs [2]. Malignancy is found in approximately 17% of patients with SCTs. Malignant SCTs usually occur in older patients (mean age 39 years) and those who have unilateral and unifocal disease (for comparison, the mean age of presentation for benign tumors is 17 years). Indices of malignancy include mitotic count greater than 3 per 10 high-power fields, size larger than 4 cm, significant nuclear atypia, tumor necrosis, and angiolymphatic invasion [6, 8, 9]. Our patient had no evidence of malignancy. Gynecomastia has been well reported in prepubertal boys with SCTs but in the context of PJS. The tumors in this context are more diffuse with calcifications, often bilateral, and may respond to medical treatment [7, 10]. SCTs in the context of Carney Complex are similarly diffuse and bilateral [11]. Also our patient had unilateral testicular mass.

In conclusion, our patient had unilateral testicular solid-cystic mass with no evidence of perioral lesions, intestinal symptoms, or family history for syndromes. Although unilateral testicular mass is very rarely reported, this patient should be followed up carefully in terms of other clinical findings of PJS as well as Carney Complex. This case was reported to remind of a very rare condition in the etiology of prepubertal gynecomastia and emphasize on the importance of careful physical examination and scrotal USG.

Conflict of Interests

The authors declare that there is no conflict of interests regarding the publication of this paper.

References

[1] R. Einav-Bachar, M. Phillip, Y. Aurbach-Klipper, and L. Lazar, "Prepubertal gynaecomastia: aetiology, course and outcome," *Clinical Endocrinology*, vol. 61, no. 1, pp. 55–60, 2004.

[2] B. Burgu, O. Aydoğdu, O. Telli et al., "An unusual cause of infantile gynecomastia: sertoli cell tumor," *Journal of Pediatric Hematology/Oncology*, vol. 33, no. 3, pp. 238–240, 2011.

[3] G. A. Ferraro, T. Romano, F. De Francesco et al., "Management of prepubertal gynecomastia in two monozygotic twins with Peutz-Jeghers syndrome: from aromatase inhibitors to subcutaneous mastectomy," *Aesthetic Plastic Surgery*, vol. 37, no. 5, pp. 1012–1022, 2013.

[4] J. H. Ross and R. Kay, "Prepubertal testis tumors," *Reviews in Urology*, vol. 6, pp. 11–18, 2004.

[5] A. Brodie, S. Inkster, and W. Yue, "Aromatase expression in the human male," *Molecular and Cellular Endocrinology*, vol. 178, no. 1-2, pp. 23–28, 2001.

[6] E. Gourgari, E. Saloustros, and C. A. Stratakis, "Large-cell calcifying Sertoli cell tumors of the testes in pediatrics," *Current Opinion in Pediatrics*, vol. 24, no. 4, pp. 518–522, 2012.

[7] M. K. Crocker, E. Gourgari, M. Lodish, and C. A. Stratakis, "Use of aromatase inhibitors in large cell calcifying sertoli cell tumors: effects on gynecomastia, growth velocity, and bone age," *Journal of Clinical Endocrinology and Metabolism*, vol. 99, no. 12, pp. E2673–E2680, 2014.

[8] S. K. Halat, L. E. Ponsky, and G. T. MacLennan, "Large cell calcifying Sertoli cell tumor of testis," *The Journal of Urology*, vol. 177, no. 6, article 2338, 2007.

[9] S. S. Kratzer, T. M. Ulbright, A. Talerman et al., "Large cell calcifying sertoli cell tumor of the testis: contrasting features of six malignant and six benign tumors and a review of the literature," *American Journal of Surgical Pathology*, vol. 21, no. 11, pp. 1271–1280, 1997.

[10] T. M. Ulbright, M. B. Amin, and R. H. Young, "Intratubular large cell hyalinizing sertoli cell neoplasia of the testis: a report of 8 cases of a distinctive lesion of the Peutz-Jeghers syndrome," *The American Journal of Surgical Pathology*, vol. 31, no. 6, pp. 827–835, 2007.

[11] B. Brown, A. Ram, P. Clayton, and G. Humphrey, "Conservative management of bilateral sertoli cell tumors of the testicle in association with the carney complex: a case report," *Journal of Pediatric Surgery*, vol. 42, no. 9, pp. e13–e15, 2007.

44

Therapeutic Hypothermia and Out-of-Hospital Cardiac Arrest in a Child with Hypertrophic Obstructive Cardiomyopathy

Nancy Spurkeland,[1] Gregory Bennett,[2] Chandran Alexander,[2] Dennis Chang,[3] and Gary Ceneviva[4]

[1]Penn State Hershey College of Medicine, Hershey, PA 17033, USA
[2]Department of Pediatrics, Hershey Medical Center, Hershey, PA 17033, USA
[3]Department of Pediatrics, Pediatric Cardiology, Hershey Medical Center, Hershey, PA 17033, USA
[4]Department of Pediatrics, Pediatric Intensive Care, Hershey Medical Center, Hershey, PA 17033, USA

Correspondence should be addressed to Gary Ceneviva; gceneviva@hmc.psu.edu

Academic Editor: Carmelo Romeo

Neurologic outcomes following pediatric cardiac arrest are consistently poor. Early initiation of cardiopulmonary resuscitation has been shown to have positive effects on both survival to hospital discharge, and improved neurological outcomes after cardiac arrest. Additionally, the use of therapeutic hypothermia may improve survival in pediatric cardiac arrest patients admitted to the intensive care unit. We report a child with congenital hypertrophic obstructive cardiomyopathy and an out-of-hospital cardiac arrest, in whom the early initiation of effective prolonged cardiopulmonary resuscitation and subsequent administration of therapeutic hypothermia contributed to a positive outcome with no gross neurologic sequelae. Continuing efforts should be made to promote and employ high-quality cardiopulmonary resuscitation, which likely contributed to the positive outcome of this case. Further research will be necessary to develop and solidify national guidelines for the implementation of therapeutic hypothermia in selected subpopulations of children with OHCA.

1. Introduction

Epidemiologic studies regarding the outcome of out-of-hospital cardiac arrest (OHCA) in children show heterogeneous results. OHCA in Netherlands resulted in 24% (12/51) survival to hospital discharge; however, larger studies in the United States, Canada, and Japan revealed overall survival rates ranging from 6.4% (40/621) to 8.5% (700/8240) [1–3]. While recovery rates from OHCA in children are low, they are even lower for those with preexisting cardiac disease [4, 5]. Although bystander cardiopulmonary resuscitation (CPR) has been associated with improved survival following cardiac arrest, prolonged CPR is associated with poor outcomes [2, 6]. Therapeutic hypothermia as a method of neuroprotection following cardiac arrest is gaining popularity within the field of pediatrics [1]. There is paucity of peer-reviewed medical literature detailing successful therapeutic hypothermia utilization in children with preexisting cardiac comorbidities [2].

We describe a 12-year-old female with a known history of hypertrophic obstructive cardiomyopathy (HOCM) who responded to therapeutic hypothermia following prolonged CPR for sudden cardiac arrest.

2. Case Report

A 12-year-old Caucasian female with a known history of HOCM (asymmetric, obstructive type) and Wolff-Parkinson-White syndrome (WPW) without supraventricular tachycardia collapsed while waiting at the school bus stop. She was unresponsive and pulseless, raising concern for cardiac arrest. Her father, a trained emergency medical technician (EMT) who witnessed the event, immediately performed CPR in the field for an estimated 30 minutes until emergency medical personnel arrived. Cardiac rhythm analysis revealed ventricular fibrillation. Manual external defibrillation (DC cardioversion) was utilized twice during transport to a local hospital, the second of which returned her to a sinus rhythm. She remained unconscious and was hemodynamically unstable, requiring endotracheal intubation, multiple normal saline intravenous boluses, and pressor therapy. She was stabilized and subsequently transferred to the PICU in our tertiary care children's hospital for further evaluation and treatment.

The patient's EKG upon admission showed a QTc of 508 milliseconds, which was prolonged from her baseline of 458 milliseconds. Due to her witnessed collapse and prompted initiation of CPR, a therapeutic hypothermia protocol was initiated with a 48-hour cooling regimen. Goal temperatures were between 32.5 and 33 degrees Celsius during cooling. The patient was maintained on antiepileptic therapy for seizure prophylaxis, as well as fentanyl and midazolam drips for appropriate sedation while undergoing therapeutic hypothermia. An EEG performed within 24 hours of admission showed "intermittent diffuse background slowing with no epileptiform discharges, focal features, or asymmetries." The patient was rewarmed at hour 48 at a rate of 1 degree Celsius every six hours over the course of the ensuing 48 hours, ultimately accomplishing euthermia between 36.5 and 37.5 degrees Celsius. Extubation trials failed on hospital day 5 due to delirium and shallow work of breathing; following CPAP trials on hospital day 10, successful extubation occurred with no gross neurologic, renal, or hepatic insults noted on clinical and laboratory evaluation. An MRI (multiplanar, multisequence MRI without contrast) of the brain at day 10 revealed no structural abnormalities or evidence of gross ischemia. An adenosine challenge was also conducted in the electrophysiology laboratory, which revealed that the cardiac preexcitation was secondary to a fasciculoventricular pathway not capable of participating in tachycardia. Therefore, it was determined that this accessory pathway did not contribute to tachycardia leading to cardiac arrest in this instance. An automated implantable cardioverter defibrillator was placed on hospital day 15. The patient was discharged on hospital day 17 with no neurological sequelae to date. Follow-up EKGs have demonstrated a return to her baseline QTc of 460 milliseconds. She has experienced no recurrent episodes of torsades de pointes, ventricular tachycardia, or ventricular fibrillation.

3. Discussion

This case correlates with existing studies that have demonstrated a survival benefit of early initiation of CPR [3]. It is theorized that cardiac arrests in children often result in poor outcomes when they occur out-of-hospital due to delays in initiation of CPR, nonavailability of advanced life support capabilities, and a lack of the necessary facilities to implement therapeutic hypothermia [4]. Early effective CPR reduces the time during which patients are hypoxic or anoxic.

Over the past half century, therapeutic hypothermia has been increasingly used as an adjunctive component of resuscitation in a variety of critically ill pediatric populations with mixed results. A multicenter, multinational randomized control trial comparing the efficacy of therapeutic hypothermia to normothermia in pediatric traumatic brain injury (TBI) patients demonstrated no mortality benefit associated with the use of hypothermia [5]. Despite documented relative successes in animal models and neonates, favorable neurologic outcomes occur in as few as one-third of pediatric patients who undergo therapeutic hypothermia after surviving cardiac arrest [6]. Other studies have reported concern regarding the use therapeutic hypothermia in patients with QTc prolongation due to the increased risk of ventricular fibrillation [7]. However, a recent report documented the successful use of therapeutic hypothermia as a means of neuroprotection in a child with OHCA and congenital long QT syndrome [8]. The use of therapeutic hypothermia in our patient who developed prolonged QTc as a result of an OHCA supports its safety in patients who may be predisposed to serious arrhythmias [9].

Much of the current peer-reviewed evidence for the utilization of therapeutic hypothermia in young children is based on patients who suffered cardiac arrest secondary to a respiratory etiology (most commonly drowning or choking) as opposed to those of cardiac origin [4]. Likewise, population based studies regarding pediatric OHCA have not mentioned the specific cardiac causes, nor the adaptation of therapeutic hypothermia in postresuscitation treatment, which further highlights the rarity of our patient's case [3, 10]. In a prospective study describing the epidemiology and outcomes after pediatric out-of-hospital cardiac arrest, only 9% (54/601) of patients suffered cardiac arrest from ventricular fibrillation [6]. To our knowledge, none of these children with documented cardiomyopathy were reported to have HOCM.

This case is an illustration of the utility of both high-quality CPR in the field and therapeutic cooling in the PICU in a child with OHCA and accompanying congenital heart disease. Continuing efforts should be made to promote and employ high-quality CPR in the general population, which likely contributed to the positive outcome in this instance. Further research is necessary to develop guidelines for routine utilization of therapeutic hypothermia in selective groups of children with OHCA like those with underlying cardiac etiology.

Abbreviations

HOCM: Hypertrophic obstructive cardiomyopathy
OHCA: Out-of-hospital cardiac arrest
TBI: Traumatic brain injury
WPW: Wolff-Parkinson-White syndrome.

Conflict of Interests

The authors have no conflict of interests to disclose. No external funding was secured for this study. The authors have no financial relationships relevant to this paper to disclose.

Authors' Contribution

Nancy Spurkeland identified the case, drafted the initial paper, reviewed and revised the paper, and approved the final paper as submitted. Gregory Bennett and Chandran

Alexander identified the case, reviewed and revised the paper, and approved the final paper as submitted. Dennis Chang and Gary Ceneviva reviewed, revised, and approved the final paper as submitted.

References

[1] Y. Okamoto, T. Iwami, T. Kitamura et al., "Regional variation in survival following pediatric out-of-hospital cardiac arrest," *Circulation Journal*, vol. 77, no. 10, pp. 2596–2603, 2013.

[2] J. J. Lin, S. H. Hsia, H. S. Wang, M. C. Chiang, and K. L. Lin, "Therapeutic hypothermia associated with increased survival after resuscitation in children," *Pediatric Neurology*, vol. 48, no. 4, pp. 285–290, 2013.

[3] P. E. Litwin, M. S. Eisenberg, A. P. Hallstrom, and R. O. Cummins, "The location of collapse and its effect on survival from cardiac arrest," *Annals of Emergency Medicine*, vol. 16, no. 7, pp. 787–791, 1987.

[4] P. M. Kochanek, E. L. Fink, M. J. Bell, H. Bayir, and R. S. B. Clark, "Therapeutic hypothermia: applications in pediatric cardiac arrest," *Journal of Neurotrauma*, vol. 26, no. 3, pp. 421–427, 2009.

[5] P. D. Adelson, S. R. Wisniewski, J. Beca et al., "Comparison of hypothermia and normothermia after severe traumatic brain injury in children (Cool Kids): a phase 3, randomised controlled trial," *The Lancet Neurology*, vol. 12, no. 6, pp. 546–553, 2013.

[6] K. D. Young, M. Gausche-Hill, C. D. McClung, and R. J. Lewis, "A prospective, population-based study of the epidemiology and outcome of out-of-hospital pediatric cardiopulmonary arrest," *Pediatrics*, vol. 114, no. 1, pp. 157–164, 2004.

[7] J. N. Khan, N. Prasad, and J. M. Glancy, "QTc prolongation during therapeutic hypothermia: are we giving it the attention it deserves?" *Europace*, vol. 12, no. 2, pp. 266–270, 2010.

[8] M. K. Aktas and A. Aguila, "Successful therapeutic hypothermia in patients with congenital long QT syndrome," *Annals of Noninvasive Electrocardiology*, vol. 16, no. 1, pp. 100–103, 2011.

[9] N. Nishiyama, T. Sato, Y. Aizawa, S. Nakagawa, and H. Kanki, "Extreme QT prolongation during therapeutic hypothermia after cardiac arrest due to long QT syndrome," *American Journal of Emergency Medicine*, vol. 30, no. 4, pp. 638.e5–638.e8, 2012.

[10] A. Bardai, J. Berdowski, C. van der Werf et al., "Incidence, causes, and outcomes of out-of-hospital cardiac arrest in children. A comprehensive, prospective, population-based study in the Netherlands," *Journal of the American College of Cardiology*, vol. 57, no. 18, pp. 1822–1828, 2011.

45

Gingival Bleeding of a High-Flow Mandibular Arteriovenous Malformation in a Child with 8-Year Follow-Up

Elvira Ferrés-Amat,[1,2,3] **Jordi Prats-Armengol,**[1,2] **Isabel Maura-Solivellas,**[3]
Eduard Ferrés-Amat,[1] **Javier Mareque-Bueno,**[1,2] **and Eduard Ferrés-Padró**[1,2]

[1]*Service of Oral and Maxillofacial Surgery, Fundació Hospital de Nens de Barcelona, Consell de Cent 437, 08009 Barcelona, Spain*
[2]*Department of Oral and Maxillofacial Surgery, Faculty of Dentistry, Universitat Internacional de Catalunya,*
Josep Trueta s/n, Sant Cugat del Vallès, 08195 Barcelona, Spain
[3]*Service of Pediatric Dentistry, Fundació Hospital de Nens de Barcelona, Consell de Cent 437, 08009 Barcelona, Spain*

Correspondence should be addressed to Elvira Ferrés-Amat; elviraferres@hospitaldenens.com

Academic Editor: Nina L. Shapiro

Intraosseous arteriovenous malformations (AVMs) in the head and neck region are uncommon. There are several types and they can have a wide range of clinical presentations. Depending on the blood flow through the AVM, the treatment may be challenging for the attending team and may lead to life-threatening hemorrhages. A clinical case report is presented. A 9-year-old girl, seen for gingival bleeding during oral hygiene, was found to have a high-flow AVM located within and around the mandible. Two-stage treatment consisted of intra-arterial embolization followed by intraoral injection of a sclerosing agent 8 weeks later. At the 8-year follow-up, imaging study showed no evidence of recurrent lesion inside or outside the bone. The final outcome is a correct occlusion with a symmetric facial result. This case shows that conservative treatment may be the first treatment option mostly in children. Arteriography and transcortical injection were enough to control the AVM.

1. Introduction

The classification of benign vascular lesions and the related terminology was confusing until Mulliken and Glowacki [1] differentiated this generic term into two entities: vascular malformations and hemangiomas (tumors). Hemangiomas are one of the most common soft tissue tumors in children [2], whereas vascular malformations occur much less frequently. The currently accepted classification was published by Mulliken and Glowacki in 1982 [1], later modified by Mulliken et al. [3], and accepted in 2014 by the International Society for the Study of Vascular Anomalies (ISSVA) http://www.issva.org/. Vascular malformations are related to an abnormality in embryonic development and are composed of ectatic vessels (venous, arteriovenous, or lymphatic vessels). They are classified according to the vessel affected and the amount of flow through the vessel: high flow

(fistulas, arteriovenous malformations, and mixed malformations) and low flow (capillary, venous, lymphatic, and mixed malformations). Vascular malformations are present from birth, but they may be asymptomatic and go undetected at that time. Most of these lesions appear in the head, neck, and trunk regions [2], and they mainly affect the skin and scalp.

Of all vascular anomalies, AVMs are the most dangerous because they can be associated with life-threatening complications. Despite their benign histology, deep lesions can produce serious systemic signs and symptoms due to extensive arteriovenous shunting and soft tissue hypertrophy. However, AVMs usually produce more subtle signs as they grow. Mandibular AVM shows a wide variety of signs and symptoms, such as dental mobility, otalgia, secondary pain due to thrombosis, facial asymmetry, and cosmetic distress [4–6]. AVMs were classified in 1990 by the International Workshop for the Study of Vascular Anomalies as follows:

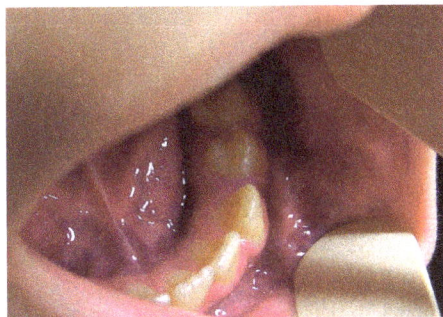

FIGURE 1: Initial intraoral picture.

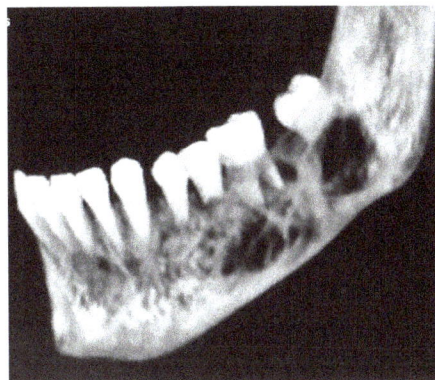

FIGURE 2: Preoperative CT scan.

stage I: cutaneous blush or warmth; stage II: bruit, audible pulsations, expanding lesion; stage III: pain, ulceration, bleeding, and infection; and stage IV: heart failure [7].

In this paper, we report a case of AVM of the mandible manifesting in the pediatric age, with a description of the clinical and imaging findings leading to the diagnosis and the strategy used for treatment.

2. Case Presentation

A 9-year-old girl was received for consultation at the Maxillofacial Unit of Hospital de Nens de Barcelona. She had been referred because of bleeding around the permanent mandibular left first molar. The child had no relevant medical history. Her mother reported gingival bleeding in the left mandible for two months. The patient presented facial asymmetry, with increased size of the lower facial third on the left side. Intraoral examination showed gingival bleeding and an ecchymotic area extending from the canine to the retromolar area (Figure 1). On palpation, the vestibular gingiva soft tissue was found to be hot and pulsatile. The volume of mandibular bone was increased compared to the right side. Furthermore, the permanent mandibular left first molar was mobile. Panoramic radiography showed a poorly delimited, multiloculated radiolucency resembling soap bubbles, displacing the permanent mandibular left second molar and expanding the mandibular cortical bone, without destruction of the dental structures. The patient was referred to Vall d'Hebrón Hospital for a complete imaging study with computed tomography (CT) and magnetic resonance angiography (MRA).

CT confirmed the multiloculated appearance, bone expansion, and preservation of the dental structures within the affected area (from the canine to the left mandibular angle, involving the entire horizontal branch of the mandible) (Figure 2). Gadolinium-enhanced MRA confirmed the diagnosis of a high-flow intra- and perimandibular AVM (Figure 3). Analytical determinations in blood were normal. The findings obtained with these examinations established the diagnosis of a high-flow CAVM (capillary arteriovenous malformation), affecting the left lower third of the face, involving the body and branch of the mandible and the masticatory muscles, mucosa, and skin.

Interventional angiography through a femoral approach was decided as a diagnostic and therapeutic option. Angiography showed a high-flow vascular malformation with

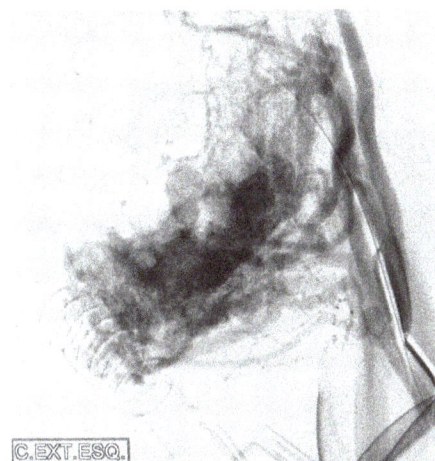

FIGURE 3: Preoperative angiography: left common carotid angiogram, lateral projection, and arterial phase showing extensive mandibular AVM with arterial supply from multiple sources and drainage into the dilated inferior alveolar vein.

branches emerging from the facial artery, the lingual artery, and the inferior alveolar nerve artery. During the procedure, several branches were sclerosed with a 40 : 60 mixture of cyanoacrylate tissue adhesive (Glubran; GEM S.r.l., Viareggio, Italy) + Lipiodol.

As only an angiographic embolization was not enough to solve the problem, a second embolization procedure with femoral access was scheduled 8 weeks later. This time in combination with an intraoral approach, transcortical puncture was used to access the interior of the mandible with a trocar under radioscopic control and angiographic support (Figure 4). An alcoholic solution of zein (Ethibloc; Ethicon, Johnson & Johnson, Switzerland) as sclerosing agent was then injected inside the body and the branch of the mandible, avoiding the tooth buds and roots, and the inferior alveolar nerve. Filling of the vascular lacuna was achieved.

Postoperative imaging showed control of the lesions with ablation of all branches. Follow-up consisted of physical examination, panoramic radiography, and MRI and CT studies. There has been no evidence of relapse to date, at 8 years of follow-up. The patient has functional occlusion with no

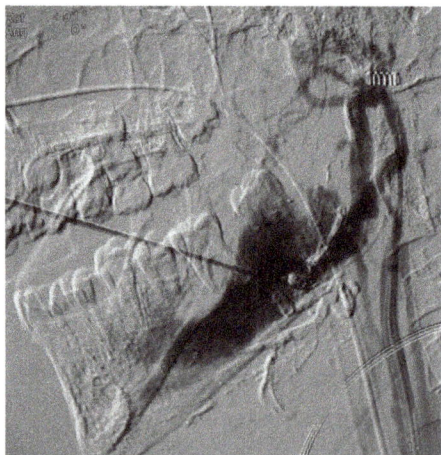

FIGURE 4: Intraoperative transcortical injection.

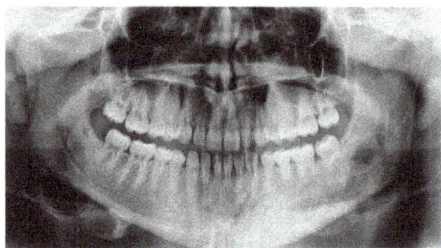

FIGURE 6: 8-year follow-up angio-CT.

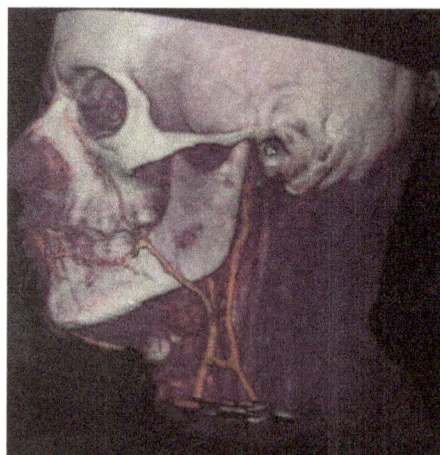

FIGURE 5: 8-year follow-up X-ray.

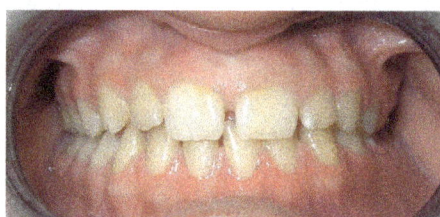

FIGURE 7: 8-year follow-up intraoral picture.

deviation of the mandible or the occlusal plane. There are no aesthetic sequelae, and her permanent mandibular left second molar has erupted correctly; although radiographically they show some root resorption they have no significant mobility (Figures 5–7).

3. Discussion

A high-flow AVM involving the mandible and surrounding soft tissue is extremely rare. The literature contains few cases and they are quite diverse; hence, the overall approach to take and therapeutic algorithm to follow in these patients remain uncertain. As reported by Corsten et al. [8], mandibular AVMs are unusual lesions that many dentists, oral and maxillofacial surgeons, head and neck surgeons, general practitioners, pediatricians, pediatric surgeons, plastic surgeons, ENT, and radiologists may not have encountered previously.

Suspicion of a maxillary or mandibular AVM should arise when the first clinical signs appear, including facial asymmetry, pain, swelling, local heat, tooth mobility, bluish discoloration of the mucosa and gums, or gingival or floor mouth bleeding in a patient with no history of predisposing factors, such as trauma or a known diagnosis of blood dyscrasia or oropharyngeal neoplasm [9]; Lamberg et al. [10] reported that intraosseous AVMs of the maxillofacial region are often diagnosed as a result of dental extraction or exfoliation, which produces torrential and life-threatening hemorrhage because the patient and physician are unaware

of the lesion [11]. It is important to alert the medical and dental community about these lesions; although they are rare, a simple radiographic study combined with clinical examination may suffice to prevent fatal consequences. Any surgical manipulation except emergency procedures to control bleeding should be postponed until the patient is first stabilized and the vascular lesion is occluded by embolization. Biopsies and dental procedures are totally contraindicated due to the risk of fatal bleeding.

The diagnosis is usually made in conjunction with clinical and radiographic investigations. The presence of a mandibular radiolucency on panoramic radiography may suggest AVM as a differential diagnosis. CT angiography shows the lesion and the feeding vessels. MRI can additionally help to differentiate between tumors and malformations. Nonetheless, angiography is the reference standard diagnostic method, although it is more invasive [9]. Regarding the imaging, MR angiography is also effective in demonstrating the vascular supply to the lesion, avoiding the use of radiation in a child. Diagnostic angiography is usually performed at the same procedure as the therapeutic embolization.

High-flow lesions are a challenge for the attending team of professionals. The standard treatment for AVM has been endovascular embolization with subsequent surgical removal of the lesion [12], but nowadays several additional treatments have been described: superselective intra-arterial embolization (SIAE), sclerotherapy, radiotherapy, bone wax packing of bone cavities and curettage, surgical resection, or combinations of these therapies [9, 11, 13–21]. Some authors have used less aggressive techniques than surgery. For example, Liu et al. [22] reported on 8 cases of central AVM of the jaw treated with direct intraosseous glue sclerotherapy. The authors considered the technique to be safe and simple and described complete devascularization and reossification after single or multiple histoacryl injections. Bergeron et al. [23] also found combined endovascular and transcutaneous angioembolization with histoacryl to be effective for mandibular AVM treatment. Mandibular AVMs are usually arterial low venous malformations with single outflow vein physiology. That is the reason why they respond so well to direct transosseous embolization of the draining vein. This effectively closes all of the arteriovenous shunts. It has a very high rate of success and permanency. However, Motamedi et al. [15] suggested that surgical treatment is needed in addition to embolization. Unfortunately, preoperative embolization does not decrease the size of the resection [16]. Segmental resection has been recommended for the treatment of extensive bone lesions. Bone reconstruction has been suggested after AVM resection in the jaws to maintain teeth and temporomandibular joint function and offer biological bases for implants and prostheses [11]. Block resection has also been used in AVMs involving the floor of the mouth or the parotid gland, lip, and cheek to avoid an obvious effect on appearance. Thus, there is considerable evidence that surgical resection is an effective but also aggressive method for the treatment of AVMs.

Recently, minimally invasive surgical management proposals have emerged, such as cleaning the cavity through the alveolar process reported by Azzolini et al. [17], the buccal window approach proposed by Rattan and Sethi [18], and the cortical holes strategy described by Brusati et al. [19]. Wang and Huang [20] proposed curettage via the intraoral approach when the lesion is confined to the bone, which is particularly useful in hospitals with limited equipment, where advanced techniques and instruments are not available. The study of Chen et al. [13] describes various treatments for AVM in the oral and maxillofacial region in 28 patients. The authors concluded that bone wax packing of the bone cavity and curettage is a simple, safe, and effective method for the treatment of AVMs of the jaws. However, radiotherapy and sclerotherapy may not be effective methods for AVMs involving the soft tissue. In 2011, Gluncic et al. [21] reported a case of mandibular AVM treated by molar extraction and direct hydroxyapatite cement infusion into the mandibular cavity, which produced complete hemostasis and AVM obliteration. Surgical ligation, at the origin of both external carotid arteries, usually precludes any further endovascular access to these malformations and should be done only if it is considered the only feasible life-saving procedure, in an emergency situation, in a hospital where endovascular techniques are not available and the patient is not stable enough to be transferred to a larger facility [24–29].

The case presented of a young patient with a mandibular mass consistent with a large and complex AVM was successfully resolved with two sclerotherapy approaches: intraarterial and a transcortical approach. Clinicians must be mindful not to consider cessation of hemorrhage as an indicator of complete cure, because vascular reconstitution can lead to regrowth of the AVM and subsequent hemorrhage. Careful follow-up of patients treated is needed before the procedure's long-term success can be assessed.

4. Conclusions

It is important to be aware of AVMs of the mandible so that the medical community and particularly dentists and pediatricians will take them into account in the differential diagnosis. The diagnosis is easily achieved with physical examination and imaging studies. Patients are usually diagnosed when the first clinical signs appear: pain, swelling, gingival bleeding, local heat, tooth mobility, or bluish discoloration of the mucosa and gums. A correct diagnosis is essential because treatment depends on it, and the proper choice of treatment is also a key factor. Patients with extensive or complex vascular anomalies should be treated by a multidisciplinary team that can provide appropriate, up-to-date treatment. Grouping of cases will facilitate clinical research in this line, with the aim of improving the therapy for this rare condition.

Conflict of Interests

The authors declare that there is no conflict of interests regarding the publication of this paper.

References

[1] J. B. Mulliken and J. Glowacki, "Hemangiomas and vascular malformations in infants and children: a classification based on endothelial characteristics," *Plastic and Reconstructive Surgery*, vol. 69, no. 3, pp. 412–422, 1982.

[2] M. C. Finn, J. Glowacki, and J. B. Mulliken, "Congenital vascular lesions: clinical application of a new classification," *Journal of Pediatric Surgery*, vol. 18, no. 6, pp. 894–900, 1983.

[3] J. B. Mulliken, P. E. Burrows, and S. F. Fishman, *Mulliken and Young's Vascular Anomalies*, Oxford University Press, 2nd edition, 2013.

[4] F. M. Enzinger and S. W. Weiss, *Soft Tissue Tumors*, Mosby, St Louis, Miss, USA, 3rd edition, 1995.

[5] E. Calonje and C. D. M. Fletcher, "Tumors of blood vessels and lymphatics," in *Diagnostic Histopathology of Tumors*, C. D. M. Fletcher, Ed., vol. 1, pp. 50–51, Churchill Livingstone, Edinburgh, UK, 1995.

[6] A. W. Barrett and P. M. Speight, "Superficial arteriovenous hemangioma of the oral cavity," *Oral Surgery, Oral Medicine, Oral Pathology, Oral Radiology, and Endodontics*, vol. 90, no. 6, pp. 731–738, 2000.

[7] M. P. Kohout, M. Hansen, J. J. Pribaz, and J. B. Mulliken, "Arteriovenous malformations of the head and neck: natural history and management," *Plastic and Reconstructive Surgery*, vol. 102, no. 3, pp. 643–654, 1998.

[8] L. Corsten, Q. Bashir, J. Thornton, and V. Aletich, "Treatment of a giant mandibular arteriovenous malformation with percutaneous embolization using histoacrylic glue: a case report," *Journal of Oral and Maxillofacial Surgery*, vol. 59, no. 7, pp. 828–832, 2001.

[9] W.-L. Chen, J.-T. Ye, L.-F. Xu, Z.-Q. Huang, and D.-M. Zhang, "A multidisciplinary approach to treating maxillofacial arteriovenous malformations in children," *Oral Surgery, Oral Medicine,*

Oral Pathology, Oral Radiology and Endodontology, vol. 108, no. 1, pp. 41–47, 2009.

[10] M. A. Lamberg, A. Tasanen, and J. Jääskeläinen, "Fatality from central hemangioma of the mandible," *Journal of Oral Surgery,* vol. 37, no. 8, pp. 578–584, 1979.

[11] N. Bagherzadegan, B. Hohlweg-Majert, T. Mücke et al., "Microvascular bone grafting: a new long-term solution for intraosseous arteriovenous malformations of the mandible in children," *Journal of Cranio-Maxillofacial Surgery,* vol. 39, no. 6, pp. 431–434, 2011.

[12] J. Lemound, P. Brachvogel, F. Götz, M. Rücker, N.-C. Gellrich, and A. Eckardt, "Treatment of mandibular high-flow vascular malformations: report of 2 cases," *Journal of Oral and Maxillofacial Surgery,* vol. 69, no. 7, pp. 1956–1966, 2011.

[13] W. Chen, J. Wang, J. Li, and L. Xu, "Comprehensive treatment of arteriovenous malformations in the oral and maxillofacial region," *Journal of Oral and Maxillofacial Surgery,* vol. 63, no. 10, pp. 1484–1488, 2005.

[14] A. C. B. R. Johann, M. C. F. Aguiar, M. A. V. do Carmo, R. S. Gomez, W. H. Castro, and R. A. Mesquita, "Sclerotherapy of benign oral vascular lesion with ethanolamine oleate: an open clinical trial with 30 lesions," *Oral Surgery, Oral Medicine, Oral Pathology, Oral Radiology and Endodontology,* vol. 100, no. 5, pp. 579–584, 2005.

[15] M. H. K. Motamedi, H. Behnia, and M. R. K. Motamedi, "Surgical technique for the treatment of high-flow arteriovenous malformations of the mandible," *Journal of Cranio-Maxillofacial Surgery,* vol. 28, no. 4, pp. 238–242, 2000.

[16] F. Angiero, S. Benedicenti, A. Benedicenti, K. Arcieri, and E. Bernè, "Head and neck hemangiomas in pediatric patients treated with endolesional 980 nm diode laser," *Photomedicine and Laser Surgery,* vol. 27, no. 4, pp. 553–559, 2009.

[17] A. Azzolini, A. Bertani, and C. Riberti, "Superselective embolization and immediate surgical treatment: our present approach to treatment of large vascular hemangiomas of the face," *Annals of Plastic Surgery,* vol. 9, no. 1, pp. 42–49, 1982.

[18] V. Rattan and A. Sethi, "Arteriovenous malformation of the mandible: successful management by buccal window approach," *British Journal of Oral and Maxillofacial Surgery,* vol. 48, no. 6, pp. e31–e33, 2010.

[19] R. Brusati, S. Galioto, F. Biglioli, and M. Goisis, "Conservative treatment of arteriovenous malformations of the mandible," *International Journal of Oral and Maxillofacial Surgery,* vol. 30, no. 5, pp. 397–401, 2001.

[20] J. Wang and H. Huang, "Intraoral curettage without presurgical endovascular embolization: a simple but controversial treatment of arteriovenous malformations of the mandible," *International Journal of Oral and Maxillofacial Surgery,* vol. 42, no. 1, pp. 133–136, 2013.

[21] V. Gluncic, R. R. Reid, F. M. Baroody, L. J. Gottlieb, and S. A. Ansari, "Hemostasis and obliteration of mandibular arteriovenous malformation through direct hydroxyapatite cement injection into the molar cavity," *Journal of NeuroInterventional Surgery,* vol. 3, no. 1, pp. 92–94, 2011.

[22] D. Liu, X. Ma, F. Zhao, and J. Zhang, "Intraosseous embolotherapy of central arteriovenous malformations in the jaw: long-term experience with 8 cases," *Journal of Oral and Maxillofacial Surgery,* vol. 67, no. 11, pp. 2380–2387, 2009.

[23] M. Bergeron, M. Cortes, Y. Dolev, and L. H. P. Nguyen, "Extensive bilateral arteriovenous malformations of the mandible successfully controlled by combined endovascular and transcutaneous angio-embolization: case report and review of the literature," *International Journal of Pediatric Otorhinolaryngology,* vol. 77, no. 1, pp. 130–136, 2013.

[24] S. A. Resnick, E. J. Russell, D. H. Hanson, and B. C. Pecaro, "Embolization of a life-threatening mandibular vascular malformation by direct percutaneous transmandibular puncture," *Head and Neck,* vol. 14, no. 5, pp. 372–379, 1992.

[25] N. Sakkas, A. Schramm, M. C. Metzger et al., "Arteriovenous malformation of the mandible: a life-threatening situation," *Annals of Hematology,* vol. 86, no. 6, pp. 409–413, 2007.

[26] A. Churojana, R. Khumtong, D. Songsaeng, C. Chongkolwatana, and S. Suthipongchai, "Life-threatening arteriovenous malformation of the maxillomandibular region and treatment outcomes," *Interventional Neuroradiology,* vol. 18, no. 1, pp. 49–59, 2012.

[27] C.-H. Yeh, Y.-M. Wu, Y.-L. Chen, and H. F. Wong, "Contralateral de novo intraosseous arteriovenous malformation in a child with arteriovenous malformation of mandible treated by endovascular embolotherapy: a case report," *Interventional Neuroradiology,* vol. 18, no. 4, pp. 484–489, 2012.

[28] C. C. de Souza Loureiro, P. C. F. Falchet, J. Gavranich Jr., and L. F. L. Leandro, "Embolization as the treatment for a life-threatening mandibular arteriovenous malformation," *Journal of Craniofacial Surgery,* vol. 21, no. 2, pp. 380–382, 2010.

[29] S. M. Manjunath, S. Shetty, N. J. Moon et al., "Arteriovenous malformation of the oral cavity," *Case Reports in Dentistry,* vol. 2014, Article ID 353580, 5 pages, 2014.

46

A Child with Lung Hypoplasia, Congenital Heart Disease, Hemifacial Microsomia, and Inguinal Hernia: Ipsilateral Congenital Malformations

Chengming Fan, Can Huang, Jijia Liu, and Jinfu Yang

Department of the Cardiothoracic Surgery, The Second Xiangya Hospital, Central South University, Middle Renmin Road 139, Changsha 410011, China

Correspondence should be addressed to Jinfu Yang; yjf19682005@sina.com

Academic Editor: Piero Pavone

A 3-year-old Chinese boy was diagnosed with ipsilateral congenital malformations: right lung hypoplasia, dextroversion of heart, atrial septal defect, hepatic vein drainage directly into the right atrium, facial asymmetry, right microtia and congenital deafness, and indirect inguinal hernia. He underwent indirect inguinal hernia repair at the age of 2. Although without any facial plastic surgery performed, he underwent a repair of atrial septal defect and recovered uneventfully. At 6-month follow-up, the patient was free from any symptom of dyspnea; his heart function returned to the first grade.

1. Introduction

Lung hypoplasia or agenesis is part of the spectrum of malformations featured by incomplete development of lung tissue and is often associated with other ipsilateral congenital malformations [1]. Congenital malformations associated with pulmonary hypoplasia may be present in any system including cardiovascular system [2], gastrointestinal system, central nervous system, and musculoskeletal system. Here we described a 3-year-old Chinese boy, who was referred to us for heart murmur in right hemithorax. Subsequently, he was found to have hypoplasia of right lung, dextroversion of heart, atrial septal defect (ASD), hepatic vein drainage directly into the right atrium through coronary sinus, facial asymmetry, microtia, and indirect inguinal hernia.

2. Case Report

A 3-year-old Chinese boy accompanied by his parents visited our outpatient clinic for a heart murmur detected at the age of 2 months. He lost hearing of his right ear from birth. He had no history of chest pain or heaviness of chest, wheeze, and dyspnea. There was no history of consanguineous marriage in their family. His birth history and perinatal period were

uneventful. Physical examination showed facial asymmetry (face and mouth deviated to right side), right microtia with aural atresia (Figure 1), a surgical scar of right indirect inguinal hernia repair, stony dullness, and absent breath sounds in the right up chest. There was grade 3/6 systolic murmur on the right parasternal border under the second rib. A chest roentgenogram showed homogeneous opacity occupying the entire right up hemithorax, hyperinflated left lung, and mediastinal shift to the right (Figure 2(a)). A 12-lead electrocardiogram showed sinus tachycardia. Echocardiogram showed dextroversion of heart and a 17 mm sized ostium secundum defect, moderate pulmonary hypertension (MPAP = 40 mmHg). Computerized tomography (CT) of the brain and chest showed a blind-ending right external acoustic meatus (Figure 2(b)), the whole heart located in the right chest, and severe right lung hypoplasia with left lung tissue compensatory hyperplasia and crossing through the mediastinum. The transverse diameter of right pulmonary artery was 7 mm without evidence of right ascending pulmonary artery. Left pulmonary artery was compensatory broadening with a diameter of 14 mm (Figure 2(c)). Hepatic vein was draining directly into the right atrium through coronary sinus (Figure 2(d)). The right side of thoracic cage was mildly collapsed, and no obvious branches of the right

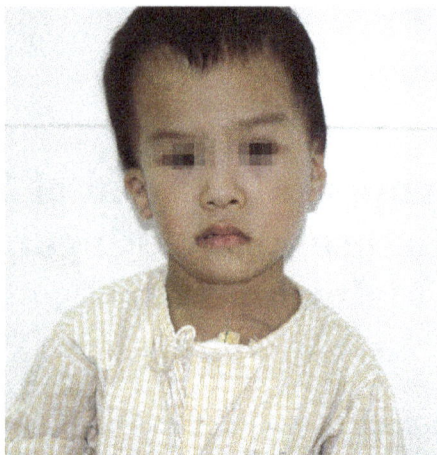

FIGURE 1: Frontal facial view showing facial asymmetry affecting the right side including microtia and downslanting zygomatic arch, jaw bone, mouth, and lips.

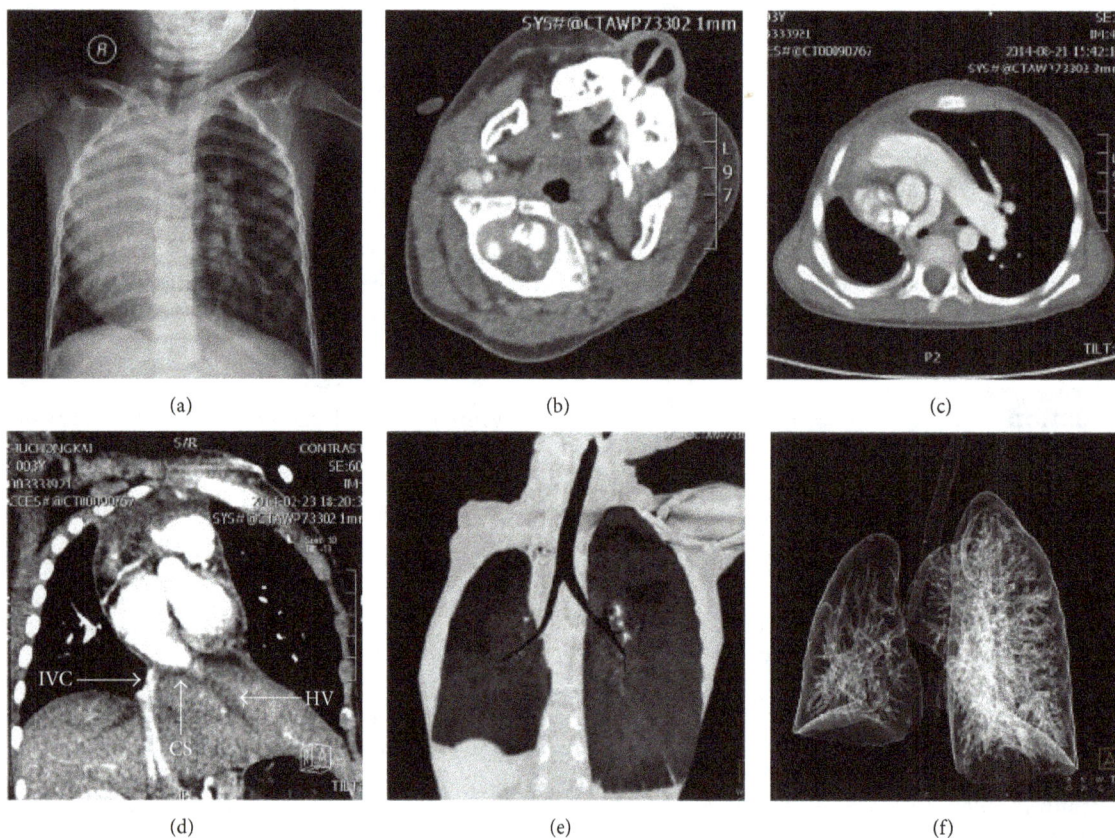

FIGURE 2: X-ray chest showing (a) a homogenous opacity occupying most of right hemithorax and compensatory hyperinflation on left side. Cranial computed tomography demonstrating (b) imperforation of right external acoustic meatus. The CECT chest in mediastinal window showing (c) right lung hypoplasia, left lung tissue crossing through the mediastinum, and hypoplastic right pulmonary artery and (d) hepatic vein that directly drains into right atrium thorough coronary sinus. CECT chest in lung window showing that (e) the right side of thoracic cage is mildly collapsed and no obvious branches of the right main bronchus could be observed. Volume-rendering computed tomography 3-dimensional reconstruction showing (f) right lung hypoplasia and a compensatory hyperplasia left lung.

main bronchus could be observed (Figures 2(e) and 2(f)). Color Doppler ultrasound examination of the abdomen and urinary system was all normal. He was diagnosed with ipsilateral congenital malformations: right lung hypoplasia, dextroversion of heart, ASD, hepatic vein drainage directly into the right atrium, facial asymmetry, right microtia with deafness, and indirect inguinal hernia. The patient underwent cardiac surgery of ASD repair 6 months after the hernioplasty of indirect inguinal hernia. Surgery progressed smoothly and no anomalous pulmonary venous connection was found. The patient was weaned from the ventilator 5 hours after surgery and discharged uneventfully on postoperative day 7. At 6-month follow-up, the patient was in good condition without the symptoms of dyspnea and palpitation. His heart function was NYHA class 1.

3. Discussion

Pulmonary agenesis is a rare malformation, which has been described as an isolated lesion or associated with other anomalies. Cardiac anomalies with pulmonary hypoplasia mainly include Ebstein's anomaly, tetralogy of Fallot (TOF), scimitar syndrome, pulmonary stenosis, and hypoplastic right heart [3, 4]. The cause of these ipsilateral congenital malformations remains unclear. Clinical presentation and the degree of respiratory compromise depend on the associated anomalies and the severity of hypoplasia. By far, there have been no effective treatment methods for pulmonary hypoplasia. In 2005, Festa et al. [2] successfully operated with a repair of total anomalous pulmonary venous connection (TAPVC) and modified Glenn anastomosis for a patient diagnosed with right lung hypoplasia associated with TOF and TAPVC. Patnaik et al. [5] reported a case of left lung hypoplasia associated with congenital pulmonary artery aneurysm and ventricular septal defect (VSD) in 2013. In order to reduce operative risks. The aneurysmal repair was performed first. The patient was discharged in stable condition leaving the VSD unclosed.

The hypoplastic right lung reported in this paper is associated with congenital heart malformation, right indirect inguinal hernia, right hemifacial microsomia, and right microtia with aural atresia. The congenital heart malformations are dextroversion of heart, ASD, and hepatic vein drainage directly into the right atrium through coronary sinus. In the literature there is no description of such ipsilateral congenital malformations. Earlier treatment of cardiac malformation and timely correction of craniofacial asymmetry and aural atresia for these congenital malformations were recommended.

Conflict of Interests

The authors declare that there is no conflict of interests regarding the publication of this paper.

References

[1] P. Collin, "Development of the thorax," in *Gray's Anatomy*, S. Standring, Ed., pp. 1013–1036, Elsevier, Philadelphia, Pa, USA, 40th edition, 2008.

[2] P. Festa, A.-A. Lamia, B. Murzi, and M. R. Bini, "Tetralogy of Fallot with left heart hypoplasia, total anomalous pulmonary venous return, and right lung hypoplasia: role of magnetic resonance imaging," *Pediatric Cardiology*, vol. 26, no. 4, pp. 467–469, 2005.

[3] M. L. Cunningham and N. Mann, "Pulmonary agenesis: a predictor of ipsilateral malformations," *American Journal of Medical Genetics*, vol. 70, no. 4, pp. 391–398, 1997.

[4] M. F. Ahamed and F. Al Hameed, "Hypogenetic lung syndrome in an adolescent: imaging findings with short review," *Annals of Thoracic Medicine*, vol. 3, no. 2, pp. 60–63, 2008.

[5] A. N. Patnaik, R. Barik, S. Babu, and A. S. Gullati, "A rare case of left lung hypoplasia associated with congenital pulmonary artery aneurysm and ventricular septal defect," *Pediatric Cardiology*, vol. 34, no. 3, pp. 748–751, 2013.

47

Subacute Sclerosing Panencephalitis in a Child with Recurrent Febrile Seizures

Ayşe Kartal,[1] Ayşegül Neşe Çıtak Kurt,[2] Tuğba Hirfanoğlu,[2] Kürşad Aydın,[2] and Ayşe Serdaroğlu[2]

[1]Department of Child Neurology, Inonu University Faculty of Medicine, Malatya, Turkey
[2]Department of Child Neurology, Gazi University Faculty of Medicine, 06500 Ankara, Turkey

Correspondence should be addressed to Ayşe Kartal; kartalays@gmail.com

Academic Editor: Piero Pavone

Subacute sclerosing panencephalitis (SSPE) is a devastating disease of the central nervous system (CNS) caused by persistent mutant measles virus infection. The diagnosis of SSPE is based on characteristic clinical and EEG findings and demonstration of elevated antibody titres against measles in cerebrospinal fluid. Subacute sclerosing panencephalitis can have atypical clinical features at the onset. Herein, we report an unusual case of subacute sclerosing panencephalitis in a child with recurrent febrile seizures. The disease progressed with an appearance of myoclonic jerks, periodic high amplitude generalized complexes on EEG, and elevated titers of measles antibodies in cerebrospinal fluid leading to the final diagnosis of subacute sclerosing panencephalitis.

1. Introduction

Subacute sclerosing panencephalitis is a progressive, fatal neurodegenerative disease caused by an aberrant measles virus in the central nervous system [1]. The typical clinical presentation of subacute sclerosing panencephalitis includes behavioral and intellectual impairment followed by myoclonia and complete neurological deterioration depending on the degree of neuroanatomical structure involvement [2]. However, the initial characteristics and clinical course of the disease can be highly variable. Different types of seizures as prominent and a first symptom of subacute sclerosing panencephalitis are also a typical clinical presentation [3, 4]. In this report, we describe a child with subacute sclerosing panencephalitis who had history of recurrent febrile seizures.

2. Case Report

A 5-year-old boy was admitted to the Pediatric Neurology Department with a history of recurrent febrile convulsions which were first seen at two months of age. For the last two months they were accompanied by axial myoclonic jerks, head drops, and decreased attention span. He was born at term by spontaneous normal delivery. The antenatal period was uneventful.

Milestones were achieved normally but he had not received any of his vaccinations, except for a dose of diphtheria, tetanus, pertussis vaccine. He also had past history of viral illness with skin rash and conjunctivitis, suggesting measles when he was 8 months old. His family history was negative for psychiatric or neurologic illnesses. His first febrile convulsion was observed at the age of 2 months a day after receiving a diphtheria, pertussis, and tetanus vaccination. This progressed to status epilepticus which lasted for 30 minutes. His second febrile generalized clonic seizure occurred 2 months later and prophylactic phenobarbital therapy was initiated. Afterwards he experienced two or more generalized clonic seizures per year, occurring mainly with fever. When he was 3 years old, treatment was supplemented with valproate due to a febrile generalized status epilepticus lasting one hour. During his fourth year, multiple febrile generalized tonic-clonic seizures of variable lateralization did not benefit from phenobarbital and valproate therapy. At the age of five, brief head nodding, myoclonic jerks, and cognitive stagnation appeared. Physical examination of the patient on admission was normal for vital signs.

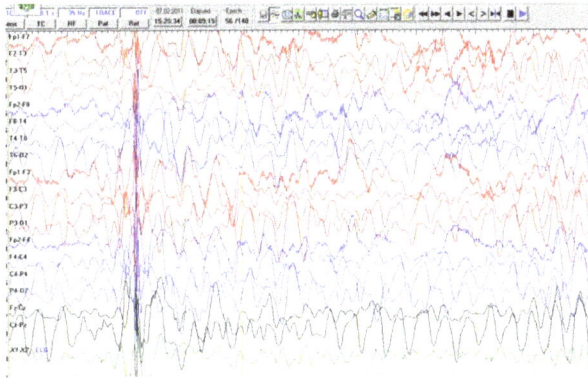

FIGURE 1: Scalp electroencephalogram showing disorganized slow background with generalized spike-wave discharges.

On neurologic examination, he was conscious but had gait ataxia, intention tremor, and myoclonic jerks. Myoclonic jerks involved mostly the head, the shoulders, and the arm. Cranial nerve and fundoscopic examinations were normal. The examination of motor system, tone, power, and reflexes was unremarkable. General examination did not reveal any abnormality. Laboratory investigations showed normal values of blood counts, chemistry, and electrolytes. Urine organic acids, tandem mass, plasma lactate, pyruvate, thyroid function tests, cerebrospinal fluid analysis, and magnetic resonance imaging were all normal. Electroencephalography (EEG) revealed a slow background with periodic generalized complexes consisting of bilaterally symmetrical, high voltage slow wave complexes which did not disappear with diazepam induction (Figure 1). As EEG picture was suggestive of subacute sclerosing panencephalitis, a sample of CSF was obtained for anti-measles antibody. The cerebrospinal fluid measles immunoglobulin G titer was higher than 1 : 1000. A diagnosis of subacute sclerosing panencephalitis was made in view of myoclonus, deterioration in cognitive function, elevated cerebrospinal fluid measles antibody levels, and periodic discharges in the EEG.

3. Discussion

SSPE is one of the most frequent causes of progressive cognitive decline in developing countries. The disease may present with varying symptoms. Uncommonly, subacute sclerosing panencephalitis may manifest with different types of seizures, such as generalized tonic-clonic seizure and myoclonic atonic seizures [5, 6]. Here, we reported a patient who presented with a history of recurrent febrile seizures, followed by deterioration in cognitive function.

This child presented with recurrent febrile seizures and a recent onset of frequent myoclonic jerks and stagnation in his cognitive status. Although this child had a history of rash illness which was suggestive of measles and he had not received MMR vaccine, we considered that was no relationship between the seizures and SSPE.

Initially, the diagnostic possibility included Dravet syndrome, but he demonstrated neither different seizures than

febrile seizures nor the characteristic cognitive deterioration, and hence those differential diagnoses were excluded. The patient developed typical features of subacute sclerosing panencephalitis-like myoclonus at 5 years of age.

In light of these findings, subacute sclerosing panencephalitis was suspected and the diagnosis of subacute sclerosing panencephalitis was confirmed by the detection of cerebrospinal fluid measles antibodies. To the best of our knowledge, even though several cases involving the association of different epileptic syndrome and subacute sclerosing panencephalitis have been reported, the association of subacute sclerosing panencephalitis and recurrent febrile seizures has not been previously reported in the literature.

The role of EEG in diagnosing both atypical and typical cases of subacute sclerosing panencephalitis has been described [7]. The classic EEG picture is characterised by periodic complexes consisting of bilaterally symmetrical, synchronous, high-voltage bursts of polyphasic, stereotyped delta waves. In the different epileptic syndromes, such as Dravet syndrome, generalized periodic epileptiform discharges can be seen [8]. Moseley et al. reported a case with Dravet syndrome and SCN1A mutation that had periodic EEG discharges [9]. In another report by Takayanagi et al., a case of a 10-month-old boy whose electroencephalogram revealed generalized periodic epileptiform discharges was subsequently found to have a de novo mutation of the SCN1A gene consistent with Dravet syndrome [10].

In conclusion, subacute sclerosing panencephalitis is a rare complication of measles infection. We strongly recommend screening for SSPE in children with new onset cognitive deterioration and myoclonic jerks. Increasing awareness of SSPE in the pediatricians and neurologists can help in the early diagnosis of the patients and prevent unnecessary investigations.

Conflict of Interests

The authors declared no potential conflict of interests with respect to the research, authorship, and/or publication of this paper.

Authors' Contribution

Ayşe Kartal and Ayşegül Neşe Çıtak Kurt wrote the paper. Kürşad Aydın, Ayşe Serdaroğlu, and Tuğba Hirfanoğlu were involved in the diagnosis and management of the patient. In addition, Kürşad Aydın edited the paper.

References

[1] R. K. Garg, "Subacute sclerosing panencephalitis," *Journal of Neurology*, vol. 255, no. 12, pp. 1861–1871, 2008.

[2] C. Campbell, S. Levin, P. Humphreys, W. Walop, and R. Brannan, "Subacute sclerosing panencephalitis: Results of the Canadian Paediatric Surveillance Program and review of the literature," *BMC Pediatrics*, vol. 5, article 47, 2005.

[3] D. Tuncel, A. E. Ozbek, G. Demirpolat, and H. Karabiber, "Subacute sclerosing panencephalitis with generalized seizure as the

first symptom: a case report," *Japanese Journal of Infectious Diseases*, vol. 59, no. 5, pp. 317–319, 2006.

[4] M. M. Cruzeiro, T. C. Vale, L. A. Pires, and G. M. Franco, "Atypical subacute sclerosing panencephalitis: case report," *Arquivos de Neuro-Psiquiatria*, vol. 65, no. 4, pp. 1030–1033, 2007.

[5] P. S. Dimova and V. S. Bojinova, "Case of subacute sclerosing panencephalitis with atypical absences and myoclonic-atonic seizures as a first symptom," *Journal of Child Neurology*, vol. 19, no. 7, pp. 548–552, 2004.

[6] R. Kravljanac, N. Jovic, M. Djuric, and L. Nikolic, "Epilepsia partialis continua in children with fulminant subacute sclerosing panencephalitis," *Neurological Sciences*, vol. 32, no. 6, pp. 1007–1012, 2011.

[7] S. Praveen-kumar, S. Sinha, A. B. Taly et al., "Electroencephalographic and imaging profile in a subacute sclerosing panencephalitis (SSPE) cohort: a correlative study," *Clinical Neurophysiology*, vol. 118, no. 9, pp. 1947–1954, 2007.

[8] R. K. Garg, "Are SCN1A gene mutations responsible for genetic susceptibility to subacute sclerosing panencephalitis?" *Medical Hypotheses*, vol. 78, no. 2, pp. 247–249, 2012.

[9] B. D. Moseley, E. C. Wirrell, and K. Nickels, "Generalized periodic epileptiform discharges in a child with Dravet syndrome," *Journal of Child Neurology*, vol. 26, no. 7, pp. 907–910, 2011.

[10] M. Takayanagi, K. Haginoya, N. Umehara et al., "Acute encephalopathy with a truncation mutation in the SCN1A gene: a case report," *Epilepsia*, vol. 51, no. 9, pp. 1886–1888, 2010.

48

Ectopic Lingual Thyroid

Khaled Khamassi, Habib Jaafoura, Fahmi Masmoudi, Rim Lahiani, Lobna Bougacha, and Mamia Ben Salah

Department of Otorhinolaryngology-Head and Neck Surgery, Charles Nicolle Hospital, Boulevard 9 Avril, 1006 Tunis, Tunisia

Correspondence should be addressed to Khaled Khamassi; khaled.khamassi@yahoo.fr

Academic Editor: Nan-Chang Chiu

Ectopy of the thyroid gland is an abnormal embryological development. Its occurrence in children is rare. In this study, we report the case of a 12-year-old girl that presented with dysphagia and nocturnal dyspnea. Magnetic resonance imaging confirmed the presence of a lingual thyroid. Thyroid scintigraphy showed intense and elective uptake of radiotracer at the base of the tongue. Hormonal tests revealed hypothyroidism. Treatment consisted of opotherapy based on levothyroxine. Evolution has been favourable and the patient showed significant improvement with reduction of the dyspnea and the dysphagia and normalization of thyroid hormone tests.

1. Introduction

Ectopy of the thyroid gland is an abnormal embryological development, defined by an aberrant localization of thyroid tissue outside the thyroid compartment. It is a very rare entity. Its frequency is estimated at 1/4000 to 1/8000 among patients with hypothyroidism and 0.3% of all diseases of the thyroid gland. It particularly affects young women. Its occurrence in children is rare. Diagnosis is mainly based on clinical examination and imaging. Treatment is mainly medical and must take into account the physiological requirements for thyroid hormones.

In this study, we report a case of lingual thyroid and we review the literature on this topic.

2. Case Report

A 12-year-old girl without past medical history consulted for high dysphagia evolving for three years. Dysphagia had worsened over the past two months and was accompanied by increasing in nocturnal dyspnea and recent onset of sleep apnea. There were neither signs of thyroid dysfunction nor alteration of general condition.

Nasofibroscopy showed a reddish oval formation, with a diameter of 2 cm, located behind the lingual V and attached to the base of the tongue. At intraoral palpation, the mass was firm, smooth, uniform, and painless, with no bleeding. Examination of the neck revealed no palpable thyroid gland in the normal pretracheal position and no cervical lymphadenopathies.

Cervical CT (Figure 1) scan showed a rounded lesion located at the base of the tongue, with heterogeneous enhancing after injection of iodine contrast medium. Thyroid compartment was empty. Magnetic resonance imaging confirmed the presence of a basilingual thyroid (Figure 2). Thyroid scintigraphy with technetium (Tc99m) showed intense and elective uptake of radiotracer at the area of the base of the tongue and no uptake in the normal thyroid location (Figure 3).

Hormonal tests showed subclinical hypothyroidism with a normal dosage of FT_4 (15.4 pmol/L) and a slight increase of TSH (5.2 IU/mL).

Treatment consisted of an opotherapy based on levothyroxine at the dose of 75 micrograms per day. Evolution has been favourable and the patient showed significant improvement in symptoms with reduction of the dyspnea and

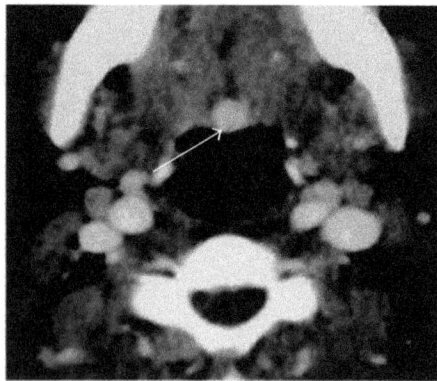

FIGURE 1: Axial CT: rounded lesion at the base of the tongue.

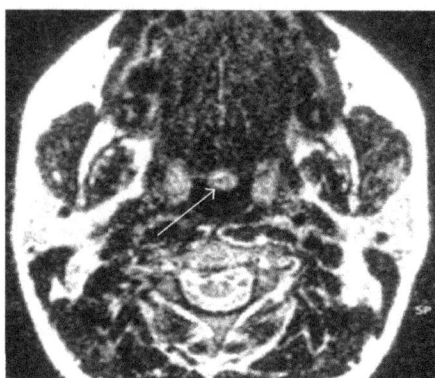

FIGURE 2: Axial MRI: lingual thyroid.

the dysphagia and normalization of thyroid hormone tests. Posttherapeutic thyroid scintigraphy showed a less intensive fixation at the base of the tongue compared to the initial scintigraphy (Figure 4).

3. Discussion

The thyroid tissue reaches the normal location in the pretracheal region by migrating caudally from the foramen cecum in the tongue base at the seventh week of fetal life. Ectopic lingual thyroid is caused by noncompletion of this migration [1, 2]. The normal thyroid gland can be seen together with ectopic thyroid tissues. A normally located thyroid is not seen in 70% of patients with lingual thyroid, as it was for our patient [3].

Lingual thyroid tissue is the most frequent ectopic location of the thyroid gland, although its clinical incidence is low with 1 in 100 000 cases occurring [4]. There are four groups of lingual thyroid: lingual, sublingual, thyroglossal, and intralaryngeal [5].

Lingual thyroid does not usually lead to any symptoms unless an increase in gland size occurs. In symptomatic cases, patients present with complaints of dysphagia, dysphonia, foreign body sensation in the throat, cough, pain, bleeding, and dyspnea [2, 5, 6]. Rarely, the lingual thyroid may cause hyperthyroidism [7] or be the site of thyroid cancer [8].

Endocrine changes such as puberty, pregnancy, and menstruation can lead to an increase in gland size and symptoms. This explains why lingual thyroid is 7-fold higher among women [3].

Biopsy is not recommended because of the risks of bleeding and infection [1, 9, 10]. On the ultrasonography, lingual thyroid is homogenous with regular contours and more echogenicity compared to tongue muscles [3]. Thyroid scintigraphy is indicated for the differential diagnosis of tongue base masses detected on physical examination or when thyroid tissue is not detected in the normal location on ultrasonography [11]. In our case, while the thyroid activity was not detected in the normal location, it was detected at the tongue base.

MRI provides valuable information about the exact size and location of the ectopic tissue and the presence of accompanying thyroglossal duct in patients for whom an operation is planned [3]. It is also helpful for determination of the posterior pharyngeal opening and the degree of narrowness in the cases with obstructive sleep apnoea syndrome (OSAS) [3, 11]. On MRI, lingual thyroid tissue is observed as either iso- or hypointense to the tongue muscles in T1-weighted sequences and more hyperintense than the tongue muscles in T2.

There are a few reports in the literature about benign oropharyngeal masses resulting in dysphagia and OSAS [12, 13]. Lipomas constitute the majority of these masses. Other masses include haemangioma, neurofibromas, and retention cysts. The gold standard test in the diagnosis of OSAS is polysomnography, with measure of the Apnoea-Hypopnoea Index [3, 12, 13].

The fact that the ectopic thyroid tissue can be the only functional thyroid tissue must be kept in mind when determining the therapeutic approach. Asymptomatic cases can be monitored with suppressive hormonal therapy aiming for reduction of ectopic tissue volume. Decrease in symptoms can occur with suppressive treatment in some cases [3]. Conservative treatment had proved its efficiency in many studies [3, 5, 9, 13, 14]. Indeed, administration of a suppressive dose of thyroid hormones aims to decrease the TSH level; therefore it can reduce the ectopic glandular volume and consequently reduce all the compressive symptoms.

Effective treatment for lingual thyroid is surgical excision, but no surgical treatment should be attempted until radioactive isotope scan has determined that there is an adequate thyroid tissue in the neck [14]. Surgical indications are important dyspnea or dysphagia, suspicion of malignancy, uncontrolled hyperthyroidism, and repetitive or severe bleeding. Transient tracheostomy may be required when surgery is indicated. Surgical excision can be made either transorally or externally with pharyngotomy through a transhyoidal approach [3, 14–16]. The surgeon has to perform meticulous homeostasis with bipolar electrocautery during tumor dissection to prevent postoperative haemorrhagic complications. Another method is transoral laser excision [17, 18]. Transoral radiofrequency ablation may also reduce the tissue volume [19]. In patients lacking thyroid tissue in the neck, lingual thyroid can be excised and autotransplanted to the muscles of neck [14, 20]

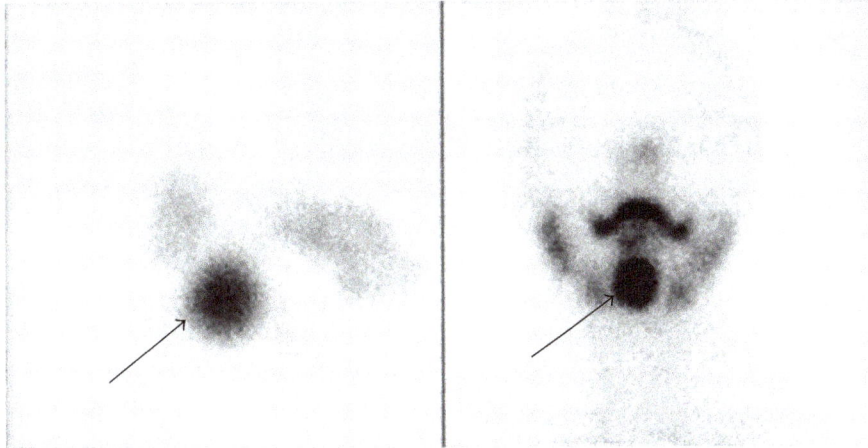

FIGURE 3: Thyroid scintigraphy: intense and elective uptake at the base of the tongue.

FIGURE 4: Posttherapeutic scintigraphy.

or they may be put under lifelong postoperative hormone replacement therapy.

An alternative treatment for patients not accepting surgical treatment or for those not appropriate for general anaesthesia is radioactive iodine therapy [1, 3, 12]. This one is not recommended in cases where there is another functional thyroid tissue.

Surgical treatment, radioactive iodine ablation, CPAP, and intraoral devices used during sleep are the treatment options for cases with severe dyspnoea or OSAS [15]. CPAP usually provides a temporary improvement of the symptoms and is not well tolerated by patients in the long term [3].

4. Conclusion

When a mass lesion is observed in the tongue base, ectopic lingual thyroid must be taken into consideration in the differential diagnosis, and the diagnosis must be verified using ultrasonography, scintigraphy, CT scan, and MRI. Therapeutic approach should be considered according to symptomatology. The risks and benefits of each treatment modality should always be discussed with the patient.

Conflict of Interests

The authors declared that there is no conflict of interests regarding this paper.

References

[1] A. Toso, F. Colombani, G. Averono, P. Aluffi, and F. Pia, "Lingual thyroid causing dysphagia and dyspnoea. Case reports and review of the literature," *Acta Otorhinolaryngologica Italica*, vol. 29, no. 4, pp. 213–217, 2009.

[2] G. Thomas, R. Hoilat, J. S. Daniels, and W. Kalagie, "Ectopic lingual thyroid: a case report," *International Journal of Oral and Maxillofacial Surgery*, vol. 32, no. 2, pp. 219–221, 2003.

[3] M. A. Babademez, E. Günbey, B. Acar, and H. P. Günbey, "A rare cause of obstructive sleep apnea syndrome: lingual thyroid," *Sleep and Breathing*, vol. 16, no. 2, pp. 305–308, 2012.

[4] S. Rabiei, M. Rahimi, and A. Ebrahimi, "Coblation assisted excision of lingual thyroid," *Indian Journal of Otolaryngology and Head and Neck Surgery*, vol. 62, no. 2, pp. 108–110, 2010.

[5] T.-T. Chiu, C.-Y. Su, C.-F. Hwang, C.-Y. Chien, and H.-L. Eng, "Massive bleeding from an ectopic lingual thyroid follicular adenoma during pregnancy," *American Journal of Otolaryngology: Head and Neck Medicine and Surgery*, vol. 23, no. 3, pp. 185–188, 2002.

[6] A. Gonciulea, D. S. Cooper, and R. Salvatori, "Lingual thyroid," *Endocrine*, vol. 46, no. 2, pp. 355–356, 2014.

[7] M. P. Abdallah-Matta, P. H. Dubarry, J. J. Pessey, and P. Caron, "Lingual thyroid and hyperthyroidism: a new case and review of the literature," *Journal of Endocrinological Investigation*, vol. 25, no. 3, pp. 264–267, 2002.

[8] R. E. Massine, S. J. Durning, and T. M. Koroscil, "Lingual thyroid carcinoma: a case report and review of the literature," *Thyroid*, vol. 11, no. 12, pp. 1191–1196, 2001.

[9] T. S. Huang and H. Y. Chen, "Dual thyroid ectopia with a normally located pretracheal thyroid gland: case report and literature review," *Head and Neck*, vol. 29, no. 9, pp. 885–888, 2007.

[10] P. Hazarika, S. A. Siddiqui, K. Pujary, P. Shah, D. R. Nayak, and R. Balakrishnan, "Dual ectopic thyroid: a report of two cases," *Journal of Laryngology and Otology*, vol. 112, no. 4, pp. 393–395, 1998.

[11] F. Giovagnorio, A. Cordier, and R. Romeo, "Lingual thyroid: value of integrated imaging," *European Radiology*, vol. 6, no. 1, pp. 105–107, 1996.

[12] T. W. Barnes, K. D. Olsen, and T. I. Morgenthaler, "Obstructive lingual thyroid causing sleep apnea: a case report and review of the literature," *Sleep Medicine*, vol. 5, no. 6, pp. 605–607, 2004.

[13] K. Taibah, M. Ahmed, E. Baessa, M. Saleem, A. Rifai, and A. Al-Arifi, "An unusual cause of obstructive sleep apnoea presenting during pregnancy," *The Journal of Laryngology & Otology*, vol. 112, no. 12, pp. 1189–1191, 1998.

[14] S. S. Kumar, D. Muthiah Selva Kumar, and R. Thirun-avukuarasu, "Lingual thyroid-conservative management or surgery? a case report," *Indian Journal of Surgery*, vol. 75, supplement 1, pp. 118–119, 2013.

[15] P. Peters, P. Stark, G. Essig Jr. et al., "Lingual thyroid: an unusual and surgically curable cause of sleep apnoea in a male," *Sleep and Breathing*, vol. 14, no. 4, pp. 377–380, 2010.

[16] B. Amr and S. Monib, "Lingual thyroid: a case report," *International Journal of Surgery Case Reports*, vol. 2, no. 8, pp. 313–315, 2011.

[17] M. A. Hafidh, P. Sheahan, N. A. Khan, M. Colreavy, and C. Timon, "Role of CO_2 laser in the management of obstructive ectopic lingual thyroids," *The Journal of Laryngology & Otology*, vol. 118, no. 10, pp. 807–809, 2004.

[18] R. Puxeddu, C. L. Pelagatti, and P. Nicolai, "Lingual thyroid: endoscopic management with CO_2 laser," *American Journal of Otolaryngology—Head and Neck Medicine and Surgery*, vol. 19, no. 2, pp. 136–139, 1998.

[19] S. D. Dasari, N. K. Bashetty, and N. S. M. Prayaga, "Radiofrequency ablation of lingual thyroid," *Otolaryngology—Head and Neck Surgery*, vol. 136, no. 3, pp. 498–499, 2007.

[20] S. Wahab, R. A. Khan, and R. Goyal, "Persistent cough in a lethargic child: watch out for lingual thyroid!," *International Journal of Pediatric Otorhinolaryngology Extra*, vol. 5, no. 1, pp. 5–8, 2010.

49

Deep Venous Thrombosis of the Leg, Associated with Agenesis of the Infrarenal Inferior Vena Cava and Hypoplastic Left Kidney (KILT Syndrome) in a 14-Year-Old Child

Sakshi Bami,[1] Yarelis Vazquez,[2] Valeriy Chorny,[1] Rachelle Goldfisher,[2] and John Amodio[2]

[1]*Department of Pediatrics, SUNY Downstate Medical Center, 450 Clarkson Avenue, Brooklyn, NY 11203, USA*
[2]*Department of Radiology, SUNY Downstate Medical Center, 450 Clarkson Avenue, Brooklyn, NY 11203, USA*

Correspondence should be addressed to John Amodio; john.amodio@downstate.edu

Academic Editor: Giovanni Montini

Agenesis of the inferior vena cava (IVC) is a rare anomaly which can be identified as incidental finding or can be associated with iliofemoral vein thrombosis. IVC agenesis has a known association with renal anomalies which are mainly confined to the right kidney. We describe a case of a 14-year-old male who presented with left leg swelling and pain. Ultrasonography confirmed the presence of left leg deep vein thrombosis (DVT). No underlying hematologic risk factors were identified. A CT scan was obtained which demonstrated absent infrarenal IVC and extensive thrombosis in the left deep venous system and development of collateral venous flow into the azygous/hemiazygous system, with extension of thrombus into paraspinal collaterals. An additional finding in the patient was an atrophic left kidney and stenosis of an accessory left renal artery. Agenesis of the IVC should be considered in a young patient presenting with lower extremity DVT, especially in patients with no risk factors for thrombosis. As agenesis of the IVC cannot be corrected, one should be aware that there is a lifelong risk of lower extremity DVT.

1. Introduction

Deep vein thrombosis occurs with a prevalence of 1 in 1000 [1]. It is seen less in younger population with an estimated incidence of 1 in 10,000. Hematologic risk factors associated with deep vein thrombosis can be congenital and/or acquired. In up to 80% of the cases of DVT, one or more risk factors can be identified [1].

Anomalies of the inferior vena cava (IVC) are an independent risk factor for DVT. These anomalies are found in 0.3–0.5% of the general population and in 0.6–2% of patients with cardiovascular defects. The most common anomalies of IVC are double IVC, left sided IVC, IVC agenesis or absence, and retroaortic left renal vein [2]. In young patients with DVT, there is an estimated higher rate of anomalies of IVC than in the general population, namely, 5% as compared to 0.5% expected [3, 4].

We describe a case of a 14-year-old male who presented with left leg swelling and pain. Ultrasonography confirmed the presence of left leg deep vein thrombosis (DVT). No

underlying hematologic risk factors were identified. CT scan was obtained which demonstrated absent infrarenal IVC and extensive thrombosis in the left deep venous system and development of collateral venous flow into the azygous/hemiazygous system, with extension of thrombus into paraspinal collaterals. An additional finding in the patient was an atrophic left kidney and stenosis of an accessory left renal artery.

2. Case Report

A 14-year-old male presented to the emergency department with complaint of left lower extremity pain for 5 days. The pain was localized to the left thigh, worsening over time despite analgesic intake. Patient also complained of swelling of the thigh, difficulty in ambulation for 2 days, and numbness for 1 day. There was no history of trauma, recent surgery, medication use, or prolonged immobilization. There was no family history of clotting or bleeding disorder or venous thromboembolism. He denies any history of smoking or illicit drug use.

Patient is a known case of type 1 diabetes mellitus diagnosed at age of 10 years, currently on insulin pump. He was diagnosed with hypertension at age 9 and is on enalapril. He was born in Jamaica, via normal spontaneous vaginal delivery at term and had shoulder dystocia at birth for which he stayed in the hospital for 10 days. A sling was applied and no other intervention was done. Patient's mother denied any other complications at birth.

On examination he was noted to have marked asymmetry between the two lower extremities. There was tense swelling of the left posterior thigh and the left calf, which was tender to palpation. No erythema, warmth, varicose veins, or ulcers were present. Peripheral pulses were palpable and equal bilaterally with normal neurological exam.

His initial laboratory results in the emergency room showed normal complete blood count, basic metabolic panel, prothrombin time, and activated partial thromboplastin time. A lower extremity ultrasound showed the left common femoral, left superficial femoral, and left popliteal vein were noncompressible and demonstrated no vascular flow, with intraluminal echogenic thrombus suggestive of deep vein thrombosis of the left lower extremity (Figure 1).

He was admitted to the pediatric floor and started on low molecular weight (LMW) heparin and warfarin after hematology consultation. His chest X-ray was normal. A thrombophilia workup was done which showed no pro-thrombin gene mutation, normal levels of Factor V Leiden, antithrombin III, and protein S. Protein C was low 51.9 (normal 55–123 units IU/dL). Low protein C in the setting of a large DVT was attributed to consumption of coagulation factors. LDH, uric acid, and homocysteine level were normal. Anticardiolipin and lupus anticoagulant were normal.

A CT of the abdomen and pelvis was done to determine the extent of the thrombosis in the pelvis. The CT showed the suprarenal IVC and the hepatic segments of the IVC were patent. There was absence of infrarenal IVC (Figure 2). There was an anomalous course of the external iliac veins communicating with lumbar veins. There was heterogeneous material within the left common femoral vein and left external iliac vein and hypodensity within the left lumbar vein consistent with thrombus (Figure 3). There were prominent azygous and hemiazygous veins. The left kidney was small in size and there was compensatory hypertrophy of the right kidney (Figure 4). The renal veins were not thrombosed and the origin of the left renal vein was normal in caliber. There was calcification of the right adrenal gland noted consistent with prior adrenal hemorrhage, the etiology of which could not be ascertained.

On review of patients past medical records it was noted that as a workup of hypertension he had a CT angiogram done which demonstrated atrophic left kidney supplied by two hypoplastic renal arteries arising from the abdominal aorta. The origin of the more inferior renal artery had a short segment of stenosis (Figure 5). The right kidney was normal. A DMSA renal scan done subsequently demonstrated left renal uptake of approximately 13% and right renal uptake of approximately 87%.

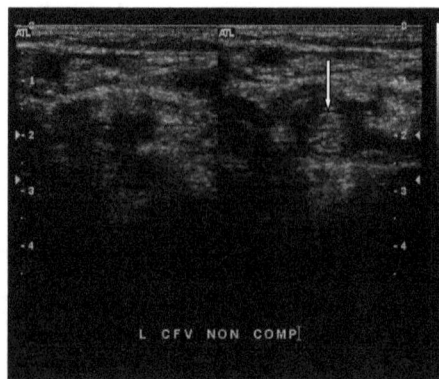

FIGURE 1: Grayscale ultrasound transverse image demonstrating a thrombus on the left common femoral vein. White arrow is pointing to the intraluminal echogenic material and noncompressibility, findings compatible with deep vein thrombosis.

The patient was continued on low molecular weight (LMW) heparin until his international normalized ratio (INR) reached more than 2. His pain and stiffness improved and he was discharged on oral warfarin therapy. Patient and mother were made aware that he may need lifelong anticoagulation therapy. In view of the fact that the patient had venous and arterial anomalies, prior to discharge the patient received a brain MRA/MRV to look for any other vascular anomalies, which were normal. A genetic evaluation was also normal. The patient is being followed by hematology team for venous thrombosis as an outpatient and is on oral warfarin therapy with therapeutic INR.

3. Discussion

The embryogenesis of IVC is complex. The normal IVC is composed of four segments: hepatic, suprarenal, renal, and infrarenal. The hepatic segment is derived from the vitelline vein. The right subcardinal vein develops into the suprarenal segment by formation of the subcardinal-hepatic anastomosis. The renal segment develops from the right suprasub-cardinal and postsubcardinal anastomoses. It is generally accepted that the infrarenal segment derives from the right supracardinal vein. In the thoracic region, the supracardinal veins give rise to the azygos and hemiazygos veins. In the abdomen, the postcardinal veins are progressively replaced by the subcardinal and supracardinal veins but persist in the pelvis as the common iliac veins [5]. Some authors propose that absence of the IVC may be a result of perinatal thrombosis or intrauterine thrombosis, with obliteration and subsequent resorbtion [6]. Without normal development of the infrarenal IVC, the iliofemoral veins drain into the azygous and hemizygous veins via anterior paravertebral collaterals. As all of the collateral vessels are much smaller in caliber with respect to the normal IVC, it is understandable that such collateral pathways may lead to chronic venous stasis and thrombosis of the lower extremity.

There are several variations in the anatomy of the IVC [5]. These include, among several, the following.

(a)   (b)

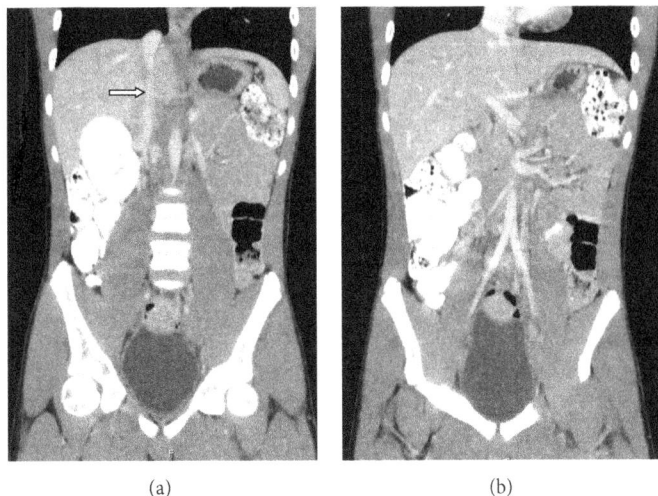

FIGURE 2: Contrast enhanced abdominopelvic CT scan. Two contiguous coronal reformations showing patent suprarenal inferior vena cava (white arrow). Note absence of the infrarenal inferior vena cava in the right image.

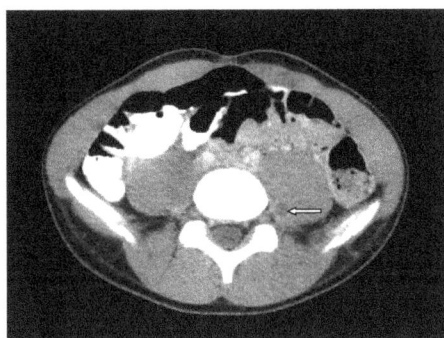

FIGURE 3: There is thrombus noted within a paraspinal collateral vein (white arrow).

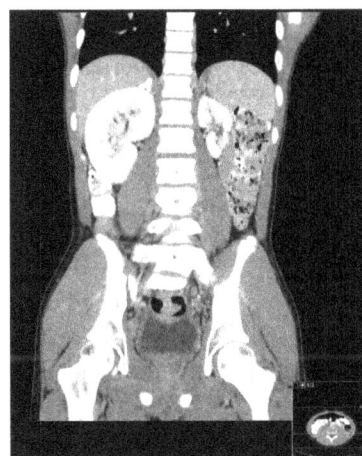

FIGURE 4: Contrast enhanced abdominopelvic CT scan. Coronal reformation demonstrating left renal hypoplasia with compensatory right renal hypertrophy. The right adrenal gland is heavily calcified.

(1) Left IVC results from regression of the right supracardinal vein with persistence of the left supracardinal vein. The prevalence is 0.2%–0.5%.

(2) Duplication of the IVC results from persistence of both supracardinal veins. The prevalence is 0.2%–3%.

(3) Azygos continuation of the IVC has also been termed absence of the hepatic segment of the IVC with azygos continuation. The prevalence is 0.6%. Agenesis of hepatic segment of IVC with azygous continuation is well defined entity in literature and is often seen in conjunction with other congenital anomalies, such the heterotaxy syndromes, specifically polysplenia.

(4) Circumaortic left renal vein results from persistence of the dorsal limb of the embryonic left renal vein and of the dorsal arch of the renal collar (intersupracardinal anastomosis). The prevalence may be as high as 8.7%.

(5) Retroaortic left renal vein results from persistence of the dorsal arch of the renal collar.

Agenesis of the infrarenal IVC is a rare anomaly, and the other associated anomaly usually involves the kidneys. The renal anomalies associated with absent IVC are mostly found to be confined to the right kidney [7]. The anomalies noted are right renal hypoplasia, aplasia, or agenesis. These anomalies are not an incidental finding and can be explained by abnormal venous embryogenesis. If there is anomalous development of the IVC which impairs venous drainage of the right metanephros, there may be aplasia or hypoplasia of the right kidney. Since the venous drainage of the left metanephros is via the gonadal vein and lumbar perforators, it is much less common to have left renal anomalies associated with IVC anomalies [8]. However, there are a few case reports in literature of absent IVC associated with left renal anomalies. Iqbal and Nagaraju [9] described a case of 54-year-old man with agenesis of the IVC and left kidney

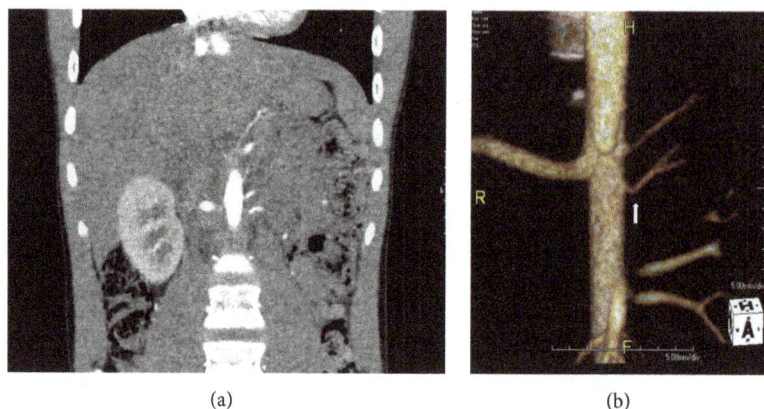

(a)   (b)

FIGURE 5: (a) Abdominal CTA coronal reformation and (b) three-dimensional reconstruction showing the left kidney supplied by two hypoplastic renal arteries originating from the aorta. The origin of the inferior left renal artery has a focal area of stenosis proximally, depicted by the white arrow.

agenesis. van Veen et al. [10] described a case of 12-year-old girl who presented with bilateral DVT and agenesis of IVC with hypoplastic left kidney. Lawless and Dangleben [11] described agenesis of the infrarenal IVC associated with left hypoplastic kidney, in a 50-year-old male. van Veen et al. [10] have proposed that the association of DVT with agenesis of the IVC and associated renal anomalies be termed "KILT" syndrome (kidney anomaly, inferior vena cava anomaly, and leg thrombosis).

The cause of the left renal hypoplasia in the case we report may be twofold; the hypoplastic arteries associated with the left kidney suggest a congenital etiology, but it is uncertain if there was a venous anomaly based on absence of the infrarenal IVC. Additionally, the renal artery stenosis associated with the most inferior renal artery may have added to the hypoplasia of the kidney and subsequently the patient's hypertension.

Patients with IVC agenesis can present with a varied clinical picture. Some can be asymptomatic and absence of the IVC is found as an incidental finding; others can present with venous thrombosis and its consequences as in our case. DVT associated with IVC agenesis usually affects young population and is often bilateral [3, 12]. It commonly involves the iliac veins and is often recurrent [13]. Although uncommonly reported, patients may also present with pulmonary embolism.

The renal veins were not thrombosed and the origin of the left renal vein was normal in caliber. Additionally, there was no evidence of a "nutcracker" phenomenon. In the nutcracker syndrome the left renal vein is compressed between the superior mesenteric artery and the aorta. Symptoms vary in this anomaly; some children are asymptomatic while others may present with hematuria, pain, and varicoceles [14].

There has not been a clear consensus in the literature about the management of patients with agenesis of the IVC and venous thrombosis. Most of the patients described have been treated with anticoagulation and elastic stockings. Few have required surgical intervention for relief of symptoms. The length of treatment with anticoagulation has also not been well described in literature. Unlike acquired risk factors which may be correctable, patients with the risk factor of absent infrarenal IVC may be at a lifelong risk for thromboembolism. More followup studies on these patients to determine their recurrence of symptoms, length of treatment, alternate treatment options, and prognosis are needed.

Conflict of Interests

The authors declare that there is no conflict of interests regarding the publication of this paper.

References

[1] J. S. Hee, T. K. Wan, Y. K. Mi, and K. C. Yun, "Combined anomaly of the right hepatic lobe agenesis and absence of the inferior vena cava: a case report," *Korean Journal of Radiology*, vol. 9, pp. S61–S64, 2008.

[2] G. Spentzouris, A. Zandian, A. Cesmebasi et al., "The clinical anatomy of the inferior vena cava: a review of common congenital anomalies and considerations for clinicians," *Clinical Anatomy*, vol. 27, no. 8, pp. 1234–1243, 2014.

[3] Y.-L. Chee, D. J. Culligan, and H. G. Watson, "Inferior vena cava malformation as a risk factor for deep venous thrombosis in the young," *British Journal of Haematology*, vol. 114, no. 4, pp. 878–880, 2001.

[4] M. Ruggeri, A. Tosetto, G. Castaman, and F. Rodeghiero, "Congenital absence of the inferior vena cava: a rare risk factor for idiopathic deep-vein thrombosis," *The Lancet*, vol. 357, no. 9254, p. 441, 2001.

[5] J. E. Bass, M. D. Redwine, L. A. Kramer, P. T. Huynh, and J. H. Harris Jr., "Spectrum of congenital anomalies of the inferior vena cava: cross-sectional imaging findings," *Radiographics*, vol. 20, no. 3, pp. 639–652, 2000.

[6] J. E. Bass, M. D. Redwine, L. A. Kramer, and J. H. Harris Jr., "Absence of the infrarenal inferior vena cava with preservation of the suprarenal segment as revealed by CT and MR venography," *American Journal of Roentgenology*, vol. 172, no. 6, pp. 1610–1612, 1999.

[7] R. J. Gil, A. M. Pérez, J. B. Arias, F. B. Pascual, and E. S. Romero, "Agenesis of the inferior vena cava associated with

lower extremities and pelvic venous thrombosis," *Journal of Vascular Surgery*, vol. 44, no. 5, pp. 1114–1116, 2006.

[8] G. Gayer, R. Zissin, S. Strauss, and M. Hertz, "IVC anomalies and right renal aplasia detected on CT: a possible link?" *Abdominal Imaging*, vol. 28, no. 3, pp. 395–399, 2003.

[9] J. Iqbal and E. Nagaraju, "Congenital absence of inferior vena cava and thrombosis: a case report," *Journal of Medical Case Reports*, vol. 2, article 46, 2008.

[10] J. van Veen, K. K. Hampton, and M. Makris, "Kilt syndrome?" *British Journal of Haematology*, vol. 118, no. 4, pp. 1199–1200, 2002.

[11] R. A. Lawless and D. A. Dangleben, "Caval agenesis with a hypoplastic left kidney in a patient with trauma on warfarin for deep vein thrombosis," *Vascular and Endovascular Surgery*, vol. 46, no. 1, pp. 75–76, 2012.

[12] M. Lambert, P. Marboeuf, M. Midulla et al., "Inferior vena cava agenesis and deep vein thrombosis: 10 patients and review of the literature," *Vascular Medicine*, vol. 15, no. 6, pp. 451–459, 2010.

[13] R. Kreidy, P. Salameh, and M. Waked, "Lower extremity venous thrombosis in patients younger than 50 years of age," *Vascular Health and Risk Management*, vol. 8, no. 1, pp. 161–167, 2012.

[14] A. K. Kurklinsky and T. W. Rooke, "Nutcracker phenomenon and nutcracker syndrome," *Mayo Clinic Proceedings*, vol. 85, no. 6, pp. 552–559, 2010.

50

Cardiac Arrest following a Myocardial Infarction in a Child Treated with Methylphenidate

Kim Munk,[1] **Lise Gormsen,**[2] **Won Yong Kim,**[1] **and Niels Holmark Andersen**[1]

[1]*Department of Cardiology, Aarhus University Hospital, Palle Juul-Jensens Boulevard 99, 8200 Aarhus N, Denmark*
[2]*Department of Psychiatry, Aarhus University Hospital, Risskov Skovagervej 2, 8240 Risskov, Denmark*

Correspondence should be addressed to Kim Munk; hindawi@kimmunk.dk

Academic Editor: Bibhuti Das

The use of psychostimulants labeled to treat attention deficit/hyperactivity disorder increases. Among side effects these drugs raise blood pressure and heart rate, and the safety has been scrutinised in recent years. Data from large epidemiological studies, including over a million person-years, did not report any cases of myocardial infarction in current users of methylphenidate, and the risk of serious adverse cardiac events was not found to be increased. We present a case with an 11-year-old child, treated with methylphenidate, who suffered cardiac arrest and was diagnosed with a remote myocardial infarction. This demonstrates that myocardial infarction can happen due to methylphenidate exposure in a cardiac healthy child, without cardiovascular risk factors.

1. Introduction

The risk of cardiovascular events and sudden death related to attention deficit/hyperactivity disorder (ADHD) medications has been scrutinized in the recent years [1–5].

In adults, the initiation of methylphenidate has been found to be associated with nearly a doubling of the rate of sudden death or ventricular arrhythmia [3]. However, in children and adolescents, large scale population studies have not found an increased cardiovascular risk in ADHD drug users [1]. Although one study reported a high hazard ratio estimate for "sudden death or ventricular arrhythmia" with methylphenidate use, the results were nonsignificant [4].

In children and adolescents, a low absolute number of cardiovascular events may explain why hazard ratios, even in large scale studies, come out nonsignificant. However, with the reported spreads in confidence intervals, one cannot rule out the possibility of an increase by as much as a tripling of the risk for serious cardiovascular events.

Mechanisms behind cardiovascular disease and methylphenidate are not fully understood. Methylphenidate increases heart rate, increases blood pressure, and potentially causes arterial vasospasms, due to the increased levels of circulating catecholamines [5, 6]. All these factors could theoretically increase cardiovascular risk [5]. There are no valid data to suggest that methylphenidate directly increases the corrected QT interval or induces arrhythmia [5, 7].

We present a case with a child treated with methylphenidate that suffered from cardiac arrest during exercise and was diagnosed with a remote myocardial infarction.

2. Case Presentation

The patient is an 11-year-old boy with attention deficit/hyperactivity disorder and Tourette syndrome. Two years prior to the current incident he had been seen by a pediatric psychiatrist over a course of time and was finally treated with methylphenidate. He was slowly uptitrated to the maximum appropriate dose of 54 mg per day (36 + 18 mg per day/body weight 50 kg), which had been ongoing ever since.

Apparently, the child had been feeling well, but a week before his admission he felt dizzy and light headed after vigorous trampoline jumping. His mother noticed he had tachycardia but thought nothing of it. The incident only lasted a few minutes and afterwards he was well.

On the day of admission, the patient had been in conflict with one of his peers. To calm down, the patient was sent to the gym court, to exercise and play ball. After a few minutes

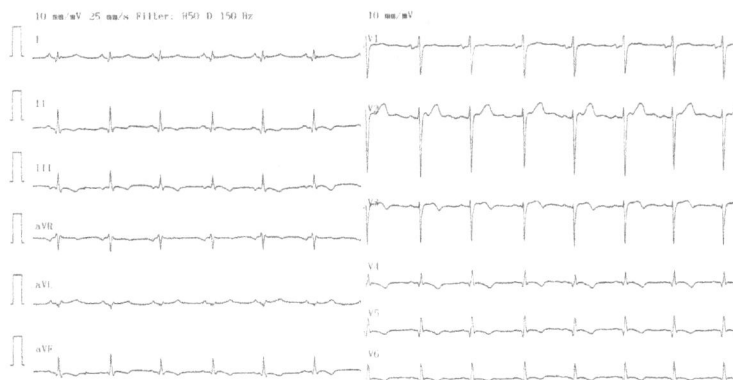

FIGURE 1: 12-lead electrocardiogram obtained on day five of the index admission. Abnormal Q-waves are seen in the left sided leads I, aVL, and V4–V6. The QTc interval was normal at 395 msec (Fredericia correction).

he left the court and fell down with cardiac arrest due to ventricular fibrillation. He was successfully resuscitated by school staff and the prehospital service.

Upon hospital arrival the child was sedated and intubated. He was circulatory stable and he was treated with hypothermia for 24 hours. A urine toxicology screening only showed traces of the anesthetics used during the resuscitation and methylphenidate according to the prescribed dose.

Both the initial ECG and the ECGs after hypothermia (Figure 1) showed Q-waves in leads I, AVL, and V4–6 and ventricular ectopic beats. The QT intervals were normal. The echocardiogram did not show any congenital defects but impaired left ventricular function due to regional wall motion abnormalities and thinning of the myocardial wall, consistent with a previous myocardial infarction in the circumflex artery area. There was only a minor increase in the troponin levels, which could be explained by the cardiac arrest, and the initial infection parameters were normal.

A coronary computed tomography angiography scan showed normal coronary artery anatomy with a dominant left coronary artery and no signs of myocardial bridging. However, a subsequent cardiac magnetic resonance scan showed clear signs of an old myocardial infarction with delayed hyperenhancement and thinning of the lateral wall of the left ventricle, corresponding to the circumflex artery supply (Figure 2).

To exclude paradox emboli, a transesophageal echocardiogram with bubble contrast was done. No atrial septal defects or mural thrombi were found. A full panel of blood coagulation tests did not reveal any coagulation disorder or hypercholesterolemia.

Before discharge, a coronary angiogram was done, which confirmed the computed tomography angiography result but also excluded abnormal coronary spasm tendency by a methylergometrine test. The patient also had an invasive electrophysiology study, which showed normal atrioventricular conduction without accessory pathways and an easily inducible sustained ventricular tachycardia, deriving from the scar tissue in the left ventricle. Subsequently, an implantable cardioverter defibrillator was implanted, and the patient was put on a low dose of metoprolol succiante (25 mg),

with a treatment plan to increase the dose at a later stage. The methylphenidate treatment was discontinued. A wide panel of genetic disorders related to tachyarrhythmia was examined, which all came out negative.

Three weeks after discharge the child was on his own in a bouncy castle on a Friday evening. After 15 minutes of exercise, he shortly felt ill and sat down but recovered quickly without any recollection of chest pain or any other discomfort. The following Monday, the defibrillator telemetry showed that the pacemaker had defibrillated an episode of ventricular fibrillation (Figure 3). Following this episode, the metoprolol succiante dosage was increased to 100 mg o.d. over two weeks.

3. Discussion

Acute myocardial infarction due to atherosclerotic plaque rupture is a leading cause of death and disability. However, in childhood and adolescence, myocardial infarction is extremely rare and other causes should be sought such as coronary artery anomalies, vasculitis, and coagulation defects. Due to the extremely rare occurrence in children, a myocardial infarction diagnosis may not be suspected and therefore overlooked. Likewise, myocardial infarction in children treated with methylphenidate is extremely rare. In two large epidemiological studies, including over half a million person-years of follow-up, of current users of attention deficit/hyperactivity disorder medications, not a single myocardial infarction was reported during treatment [1, 4]. The boy in this case report presented with cardiac arrest without any prior complaints about chest discomfort or shortness of breath. The only symptom was the short exertion induced tachycardia episode a week before the major event. Had this been presented for a physician, it is unlikely that it would have led to further diagnostic workup. In retrospect this episode was most likely caused by ventricular tachycardia.

The large epidemiological studies on methylphenidate are based on reported diagnoses, among which this boy's myocardial infarction diagnosis probably would never have appeared. Instead, he suffered from cardiac arrest and would

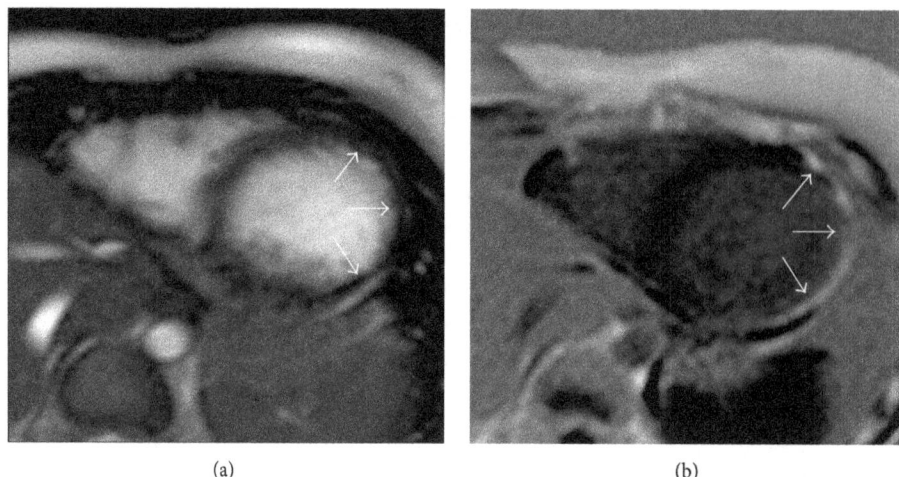

(a)   (b)

FIGURE 2: Cardiac magnetic resonance (CMR) imaging showing short-axis views in diastole (a) by cine CMR and (b) by late gadolinium enhancement imaging. Arrows indicate myocardial wall thinning and late gadolinium enhancement in the circumflex artery area consistent with myocardial necrosis and scar formation.

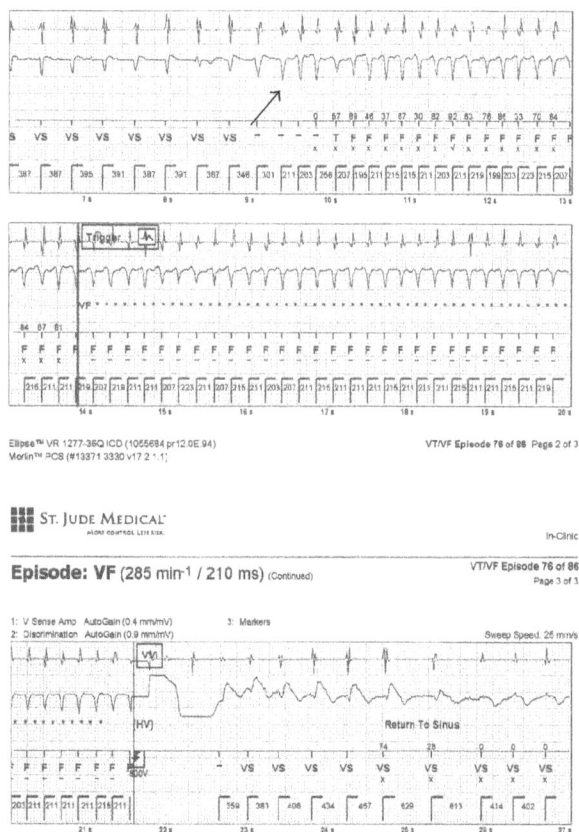

FIGURE 3: Reading from the implantable cardioverter defibrillator showing onset of ventricular fibrillation (arrow) at an average cycle length of 210 ms corresponding to a rate of 285 per minute. After the first shock (HV) delivered by the defibrillator, sinus rhythm is restored.

have been classified as sudden cardiac death, had he not been resuscitated.

When the boy was admitted, the first assumption was a primary arrhythmia. However the ECG clearly indicated regional myocardial necrosis and the echocardiogram showed thinning of the myocardial wall. The CMR scan clearly indicated that the myocardial infarction was of an older date (more than weeks) due to thinning of the myocardium and an adversely remodeled left ventricle.

Currently there is no recommendation in Denmark or by the FDA to obtain ECG before and during methylphenidate treatment, explaining why there was no ECG prior to treatment. Theoretically, there may be more children with undiagnosed myocardial infarctions among methylphenidate users that are missed, if routine ECGs are not obtained on a regular basis. In the present case, the Q-waves in the ECG would have disclosed that the child had developed heart disease. Whether this would have altered the course is speculative.

Obviously it may be questioned if the myocardial infarction actually developed prior to methylphenidate treatment and if it really was the cause. It is now two years since the index admission. The boys present clinical situation is quite concerning. Despite high dose ACE-inhibitors and beta-blockers his left ventricle has further adversely remodeled from an initial internal diastolic diameter of 5.4 cm to 7.2 cm on the latest echocardiography. His ejection fraction has deteriorated to 35%. He is in heart failure class II. He recently underwent two VT ablations due to long lasting tachycardia episodes and therapies from the ICD. Therefore it is unbelievable that this boy was started on methylphenidate after the huge myocardial infarct. He would have been in overt heart failure which would have been noticed. Children do not develop huge myocardial infarcts without a cause. This young boy has been very thoroughly examined. He did not suffer from hypertension or hypercholesterolemia, and there was no coronary artery anomaly, no myocardial bridging, no coagulation defects, no PFO, and no abnormal coronary spasm tendency to explain his myocardial infarct.

Furthermore, the dosage of methylphenidate was uptitrated correctly to an appropriate dosage and there was not any suspicion of abuse. The only thing that points out is the methylphenidate treatment, which FDA recognizes can cause heart attacks in adults.

Randomized trials show that ADHD drugs reduce symptoms significantly, compared to placebo [8], and improve children's learning and academic achievement modestly [9]. At present, the use of ADHD drugs is increasing. For this reason, even though registry studies do not show associations with cardiovascular events in children, it is important to closely monitor and report cardiovascular events to ensure that this treatment remains well controlled, efficient, and safe.

In conclusion, myocardial infarction and sudden cardiac death are extremely rare among children during treatment with methylphenidate. However, the present case shows that myocardial infarction can happen due to methylphenidate exposure in a cardiac healthy child, without any other cardiovascular risk factor.

Conflict of Interests

The authors declare that there is no conflict of interests regarding the publication of this paper.

References

[1] W. O. Cooper, L. A. Habel, C. M. Sox et al., "ADHD drugs and serious cardiovascular events in children and young adults," *The New England Journal of Medicine*, vol. 365, no. 20, pp. 1896–1904, 2011.

[2] S. E. Nissen, "ADHD drugs and cardiovascular risk," *The New England Journal of Medicine*, vol. 354, no. 14, pp. 1445–1448, 2006.

[3] H. Schelleman, W. B. Bilker, S. E. Kimmel et al., "Methylphenidate and risk of serious cardiovascular events in adults," *The American Journal of Psychiatry*, vol. 169, no. 2, pp. 178–185, 2012.

[4] H. Schelleman, W. B. Bilker, B. L. Strom et al., "Cardiovascular events and death in children exposed and unexposed to ADHD agents," *Pediatrics*, vol. 127, no. 6, pp. 1102–1110, 2011.

[5] N. D. Volkow, G.-J. Wang, J. S. Fowler et al., "Cardiovascular effects of methylphenidate in humans are associated with increases of dopamine in brain and of epinephrine in plasma," *Psychopharmacology*, vol. 166, no. 3, pp. 264–270, 2003.

[6] A. N. Westover and E. A. Halm, "Do prescription stimulants increase the risk of adverse cardiovascular events? A systematic review," *BMC Cardiovascular Disorders*, vol. 12, article 41, 2012.

[7] F. M. C. Besag and G. Stiefel, "Cardiovascular effects of methylphenidate, amphetamines and atomoxetine in the treatment of attention-deficit hyperactivity disorder," *Drug Safety*, vol. 33, no. 10, pp. 821–842, 2010.

[8] M. Rösler, M. Casas, E. Konofal, and J. Buitelaar, "Attention deficit hyperactivity disorder in adults," *World Journal of Biological Psychiatry*, vol. 11, no. 5, pp. 684–698, 2010.

[9] V. Prasad, E. Brogan, C. Mulvaney, M. Grainge, W. Stanton, and K. Sayal, "How effective are drug treatments for children with ADHD at improving on-task behaviour and academic achievement in the school classroom? A systematic review and meta-analysis," *European Child and Adolescent Psychiatry*, vol. 22, no. 4, pp. 203–216, 2013.

51

Massive Gastric Hemorrhage due to Dieulafoy's Lesion in a Preterm Neonate: A Case Report and Literature Review of the Lesion in Neonates

Christos Salakos,[1,2] **Panayiota Kafritsa,**[3] **Yvelise de Verney,**[2]
Ariadni Sageorgi,[4] **and Nick Zavras**[1]

[1]*Department of Pediatric Surgery, ATTIKON University Hospital, 1 Rimini Street, Haidari, 12462 Athens, Greece*
[2]*Department of Pediatric Surgery, "IASO" Maternity and Children's Hospital, 37-39 Kifisias Street, Marousi, 15123 Athens, Greece*
[3]*Department of Gastroenterology, "IASO" Maternity and Children's Hospital, 37-39 Kifisias Street, Marousi, 15123 Athens, Greece*
[4]*Neonatal Intensive Care Unit, "IASO" Maternity and Children's Hospital, 37-39 Kifisias Street, Marousi, 15123 Athens, Greece*

Correspondence should be addressed to Nick Zavras; nzavras@med.uoa.gr

Academic Editor: Denis A. Cozzi

Dieulafoy's lesion is an extremely rare cause of upper gastrointestinal bleeding in the neonatal age group. Till now, only 6 cases of Dieulafoy's lesion in neonatal period have been reported in the international literature. Herein, we report an extremely rare case of Dieulafoy's lesion in a preterm neonate.

1. Introduction

Dieulafoy's lesion (DL) is a distinct entity characterized by the presence of a large artery located under the muscularis mucosa and usually protruding into the gastric lumen [1]. The lesion accounts for 0.3% to 6.7% of the upper gastrointestinal (GI) tract bleeding cases in adults [2]. However, its exact prevalence in the pediatric population is unknown as most published studies concern case reports. In a recent review of the English language literature, the authors identified 28 pediatric cases with DL, among whom there were two full-term neonates and one preterm. All these neonates manifested the disease on the 1st, 3rd, and 4th postnatal day, respectively [3–5].

Herein, we describe a preterm neonate with DL. A brief review on neonatal cases is discussed.

2. Case Report

A preterm male neonate was born as twin B after an IVF pregnancy to a 36-year-old gravida 1, para 2 mother at 26^{+1}-week gestation, due to idiopathic preterm labor. His birth weight was 1010 g (90th percentile), and his length and head circumference were 34 cm (50th percentile) and 25.4 cm (90th percentile), respectively. Apgar scores were 4 at 1 minute and 6 at 5 minutes. The neonate was intubated to increase respiratory efforts and he was transferred to the neonatal intensive care unit (NICU). He remained on mechanical ventilation for 36 days. On day 65 of hospitalization (postconceptual age: 34^{+5} weeks, weight 2020 g), he presented with a massive oral hematemesis and was transferred to the NICU yet again. On examination, he was pale and displayed mild abdominal distention. Initial laboratory examinations showed hemoglobin of 10 g/dL (13.5–19.5 g/dL); hematocrit 29.3% (40–64%); WBC 5,050 cells/μL (10.000–26000 cells/μL); and platelet count 190,000/μL (150,000–400,000/μL). The coagulation tests were normal. After a one-blood volume transfusion, esophagogastroduodenoscopy (EGD) was performed with an Olympus GIF-N180 neonatal endoscope, which identified the presence of a big blood clot in the fundus, adherent to the gastroesophageal junction without signs of active bleeding (Figure 1). However, despite the efforts, the blood clot could not be reached even in full retroflexion. A second endoscopy was performed the following day after a massive

TABLE 1: Published cases of Dieulafoy's lesion in the neonatal age group.

Authors	GA	Sex	Age	Site	Diagnosis	Treatment	Recurrence	Outcome
Lee et al. [4]	Full-term	M	3 d	Stomach	Endoscopy	Hemostatic clip	No	Successful
Koo et al. [7]	Full-term	M	1 d	Stomach	Endoscopy	Endoscopic epinephrine injection	No	Successful
Koo et al. [7]	Full-term	F	1 d	Stomach	Endoscopy	Endoscopic epinephrine injection	No	Successful
Lee et al. [8]	Full-term	M	1 d	Stomach	Endoscopy	Hemostatic clip	No	Successful
Polonkai et al. [5]	Late preterm	M	5 d	Stomach	Endoscopy	Hemostatic clip	No	Death
Zavras et al. [3]	Full-term	M	1 d	Stomach	Endoscopy	Thermocoagulation	No	Successful
Present case	Preterm	M	65 d	Stomach	Laparotomy	Laparotomy	No	Successful

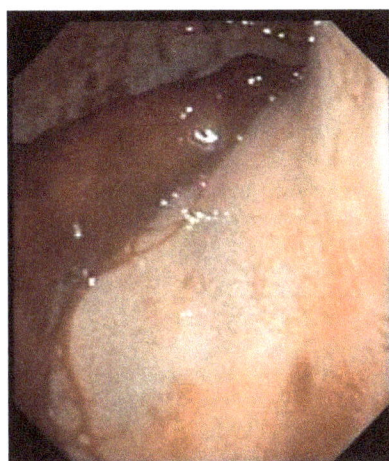

FIGURE 1: A big blood clot adherent to the gastroesophageal junction was seen in the 1st endoscopy. The clot could not be reached by endoscopy.

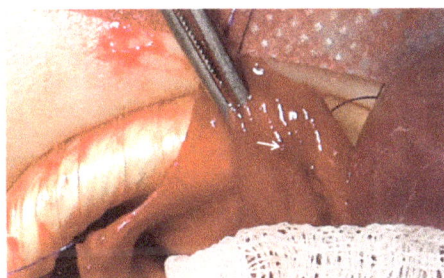

FIGURE 2: A spurting arterial vessel was seen after gastrotomy (white arrow).

hematemesis and a further drop in the levels of hemoglobin and hematocrit (8.6 g/dL and 25.1%, resp.). However, the presence of a pool of blood prevented the endoscope from visualizing the source of bleeding. Again, the site of bleeding could not be approximated. An emergency laparotomy with gastrotomy was carried out which revealed a spurting arterial vessel that was ligated at a distance of less than 3 cm from the gastroesophageal junction (Figure 2). The infant had

an uneventful recovery. No recurrence of bleeding was noted during 8 months of follow-up.

3. Discussion

DL lesion is extremely rare in the neonatal age group. Relevant articles in the international literature, dating from the first case reported in 1968 [6] to present, were retrieved from PubMed, SCOPUS, and Medline using the key words Dieulafoy's lesion, caliber persistent artery, neonates, and children. We found only three cases in the English literature [3–5] and another three in the Asian literature [7, 8]. All but one neonate were full-term, with a male/female ratio 5 : 1 (Table 1). To our knowledge, this case is the second to be described in a preterm male neonate.

Although DL was first reported by Gallard in 1884 [9], it carries the name of Dieulafoy who reported the lesion in three patients with upper gastrointestinal bleeding [10]. He called it "exulceratio simplex," characterised by an oval or elliptical shaped acute ulcerative process with dimensions of 2–5 mm. Regardless of the age of the patient, the lesion is usually located in the upper stomach 6 cm below the esophagogastric mucosa [11], but it can also be found anywhere within the entire GI tract from the esophagus to the rectum, or at sites outside the GI tract, such as the bronchi [12]. In the reviewed cases, including our own, DL was located in the stomach in all neonates (Table 1).

The clinical presentation more commonly includes a painless and massive upper GI hemorrhage, possibly recurrent [12]. Hemodynamic instability may be involved [12]. The pathogenesis of DL is not clearly understood. Among various causes, the hypothesis of a congenital origin seems to be the most acceptable [13]. According to this theory, the bleeding artery maintains its initial diameter as it enters the gastric wall rather than decreasing [13]. This abnormality renders the vessel prone to massive bleeding. The congenital anomaly is supported by reported cases of neonates.

Endoscopy is the first method of diagnosis in DL, and the diagnostic criteria are well established [14]. In cases of gastric DL in both the adult and pediatric population, the success rate ranges between 70% and 80% [11, 14], though repeated endoscopies may be required to establish the diagnosis [14]. Similarly, in the cases listed here (Table 1), the success rate of endoscopic diagnosis was as high as 85.7%. However, in our case, two endoscopic investigations failed to localize the source of bleeding due to the presence of a clot in the first endoscopy and active bleeding in the second; thus, a gastrotomy was performed to identify the source of bleeding.

So far, there is not a general agreement on the management of DL [14]; hence, the choice of treatment relies on the location of the DL and suitable skills. It is worth saying that advancements in endoscopic procedures, even in neonates, have limited the use of surgical intervention. A success rate reaching 98% has been reported with various endoscopic modalities, including the hemoclip, injection of sclerosants, thermocoagulation, or band ligation [3, 15]. In neonatal case series (Table 1), successful hemostasis was achieved with a hemoclip in three patients, injection of epinephrine in two patients, and thermal coagulation in one patient. Recently, surgical intervention was reserved only for cases deemed unmanageable with endoscopic procedures [3]. In our case, the site of the DL was very close to the gastroesophageal junction and was covered with blood. Consequently, an open laparotomy was decided. No recurrence was noted in our listed cases, and death was reported in just one patient [5] due to coexistent lesions.

The present case illustrates a very rare case of DL in a preterm neonate. Although endoscopy is considered the first diagnostic tool of intervention, in the paediatric population, the management of DL may be very difficult. The lack of fine endoscope and the tiny size of the stomach pose a challenge for endoscopic procedures. Notably, in the cases of recurrent massive bleeding of upper GI, an open approach should be promptly carried out to determine and treat DL.

Conflict of Interests

The authors declare that there is no conflict of interests regarding the publication of this paper.

References

[1] H. L. Karamanoukian, D. T. Wilcox, E. I. Hatch, R. Sawin, and P. L. Glick, "Dieulafoy's disease in infants," *Pediatric Surgery International*, vol. 9, no. 8, pp. 585–586, 1994.

[2] H. F. Reilly III and F. H. Al-Kawas, "Dieulafoy's lesion: diagnosis and management," *Digestive Diseases and Sciences*, vol. 36, no. 12, pp. 1702–1707, 1991.

[3] N. Zavras, C. Siafakas, G. Pergamalis, Y. de Verney, M. Clavdianou, and C. Salakos, "Successful diagnosis and treatment of Dieulafoy's lesion with endoscopy and thermocoagulation in a full-term neonate: report of a case and literature review," *Journal of Pediatric Surgery Case Reports*, vol. 2, no. 5, pp. 250–253, 2014.

[4] Y. J. Lee, J. M. Oh, S. E. Park, and J. H. Park, "Successful treatment of a gastric Dieulafoy's lesion with a hemoclip in a newborn infant," *Gastrointestinal Endoscopy*, vol. 57, no. 3, pp. 435–436, 2003.

[5] E. Polonkai, A. Nagy, I. Csízy et al., "Pyloric atresia associated with Dieulafoy lesion and gastric dysmotility in a neonate," *Journal of Pediatric Surgery*, vol. 46, no. 10, pp. E19–E23, 2011.

[6] N. P. Rossi, E. W. Green, and J. D. Pike, "Massive bleeding of the upper-gastrointestinal tract due to Dieulafoy's erosion," *Archives of Surgery*, vol. 97, no. 5, pp. 797–800, 1968.

[7] Y. H. Koo, J. S. Jang, J. H. Cho et al., "Endoscopic injection treatment for gastric dieulafoy lesion in two newborn infants," *The Korean Journal of Gastroenterology*, vol. 46, no. 5, pp. 413–417, 2005.

[8] Y. W. Lee, J. H. Shin, M. Y. Chang, and J. Y. Kim, "Endoscopic hemoclipping treatment for gastric Dieulafoy lesion in a newborn," *Korean Journal of Pediatric Gastroenterology and Nutrition*, vol. 14, no. 4, pp. 393–397, 2011.

[9] T. Gallard, "Aneurysmes miliaires de l'estomac donnant lieu à des hematemesis mortelles," *Bulletins et Mémoires de la Société Médicale des Hôpitaux de Paris*, vol. 1, pp. 84–91, 1884.

[10] G. Dieulafoy, "Exulceratio simplex: l'intervention chirurgicale dans les hematemesis foundroyantes consecutive à l'exulceration simplex de l'estomac," *Bulletin de l'Académie Nationale de Médecine*, vol. 39, pp. 49–84, 1898.

[11] M. Itani, T. Alsaied, L. Charafeddine, and N. Yazbeck, "Dieulafoy's lesion in children," *Journal of Pediatric Gastroenterology and Nutrition*, vol. 51, no. 5, pp. 672–674, 2010.

[12] M. M. Linhares, B. H. Filho, V. Schraibman et al., "Dieulafoy lesion: endoscopic and surgical management," *Surgical Laparoscopy, Endoscopy and Percutaneous Techniques*, vol. 16, no. 1, pp. 1–3, 2006.

[13] D. Voth, "Zur Pathogenese ungerwöhnlischer, artellier mangendlutungen," *Die Medizinische Welt*, vol. 19, pp. 1095–1097, 1962.

[14] M. Baxter and E. H. Aly, "Dieulafoy's lesion: current trends in diagnosis and management," *Annals of The Royal College of Surgeons of England*, vol. 92, no. 7, pp. 548–554, 2010.

[15] W. Lim, T. O. Kim, S. B. Park et al., "Endoscopic treatment of dieulafoy lesions and risk factors for rebleeding," *Korean Journal of Internal Medicine*, vol. 24, no. 4, pp. 318–322, 2009.

52

Postinjection Muscle Fibrosis from Lupron

Erica Everest,[1,2] Laurie A. Tsilianidis,[1,2] Nouhad Raissouni,[1,2] Tracy Ballock,[1,2] Terra Blatnik,[1,2] Anzar Haider,[1,2] Douglas G. Rogers,[1,2] and B. Michelle Schweiger[1,2]

[1]Cleveland Clinic, 9500 Euclid Avenue, Cleveland, OH 44195, USA
[2]Case Western Reserve University School of Medicine, 10900 Euclid Avenue, Cleveland, OH 44106, USA

Correspondence should be addressed to Erica Everest; ericaeverest@gmail.com

Academic Editor: Giovanni Montini

We describe the case of a 6.5-year-old girl with central precocious puberty (CPP), which signifies the onset of secondary sexual characteristics before the age of eight in females and the age of nine in males as a result of stimulation of the hypothalamic-pituitary-gonadal axis. Her case is likely related to her adoption, as children who are adopted internationally have much higher rates of CPP. She had left breast development at Tanner Stage 2, adult body odor, and mildly advanced bone age. In order to halt puberty and maximize adult height, she was prescribed a gonadotropin releasing hormone analog, the first line treatment for CPP. She was administered Lupron (leuprolide acetate) Depot-Ped (3 months) intramuscularly. After her second injection, she developed swelling and muscle pain at the injection site on her right thigh. She also reported an impaired ability to walk. She was diagnosed with muscle fibrosis. This is the first reported case of muscle fibrosis resulting from Lupron injection.

1. Background

Lupron (leuprorelin acetate) is a gonadotropin releasing hormone analog (GnRHa). GnRH is normally released in a pulsatile manner, which can be interrupted by a constant serum level of an agonist. Resultant downregulation of the GnRH receptors reduces the amounts of estradiol and testosterone produced [1]. This medication is indicated for prostate cancer, endometriosis, uterine fibroids, and central precocious puberty, the condition of our patient [2]. GnRHas are the first-line treatment for central precocious puberty (CPP) [3].

Precocious puberty is early sexual maturation, before the age of eight in girls and the age of nine in boys [4]. There are two types: central (gonadotropin-dependent) and peripheral (gonadotropin-independent) types. CPP results from premature activation of the hypothalamic-pituitary-gonadal axis. CPP is concerning, because premature fusion of the epiphyseal growth plates decreases adult height and because early development may cause psychosocial issues [5, 6]. Interestingly, CPP is more prevalent in children who were adopted internationally, which is the case for our patient. These children are ten to twenty times more likely to develop precocious puberty. It is hypothesized that early nutritional deficits followed by rapid weight gain after adoption trigger the endocrine changes and physical growth of puberty prematurely [7, 8] However, the condition may still be idiopathic in nature, because idiopathic central precocious puberty makes up 90% of cases in females. Males are more likely to have pathological causes for central precocious puberty [1].

Established Facts

  (i) Gonadotropin releasing hormone analogs are the standard of care for central precocious puberty [3].

  (ii) Injection site reactions are common from Lupron administration [9].

Novel Insights

  (i) This is the first reported case of muscle fibrosis from a Lupron injection.

We report a case of a seven-year-old girl with muscle fibrosis of the right thigh following an injection of Lupron to treat her precocious puberty. A review of the literature reveals no previous reports of muscle fibrosis resulting from an intramuscular injection of Lupron.

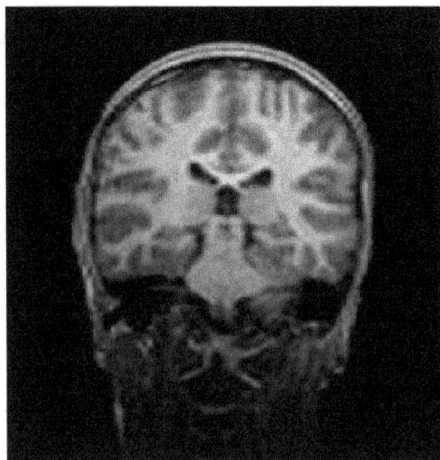

FIGURE 1

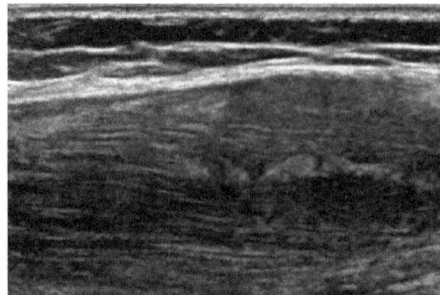

FIGURE 2

2. Case Presentation

A six-year-eleven-month-old female presented to the Pediatric Endocrinology Clinic with signs of early puberty. Her mother noticed her daughter having adult body odor two months prior and development of her left breast (Tanner Stage 2) one month prior to the appointment. The patient denied any vaginal bleeding or discharge. She also denied pubic and axillary hair development, as well as any acne. Review of systems revealed increased thirst, while her physical exam was unremarkable. Her height and weight were at the 64th percentile for her age. This is an increase from the 14th percentile at the age of four, at which time she was adopted internationally. An X-ray to determine bone age was performed and showed bones between seven years ten months and eight years ten months of age by standards of Greulich and Pyle [10].

Laboratory data showed that the testosterone level was elevated at 12 ng/dL (0–9 ng/dL for Tanner Stage 1 females), and the hydroxyprogesterone level was elevated at 1.4 ng/mL (0.0–0.3 ng/mL). (A hydroxyprogesterone under 2 ng/mL and a testosterone that is not substantially higher than normal make congenital adrenal hyperplasia unlikely. However, the body odor suggested testing). The luteinizing hormone level of 2.0 mU/mL was consistent with CPP (diagnostic criteria is LH > 0.3 mU/mL). Follicle stimulating hormone was elevated at 4.5 mU/mL (0.0–4.0 mU/mL in prepubescent females) and estradiol 17B was also in the pubertal range at 39 pg/mL (<30 pg/mL). DHEA-S was normal at 28.6 ug/dL (0.0–37.0 ug/dL).

Given her increased growth velocity, thelarche, body odor, mildly advanced bone age, and gonadotropins and estradiol in pubertal ranges, she was diagnosed with CPP. She was given an MRI of her pituitary gland to rule out intracranial pathology as the cause of her precocious puberty (see Figure 1). The posterior T1 bright spot was present. The pituitary was homogenous in signal but was enlarged at 8 mm in the craniocaudal dimension. It had a convex superior margin, and no mass effect was noted. Overall, the pituitary gland was enlarged, but with no lesions to suggest

an adenoma. We recommended injections of Lupron to halt puberty and prescribed Lupron Depot-Ped, 3 months 11.25 mg. We planned for her to return in five months, at which point she would have received two Lupron injections.

She received her first Lupron injection two weeks after the appointment. It was administered IM in the right vastus lateralis muscle. The patient tolerated the injection well, and she returned for a second injection in three months in the same location in her right thigh. At the time, the patient appeared to tolerate this injection well also. However, three weeks after the second injection, the patient had an appointment with a pediatric orthopedic surgeon. The reason for the visit was a lump on and swelling of her right thigh at the injection site. The lump measured 5 × 5 cm and was not tender to palpation. She reports pain in her right leg and trouble walking. She rated the pain as a 5 on a 0 to 10 scale with daily activities and with exercise. Her knee flexion was only fifteen degrees. Her right extremity showed no deformity. Ultrasound revealed no cellulitis or abnormal fluid collection at the injection site on her right thigh (see Figure 2). The lack of fluid indicated that this was not an abscess. She was diagnosed with muscle fibrosis based on the severe restriction of knee flexion due to lack of muscle excursion following the injection, as well as the presence of a mass at the injection site. She was instructed to have physical therapy.

3. Discussion

Muscle fibrosis and contracture following an intramuscular injection occurs most commonly in the anterior and lateral thigh [11]. Muscle fibrosis usually presents as atrophy, dimpling, reduced range of motion, and abnormal gait [12]. The major symptoms are recurrent dislocation of the patella and limitation of flexion of the knee. The contractures may form within weeks but also may take months to years after an injection [11]. These deformities may be coming later in our patient, since the diagnosis was merely weeks after the injection. For cases in which the diagnosis is made early or the fibrosis is mild, physical therapy and casting may be helpful [13]. However, these treatments are usually unhelpful in established cases. Surgery is often required and can create substantial improvement, especially when performed before there is permanent damage to the knee joint [14]. Since our patient was diagnosed quickly and began physical therapy, it is possible that this will prevent the muscle deformity from ever happening.

Thus far, there have been no reported cases of muscle fibrosis following an injection of Lupron. Treatment-related adverse effects occurred in 29% of patients dosed at 11.25 mg over three years in a long-term safety and efficacy study [9]. Common side effects at the injection site are pain and abscess, which occur in 5–15% of patients [5]. Also, there is the potential for acne, rash, blisters, facial swelling, weight gain, altered mood, headache, flushes and sweating, and vaginal symptoms, such as vaginitis, bleeding, and discharge [2].

The depot suspension of leuprolide acetate consists of microspheres of the drug within a biodegradable copolymer of lactic and glycolic acids [15]. With regard to the adverse effects of sterile abscess formation, it is believed that the cause is a reaction to the inert polymer rather than to the drug itself. The chance of having a reaction to these materials is estimated to be 3 to 13 per 100 children [16]. Given that patients have been successfully treated with the daily non-depot form of leuprolide acetate following an adverse reaction to the depot form, it seems as if the polymer was the component causing the problem [17]. However, there also have been cases reported of people with prostate cancer who have become resistant to GnRHa therapy following a sterile abscess formation [18, 19].

Although muscle fibrosis is a rare side effect of the Lupron depot injection, there are a substantial number of adverse effects reported at the injection site. Parents should be advised to monitor their child's injection site for abnormalities, even up to a few weeks or months afterward. Moreover, if they report any symptoms that resemble muscle fibrosis, they should be advised to seek medical care promptly.

4. Conclusion

This report describes the first case of muscle fibrosis of the thigh following an injection of Lupron Depot-Ped. The patient is a seven-year-old female being treated for central precocious puberty.

Conflict of Interests

The authors declare that there is no conflict of interests regarding the publication of this paper.

References

[1] J. S. Fuqua, "Treatment and outcomes of precocious puberty: an update," *Journal of Clinical Endocrinology and Metabolism*, vol. 98, no. 6, pp. 2198–2207, 2013.

[2] Lupron Depot, leuprolide acetate for depot suspension, 2013, http://www.lupron.com/.

[3] S. R. Johnson, R. C. Nolan, M. T. Grant et al., "Sterile abscess formation associated with depot leuprorelin acetate therapy for central precocious puberty," *Journal of Paediatrics and Child Health*, vol. 48, no. 3, pp. E136–E139, 2012.

[4] P. S. N. Menon and M. Vijayakumar, "Precocious puberty—perspectives on diagnosis and management," *Indian Journal of Pediatrics*, vol. 81, no. 1, pp. 76–83, 2014.

[5] J. C. Carel, E. A. Eugster, A. Rogol, L. Ghizzoni, and M. R. Palmert, "Consensus statement on the use of gonadotropin-releasing hormone analogs in children," *Pediatrics*, vol. 123, no. 4, pp. e752–e762, 2009.

[6] J.-C. Carel, N. Lahlou, M. Roger, and J. L. Chaussain, "Precocious puberty and statural growth," *Human Reproduction Update*, vol. 10, no. 2, pp. 135–147, 2004.

[7] L. Soriano-Guillén, R. Corripio, J. I. Labarta et al., "Central precocious puberty in children living in Spain: incidence, prevalence, and influence of adoption and immigration," *Journal of Clinical Endocrinology and Metabolism*, vol. 95, no. 9, pp. 4305–4313, 2010.

[8] G. Teilmann, C. B. Pedersen, N. E. Skakkebæk, and T. K. Jensen, "Increased risk of precocious puberty in internationally adopted children in Denmark," *Pediatrics*, vol. 118, no. 2, pp. 391–399, 2006.

[9] P. Lee, K. Klein, N. Mauras et al., "36-month treatment experience of 2 doses of leuprolide acetate 3-month depot for children with central precocious puberty," *The Journal of Clinical Endocrinology & Metabolism*, vol. 99, pp. 3153–3159, 2014.

[10] W. W. Greulich and S. I. Pyle, *Radiographic Atlas of Skeletal Development of Hand Wrist*, vol. 2, Stanford University Press, Stanford, Calif, USA, 1971.

[11] P. S. Bergeson, S. A. Singer, and A. M. Kaplan, "Intramuscular injections in children," *Pediatrics*, vol. 70, no. 6, pp. 944–948, 1982.

[12] N. A. Mir, S. M. Ahmed, and J. A. Bhat, "Post-injection gluteal fibrosis: a neglected problem," *JK Science*, vol. 4, no. 3, pp. 144–146, 2002.

[13] R. Jerotic, G. Rikolic, S. Rejie et al., "Rehabilitation of post-injection contractures in children," *Srpski Arhiv za Celokupno Lekarstvo*, vol. 103, p. 59, 1975.

[14] E. V. Alvarez, M. Munters, L. S. Lavine, H. Manes, and J. Waxman, "Quadriceps myofibrosis: a complication of intramuscular injections," *The Journal of Bone & Joint Surgery—American Volume*, vol. 62, no. 1, pp. 58–60, 1980.

[15] Abbott Laboratories, *Lupron Depot Ped (leuprolide acetate for depot suspension)*, Abbott Laboratories, North Chicago, Ill, USA, 2008, http://www.rxabbvie.com/pdf/lupronpediatric.pdf.

[16] G. Tonini, S. Marinoni, V. Forleo, M. Rustico, E. K. Neely, and D. M. Wilson, "Local reactions to luteinizing hormone releasing hormone analog therapy," *The Journal of Pediatrics*, vol. 126, no. 1, pp. 159–160, 1995.

[17] E. K. Neely, R. L. Hintz, B. Parker et al., "Two-year results of treatment with depot leuprolide acetate for central precocious puberty," *Journal of Pediatrics*, vol. 121, no. 4, pp. 634–640, 1992.

[18] T. J. Daskivich and W. K. Oh, "Failure of gonadotropin-releasing hormone agonists with and without sterile abscess formation at depot sites: insight into mechanisms?" *Urology*, vol. 67, no. 5, pp. 1084.e15–1084.e17, 2006.

[19] E. A. Curry III and C. J. Sweeney, "Resistance to luteinizing hormone releasing hormone agonist therapy for metastatic prostate cancer," *Journal of Urology*, vol. 168, no. 1, p. 193, 2002.

53

Acute Kidney Injury Complicated Epstein-Barr Virus Infection in Infancy

Gamze Ozgurhan,[1] **Mustafa Ozcetin,**[1] **Aysel Vehapoglu,**[2]
Zeynep Karakaya,[1] **and Fatih Aygun**[3]

[1]*Department of Pediatrics, Suleymaniye Maternity and Children's Training and Research Hospital, Istanbul, Turkey*
[2]*Department of Pediatrics, Bezmialem Vakif University Medical School, Istanbul, Turkey*
[3]*Department of Pediatric Intensive Care, Istanbul University Cerrahpasa Medical School, Istanbul, Turkey*

Correspondence should be addressed to Gamze Ozgurhan; gamzeozgurhan@yahoo.com

Academic Editor: Nina L. Shapiro

Infectious mononucleosis is an acute lymphoproliferative disorder caused by the Epstein-Barr virus (EBV) and seen most commonly in children and young adults. Clinical presentation of the disease is characterized by fever, tonsillopharyngitis, lymphadenopathy, and hepatosplenomegaly, whereas serological findings of this benign disorder include positive heterophilic antibody formation (transient increase in heterophilic antibodies) and prominence of hematological lymphocytosis of more than 10% of atypical lymphocytes. An EBV infection is usually asymptomatic in childhood, but acute kidney injury can be a rare complication during its course. Most cases recover from the disease completely. Early recognition of EBV infection and estimation of its complication are important for its prognosis. In light of previous literature, we discuss the case evaluated as an EBV infection complicated by acute kidney injury in early childhood and results of tubulointerstitial nephritis shown on a renal biopsy that was later diagnosed as an EBV infection by serological examination.

1. Introduction

The Epstein-Barr virus (EBV) affects almost all the systems of the body and therefore has a broad spectrum of clinical outcomes. It was discovered by Epstein, Achong, and Barr on microscopic examination of cell cultures obtained from Burkitt lymphoma 50 years ago [1]. In 1968, EBV was demonstrated as a causative agent for heterophile-positive infectious mononucleosis. In the 1970s, it was found in certain tissues of nasopharyngeal carcinoma patients. Finally in the 1980s, a correlation between EBV and oral hairy leukoplakia and non-Hodgkin's lymphoma was proven in patients with AIDS [2]. The most common clinical feature seen in adults and adolescents with infectious mononucleosis is a triad of fever, sore throat, and lymphadenopathy. Serological tests showing positive heterophilic antibodies and peripheral lymphocytosis with atypical lymphocytes have been determined [3]. In infants and young children, nonspecific and subclinical symptoms are usually observed [4]. In some cases, a primary

EBV infection remains silent and clinically atypical until this period. Clinical signs related to almost all affected organs of the body appear as an atypical type of infection with EBV. Diagnosis is made by specific serological tests [5]. Healthy cases generally recover from primary EBV infection completely. However, it can be complicated by renal, cardiac, pulmonary, neurological, and hematological problems [6]. Acute kidney injury related to acute EBV infection has been rarely demonstrated in the literature [7, 8]. In the light of the literature, we discuss here a case of acute kidney injury related to EBV infection in a 13-month-old male patient.

2. Case

A previously healthy 13-month-old male patient was admitted to the hospital presenting four days of fever and rash. Before admission, the patient had used amoxicillin and clavulanic acid treatment in an appropriate dose for an upper respiratory tract infection, but the fever did not subside and his body temperature increased to 40°C with shivering. He had no complaints other than fatigue. His past history and family history were unremarkable.

On physical examination, he appeared fatigued with body weight of 9750 g (25 p); height of 76 cm (25–50 p); axillary temperature of 39.8°C; blood pressure of 100/60 mmHg; heart rate of 130/min; and respiratory rate within normal range. Lymphadenopathy and organomegaly were not present. There were no respiratory, cardiovascular, gastrointestinal, or neurological signs, but fever, mild hyperemia of pharynx, maculopapular rash that blanches under pressure, and some petechial rashes on lower limbs.

On total blood count, Hb was 10.4 g/dL and WBC was 17,060/mm^3 (36.2% neutrophil, 48.4% lymphocytes, and 11% atypical lymphocytes), and PLT count was found normal (309,000/mm^3). Liver function and renal function tests and serum electrolytes were found normal. Due to the presence of persistent fever and rash, viral serological tests for isolation of etiological agent (TORCH, parvovirus, EBV VCA IgM, and EBV VCA IgG), monospot tests, rose bengal tests, tube agglutination tests for *Brucella*, urine, and stool analysis, and blood cultures were investigated. On examination, direct stool smear was normal. Urine analysis showed no significant results other than (+) proteinuria, 7 leucocytes, and 2 erythrocytes. For differential diagnosis and exclusion of atypical Kawasaki disease, an echocardiogram was performed and found normal. Monospot tests, rose bengal tests, and tube agglutination tests for *Brucella* were negative.

On the fourth day of admission, due to low urine output and bilateral orbital edema, laboratory tests were repeated with results as follows: WBC: 16,600/mm^3, hemoglobin: 10 g/dL, and PLT: 173,000/mm^3. Serum electrolytes include sodium: 135 mEq/L; potassium: 7.09 mEq/L; chlorine: 107 mEq/L; bicarbonate: 11.5 mEq/L; urea: 181 mg/dL; creatinine: 4.1 mg/dL; calcium: 7.3 mg/dL; albumin: 2.95 g/dL; uric acid: 3.11 mg/dL; and mild elevation of transaminases (aspartate aminotransferase: 170 U/L and alanine aminotransferase: 79 U/L). Bilirubin and alkaline phosphatase were found to be normal. All types of cultures sent were found sterile.

An abdominal ultrasound showed the right and left kidney long axes to be 82 mm and 83 mm, respectively, and increased in length (>95th percentile for age). Both kidneys had grades 1-2 parenchymal hyperechogenicity. Sonography showed free collections at various sites, including perihepatic, perisplenic, and lower quadrant of the abdomen with the largest site measuring 8 mm.

The first attempt for treatment was fluid restriction (urine output + insensible losses), sodium bicarbonate (1 mEq/kg), and calcium gluconate (1 mL/kg). Later, the patient developed oligoanuria, features of acute kidney injury, and metabolic acidosis; therefore, hemodialysis treatment in the pediatric intensive care unit was applied. Serological testing for EBV VCA IgM and EBV VCA IgG performed at admission was positive. Hence EBV nuclear antigen (EBNA) was checked and found to be negative. No evidence for acute infection was determined in other serological tests. ASO was found

negative. C3 complement level was normal. Early examination of renal biopsy material showed intense and mixed tubulointerstitial inflammatory infiltration rich with T cells and histiocytes. Immunofluorescence studies for IgG, IgA, IgM, C3, fibrinogen, C19, kappa, and lambda were negative. Immunohistochemical studies for CMV, EBV, HSV I/II, and parvovirus were also found negative.

Due to the presence of peripheral atypical lymphocytosis and positive serological tests for EBV, the case was evaluated as acute kidney injury related to interstitial nephritis secondary to atypical EBV infection in early childhood. The patient needed sequential hemodialysis due to acute kidney injury and metabolic acidosis and complete recovery of renal functions (urea: 29 mg/dL; creatinine: 0.4 mg/dL; sodium: 138 mEq/L; potassium: 4.6 mEq/L) occurred in about one month.

3. Discussion

The Epstein-Barr virus usually appears as infectious mononucleosis in adolescents and adults, whereas it has asymptomatic and nonspecific symptoms in infants and children [2–4]. We present a case where a 13-month-old infant, who had been under treatment for acute infection, developed acute kidney injury and was duly followed up in pediatric intensive care unit.

Infectious mononucleosis, when it has significant clinical features, presents as a triad of fever, lymphadenopathy, and pharyngitis in half of the patients. Rarely being atypical, it can be complicated with pneumonia, shock, blood dyscrasias, fulminant hepatitis, encephalitis, carditis, arthritis, uveitis, and pancreatitis [1]. These rare features make the diagnosis of infectious mononucleosis and its differential diagnosis for Kawasaki disease difficult, especially in early phases of the infection. So far, one of the rarest complications caused by infectious mononucleosis is acute kidney injury. In our case, atypical features of infectious mononucleosis with development of acute kidney injury requiring sudden hemodialysis and diagnosis as EBV infection using serological tests are represented. Typical laboratory findings of infectious mononucleosis are atypical lymphocytosis (>10%) with absolute lymphocytosis, positive heterophilic antibodies, and mild-to-moderate elevation of serum aminotransferases. The presented case demonstrated 17060 leucocytes and 11% atypical lymphocyte count. Heterophilic antibody response is not generated well in children under 10, a well-known reaction also in line with the response in our case.

Serological profiles of EBV antibodies are quite characteristic and necessary for diagnosis of atypical infections [9]. In our case, there were no particular signs of EBV infection and diagnosis was based on serological examination and elevation of both EBV VCA IgM and EBV VCA IgG. It is expected that EBV infection coupled with amoxicillin use can cause a rash, which was also the case with our patient.

In EBV infections, a true renal parenchymal involvement is rarely found, although abnormalities in urine sediment can be seen in 5–15% of cases [10, 11]. Wechsler et al. [12] reported that 17 out of 556 cases presented abnormalities in urine analysis such as microscopic hematuria and proteinuria without renal parenchymal involvement. Lee and Kjellstrand described 14% of proteinuria and 11% of hematuria in 128 EBV-infected cases [13]. In another study, where a series of cases of infectious mononucleosis without clinical findings related to renal illness are studied, swelling in glomerular cells and focal interstitial mononuclear infiltration in renal biopsy are found in 12 out of 13 patients [14].

Rhabdomyolysis and hepatic failure are the leading causes of EBV-related acute kidney injury [7]. In some cases, isolated tubulointerstitial nephritis, mesangial proliferation, and tubular necrosis result in kidney injury as well [7, 8, 13]. Mayer et al. examined EBV-associated kidney injury cases and found 3 with rhabdomyolysis, 2 with glomerulonephritis, 1 with minimal change disease, 1 with hemolytic uremic syndrome, and 1 with interstitial nephritis relevant acute kidney injury out of 13 cases with ages ranging from 4 to 18 years. In the majority of these cases, kidney injury patients had recovered completely within one to two weeks, whereas only one patient required dialysis. In case of the patient with interstitial nephritis, the patient required renal transplantation despite treatment with prednisolone [7]. In 14 patients with glomerular abnormalities with infectious mononucleosis, Ramelli et al. found the glomerular pathology being quite diverse, ranging from minimal change to focal sclerosis, and proliferative or sclerosing glomerulonephritis [15].

Tubulointerstitial nephritis is an unusual cause of acute kidney injury in pediatric patients. Greising et al. reported 7% of child patients having tubulointerstitial nephritis among all who went on renal biopsy. In this series, FSGS and interstitial nephritis were detected during renal biopsy in the case of a 15-year-old patient with acute mononucleosis [16]. Ellis et al. linked only two cases out of 13 TIN patients between 5 and 16 years old with nonspecific viral infections [17]. In our case, acute kidney injury is found to emerge due to interstitial nephritis. Although it appeared in early childhood, the patient required hemodialysis as acute kidney injury and metabolic acidosis developed, and his renal functions recovered completely within one month.

In summary, it should be kept in mind that, in early childhood, unexpected and abrupt emergence of acute kidney injury features in cases with fever can be caused by EBV as an etiological agent; therefore, serological tests should be performed. Renal biopsy done in early periods of the disease can further clarify the diagnosis by determining classical tubular cell infiltration.

Conflict of Interests

The authors declare that there is no conflict of interests regarding the publication of this paper.

References

[1] J. I. Cohen, "Epstein-Barr virus infection," *The New England Journal of Medicine*, vol. 343, no. 7, pp. 481–492, 2000.

[2] W. A. Durbin and J. L. Sullivan, "Epstein-Barr virus infection," *Pediatrics in Review*, vol. 15, no. 2, pp. 63–68, 1994.

[3] J. Peter and C. G. Ray, "Infectious mononucleosis," *Pediatrics in Review*, vol. 19, no. 8, pp. 276–279, 1998.

[4] R. J. Schaller and F. L. Counselman, "Infectious mononucleosis in young children," *The American Journal of Emergency Medicine*, vol. 13, no. 4, pp. 438–440, 1995.

[5] C. V. Sumaya and Y. Ench, "Epstein-Barr virus infectious mononucleosis in children. I. Clinical and general laboratory findings," *Pediatrics*, vol. 75, no. 6, pp. 1003–1010, 1985.

[6] K. Taga, H. Taga, and G. Tosato, "Diagnosis of atypical cases of infectious mononucleosis," *Clinical Infectious Diseases*, vol. 33, no. 1, pp. 83–88, 2001.

[7] H. B. Mayer, C. A. Wanke, M. Williams, A. W. Crosson, M. Federman, and S. M. Hammer, "Epstein-Barr virus-induced infectious mononucleosis complicated by acute renal failure: case report and review," *Clinical Infectious Diseases*, vol. 22, no. 6, pp. 1009–1018, 1996.

[8] V. F. Norwood and B. C. Sturgill, "Unexplained acute renal failure in a toddler: a rare complication of Epstein-Barr virus," *Pediatric Nephrology*, vol. 17, no. 8, pp. 628–632, 2002.

[9] C. V. Sumaya, "Epstein-Barr virus infections in children," *Current Problems in Pediatrics*, vol. 17, no. 12, pp. 677–745, 1987.

[10] R. J. Hoagland, "The clinical manifestations of infectious mononucleosis: a report of two hundred cases," *The American Journal of the Medical Sciences*, vol. 240, no. 7, pp. 55–63, 1960.

[11] J. E. Stevens, "Infectious mononucleosis: a clinical analysis of 210 sporadic cases," *Virginia Medical Monthly*, vol. 79, no. 2, pp. 74–80, 1952.

[12] H. F. Wechsler, A. H. Rosenblum, and C. T. Sills, "Infectious mononucleosis; report of an epidemic in an army post," *Annals of Internal Medicine*, vol. 25, no. 1, p. 113, 1946.

[13] S. Lee and C. M. Kjellstrand, "Renal disease in infectious mononucleosis," *Clinical Nephrology*, vol. 9, no. 6, pp. 236–240, 1978.

[14] J. H. Peters, J. Flume, and D. Fuccillo, "Nephritis in infectious mononucleosis," *Clinical Research*, vol. 10, p. 254, 1962.

[15] G. P. Ramelli, C. Marone, and B. Truniger, "Akutes Nierenversagen bei infecktioser Mononukleose," *Schweizerische Medizinische Wochenschrift*, vol. 120, pp. 1590–1594, 1990.

[16] J. Greising, H. Trachtman, B. Gauthier, and E. Valderrama, "Acute interstitial nephritis in adolescents and young adults," *Child Nephrology and Urology*, vol. 10, no. 4, pp. 189–195, 1990.

[17] D. Ellis, W. A. Fried, E. J. Yunis, and E. B. Blau, "Acute interstitial nephritis in children: a report of 13 cases and review of the literature," *Pediatrics*, vol. 67, no. 6, pp. 862–870, 1981.

54

Giant Ovarian Cyst Masquerading as Massive Ascites in an 11-Year-Old

Shaza Ali Mohammed Elhassan, Shabina Khan, and Ahmed El-Makki

Hamad Medical Corporation, P.O. BOX 3050, Doha, Qatar

Correspondence should be addressed to Shaza Ali Mohammed Elhassan; alishaza222@gmail.com

Academic Editor: Pauline M. Chou

We are presenting a unique case of an 11-year-old girl admitted for investigation of progressive abdominal distention of more than one-year duration. Due to the complete cystic nature of the mass and its enormous size, it was not visualized by the ultrasound and was reported as massive ascites. MRI and postoperative histopathology confirmed a diagnosis of giant serous cystadenoma of the right ovary. She underwent a right ovarian cystectomy with complete preservation of both ovaries and fallopian tubes and is doing well on outpatient follow-up.

1. Introduction

Although an ovarian cyst detected in an adolescent girl is most likely a physiological or functional cyst [1], it still deserves a thorough evaluation as up to 15% of all cystic ovarian lesions prove to be neoplastic [2, 3]. Neoplastic lesions of the ovary are classified based on the anatomic tissue from which they originate—germ cell tumors, epithelial cell tumors, and stromal cell tumors [4]. The epithelial cell tumors (serous or mucinous cystadenomas) are most commonly encountered in the fourth or fifth decade of life, but they should also be considered to be differential diagnoses in pediatric patients given that they are the second most common benign ovarian tumor in adolescents [4]. These tumors can reach giant proportions and very few cases of giant serous cystadenomas in adolescents have been reported. We present one such case of an 11-year-old girl who was admitted to our hospital for investigation of progressive abdominal distention of one-year duration. Due to the complete cystic nature of the mass and its enormous size, it was not visualized by the ultrasound and was reported as massive ascites. MRI and postoperative histopathology confirmed a diagnosis of serous cystadenoma of the right ovary.

2. Case Report

Our case is an 11-year-old Sudanese girl, residing in Qatar, who presented to the pediatric outpatient department with an 18-month history of progressive abdominal distention. The parents had been attributing the abdominal distention to weight gain, especially as the child remained otherwise asymptomatic. They had in fact been encouraging the girl to lose weight. The parents sought medical advice at a local health center, due to flu-like symptoms. The examination at the health center was impressive for signs of massive abdominal distention and she was admitted to our tertiary care hospital promptly for further investigations with a preliminary diagnosis of ascites. Apart from the progressive abdominal distention, there was no other contributory history suggestive of any underlying malignancy, liver disease, heart failure, or undiagnosed renal problems. The girl did not complain of any abdominal pain, constipation, urinary retention, or respiratory distress secondary to her abdominal distention. Our patient had achieved menarche 1 year ago with infrequent menstrual cycles; her first day of the last menstrual period was two weeks prior to her admission. There was no history of menorrhagia or dysmenorrhea.

Upon examination, the child was noted to be in good general condition with normal vital signs for age and in no apparent pain or distress. Her weight was 64.5 kg, which was above the 95th centile for her age. Apart from the massive abdominal distention, she was thin built. Her general examination did not reveal any clubbing, pallor, icterus, peripheral edema, or lymphadenopathy. There were no stigmata of chronic liver disease. Abdominal examination revealed a huge uniformly distended abdomen (maximum diameter was 105 cm), extending from the pelvis to the xiphisternum with full flanks. There were no visible dilated veins on the abdomen. Palpation did not reveal any tenderness or masses; fluid thrill was positive. She had normal female genitalia. Her respiratory, cardiovascular, and nervous system examinations were unremarkable. A bedside urine dipstick did not reveal any proteinuria.

As the physical findings detected a fluid thrill, her preliminary investigations were directed towards finding a likely explanation for what seemed like a massive ascites. Her preliminary laboratory work-up which included a complete blood count, peripheral smear, serum electrolytes, renal and liver functions tests were within normal. As our patient did not show any signs of chronic liver or renal disease, there was a strong concern among the treating physicians that the presumed ascites could be secondary to an underlying abdominal malignancy. At this stage, the pediatric oncology team was consulted and tumor markers which included Ca125 (6 U/mL), CEA 0.7 microgram/L, alpha-fetoprotein (<1.7 IU/mL) and beta-hCG (<5 IU/L) along with Uric acid 297 micromol/L, and LDH (174 U/L) were ordered, all of which were within normal limits.

An urgent transabdominal ultrasonogram of the abdomen confirmed the suspicion of massive ascites (Figure 1). The possibility of requiring a diagnostic paracentesis was discussed with the family once the MRI of the abdomen and pelvis reasonably ruled out any underlying malignancy.

The MRI of the abdomen and the pelvis (Figure 2) revealed that what was visualized as massive ascites by the sonographer was in fact a large homogenous well defined unilocular huge cystic abdominopelvic mass which measured $39 \times 29 \times 18$ cm in dimension, occupying the entire abdomen and pelvis and bulging into the anterior abdominal wall. No solid component could be noted within the mass lesion. No loculation or septation was seen given the likelihood of serous cyst adenoma of the right ovary.

A lower abdominal midline incision was made revealing the peritoneum. An elliptical incision is carefully made through the ovarian cortex to the cyst wall.

When the cyst wall was reached, blunt and sharp dissection using surgical scissors was used to separate the cyst wall from the surface of the ovary. Intraoperative visualization did not reveal any abnormality of the left adnexal structures. The cyst was aspirated prior to its delivery and gave 13000 milliliters of fluid. The patient underwent right ovarian cystectomy with complete preservation of both ovaries and fallopian tubes. It weighed 13 kg and contained 13 liters of fluid. (Figure 3) Histopathological examination of the cyst revealed simple tubal-type epithelium confirming

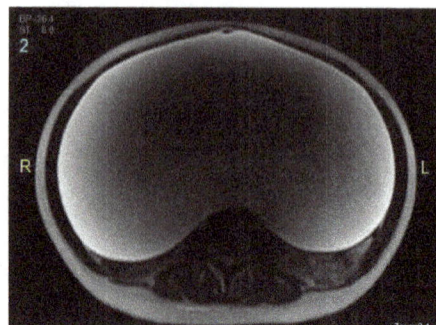

FIGURE 1: Abdominal ultrasound.

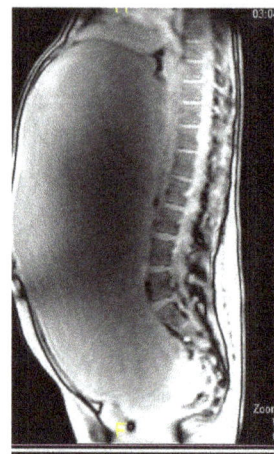

FIGURE 2: MRI abdomen.

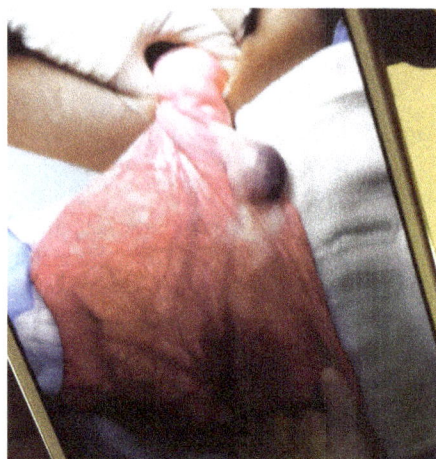

FIGURE 3: Intraoperative cystectomy.

the diagnosis of a serous cystadenoma of the right ovary, consistent with the preoperative MRI diagnosis.

Our patient did well after surgery and was discharged on the fourth postoperative day. Her discharge weight was 48 kg. Upon follow-up a week after her surgery she showed an excellent recovery and will continue to have regular follow-up in our outpatient clinic with an ultrasound examination every three months for early detection of any recurrence.

3. Discussion

An ovarian mass in pediatrics may represent the commoner physiological functional ovarian cyst or be a benign or rarely malignant tumor [1]. The most common ovarian tumors encountered in pediatric practice are germ cell tumors, which account for about two-thirds of ovarian tumors in this age group [5]. Surface epithelial tumors including serous cyst adenomas are rare in pediatrics [4] with a reported international incidence of around 15–20% of all pediatric ovarian masses [6]. Compared to their adult counterparts, fortunately, 90% of ovarian masses seen in the pediatric and adolescent population are benign [7]. Differential diagnoses of ovarian masses in adolescence include cyst formation, ovarian torsion, benign or malignant ovarian neoplasm, and involvement of the ovary in lymphoma, leukemia, or metastatic disease [8].

As general pediatricians, we need to acknowledge that ovarian masses in general in our patient population are by no means uncommon [9] and can have a varied presentation. They may present as vague abdominal pain, acute abdomen, and an asymptomatic pelviabdominal mass, with features of hormonal derangement, or be discovered incidentally on a routine imaging [2]. On the other hand, ovarian tumors that reach giant proportions of greater than 15 cm are quite rare in this population [2]. Our patient was diagnosed with a giant serous cyst adenoma, and to date very few such cases have been reported in literature in adolescents ranging from the age of 13 to 19 years [10–16]. Our patient, who achieved menarche at age 10, was 11 years at the time of diagnosis and perhaps represents one of the youngest cases of giant serous cyst adenoma reported. Postpubertal estrogen and progesterone hormone levels are postulated to play a role in the pathogenesis of surface epithelial tumors, which might explain why the reported cases are mostly 13 years or older [5].

Giant ovarian tumors can be present as asymptomatically increasing abdominal girth [2] or be accompanied by symptoms of nausea, vomiting, weight loss or increased urinary frequency, urinary retention, constipation, and dyspnea due to pressure effects [17]. Despite being asymptomatic, giant ovarian tumors have potential for serious complications such as torsion, suppuration, obstruction, and perforation necessitating urgent admission [18]. Ultrasonography is considered the initial imaging modality for ovarian masses [4].

Our patient is unique not only in terms of her age, but also as she posed a diagnostic challenge in many aspects. Firstly, she presented with a huge asymptomatic abdominal distention, which upon initial clinical assessment was presumed to be massive ascites. Moreover, ultrasound of the pelvis and abdomen, in our case, confirmed this clinical diagnosis of massive ascites without delineating a possible cause, necessitating an urgent MRI, which led to the final diagnosis of a giant ovarian mass. If management was undertaken in our patient on the basis of ultrasound diagnosis alone (namely, paracentesis for the presumed ascites), it may have led to erroneous transabdominal aspiration of the undiagnosed ovarian cyst. If paracentesis was undertaken in this patient it could lead to infection, bleeding, and increased peritoneal adhesion, thus making surgical cystectomy more challenging [19]. Ultrasound alone, being operator dependent, should perhaps be interpreted in caution in such patients in whom there is no clear diagnosis based on history and examination. Moreover, our case highlights the fact the pediatrician needs to entertain the diagnosis of a giant ovarian tumor early on in pediatric patients who present with a huge abdominal mass with a noncontributory history or exam, regardless of the rarity of the condition.

Giant ovarian tumors have become rare in current medical practice, as most cases are discovered early during routine check-ups. In our case, the patient's family did not seek medical advice for 1.5 years, as they assumed that the increased abdominal girth was due to weight gain and put her on an intense diet and exercise regime. The patient's weight at admission was 67 Kg and at one week postsurgery was 55 Kg. Teaching families and raising awareness are extremely important aspects in such cases.

As pediatricians are often the first physicians who encounter such cases, they should be aware of asymptomatic ovarian tumors as a differential diagnosis for massive abdominal distension, given that they are the largest tumors found in the human body [20].

If the pure cystic mass reaches an enormous size and the tumor markers are within normal limits, as in our patient, serous or mucinous cyst adenomas should be considered in the differential diagnosis in adolescent patient [2]. Management of these cases is usually by conservative surgery including cystectomy or unilateral salpingoooophorectomy, which are adequate for benign lesions. After conservative surgery, the patients must be followed up carefully because some tumors recur, especially if not completely removed during surgery.

According to literature review by Patel et al. [2], 7 cases of giant cell serous cyst adenoma from case reports in adolescent ranging from 13 to 19 years, the maximum weight of 29 kg, most presented with increased abdominal girth but otherwise were asymptomatic between 6 months and 2 years. One case presented as acute abdomen and another with palpable abdominal mass with pressure symptoms, that is, nausea, vomiting, constipation, dyspnea, and abdominal distention. The mode of the treatment for these patients varied, three of them underwent cystectomy with complete preservation of the affected ovary and adnexal structures, the other three underwent cystectomy with removal of ovary, and the remaining one patient underwent open cystectomy with salpingectomy [10–16]. Our patient had fertility preserving surgery, that is, cystectomy with complete preservation of the ovaries, as it is the preferred modality of treatment in this age group. Management of this pathology and fertility-conserving treatment need careful follow-up because of the possibility of recurrence and malignant transformation.

4. Conclusion

As rare as giant ovarian tumors are, pediatricians should be aware of its presentation and should include ovarian masses in their differential diagnosis of abdominal distention. Pediatricians should raise families' awareness for seeking medical advice early in case of persistent abdominal distention. Ultrasound should not be the only imaging modality especially in case of massive ovarian cysts as it may mimic ascites. This case report emphasizes the paramount importance of considering ovarian masses in the differential diagnosis of a patient who has abdominal distention without symptoms or signs of liver, renal, or cardiac diseases. It is also vital to raise awareness among the population to seek medical advice as early as possible to avoid complications such as ovarian torsion, rupture, and eventually infertility in such young age group. Fertility-conserving treatments, as in our patient, need careful follow-up because of the possibility of recurrence in the remaining ovary or malignancy transformation.

Conflict of Interests

The authors declare that there is no conflict of interests regarding the publication of this paper.

References

[1] K. S. H. de Silva, S. Kanumakala, S. R. Grover, C. W. Chow, and G. L. Warne, "Ovarian lesions in children and adolescents—an 11-year review," *The Journal of Pediatric Endocrinology & Metabolism*, vol. 17, no. 7, pp. 951–957, 2004.

[2] N. Patel, G. Dupuis, and R. Wild, "Giant ovarian cyst in an adolescent with PCOS," *Canadian Family Physician*, vol. 12, no. 12, pp. 559–562, 2013.

[3] E. Hassan, G. Creatsas, E. Deligeorolgou, and S. Michalas, "Ovarian tumors during childhood and adolescence: a clinicopathological study," *European Journal of Gynaecological Oncology*, vol. 20, no. 2, pp. 124–126, 1999.

[4] I. Ciftci, T. Sekmenli, and S. Ugras, "Ovarian huge serous cystadenoma in adolescent girl: a case report," *National Journal of Medical Research*, vol. 3, no. 2, pp. 187–189, 2013.

[5] N. K. Bhattacharyya, A. De, P. Bera, S. Mongal, S. Chakraborty, and R. Bandopadhyay, "Ovarian tumors in pediatric age group—a clinicopathologic study of 10 years cases in West Bengal, India," *Indian Journal of Medical and Paediatric Oncology*, vol. 31, no. 2, pp. 54–57, 2010.

[6] D. Grapsa, E. Kairi-Vassilatou, D. Hasiakos, and A. Kondi-Pafiti, "Ovarian mucinous cystadenoma with extended calcification in an 11-year-old girl: case report and review of the literature," *Clinical and Experimental Obstetrics and Gynecology*, vol. 33, no. 3, pp. 181–182, 2006.

[7] R. E. Behrman, " Overview of pediatrics," in *Nelson Textbook of Pediatrics*, R. E. Behrman, R. M. Kliegman, and H. B. Jenson, Eds., p. 15, Saunders, Philadelphia, Pa, USA, 17th edition, 2005.

[8] E. H. Quint and Y. R. Smith, "Ovarian surgery in premenarchal girls," *Journal of Pediatric and Adolescent Gynecology*, vol. 12, no. 1, pp. 27–29, 1999.

[9] Oumachigui, K. L. Narasimhan, K. S. Reddy et al., "A clinicopathologic study of ovarian tumors in children," *Journal of Obstetrics & Gynaecology*, vol. 140, pp. 441–445, 1991.

[10] C. T. Westfall and R. J. Andrassy, "Giant ovarian cyst: case report and review of differential diagnosis in adolescents," *Clinical Pediatrics*, vol. 21, no. 4, pp. 228–230, 1982.

[11] A. Fimmanò, E. Coppola Bottazzi, and C. Cirillo, "Giant bilateral ovarian cysts in an adolescent masked by obesity and mimicking ascites: a case report," *Chirurgia Italiana*, vol. 56, no. 5, pp. 711–715, 2004.

[12] M. E. Coccia, F. Rizzello, G. L. Bracco, and G. Scarselli, "Seven-liter ovarian cyst in an adolescent treated by minimal access surgery: laparoscopy and open cystectomy," *Journal of Pediatric Surgery*, vol. 44, no. 6, pp. E5–E8, 2009.

[13] W. E. Khalbuss and B. Dipasquale, "Massive ovarian edema associated with ovarian serous cystadenoma: a case report and review of the literature," *International Journal of Gynecological Cancer*, vol. 16, supplement 1, pp. 326–330, 2006.

[14] R. Vecchio, V. Leanza, F. Genovese et al., "Conservative laparoscopic treatment of a benign giant ovarian cyst in a young woman," *Journal of Laparoendoscopic & Advanced Surgical Techniques A*, vol. 19, no. 5, pp. 647–648, 2009.

[15] N. D. Tofteland, M. Stuart-Hilgenfeld, R. Hunt et al., "Index of suspicion, case 1: hemoptysis, dyspnea, and hematuria, case 2: rash and headache in a wrestler, case 3: abdominal distention in a teenage girl," *Pediatrics in Review*, vol. 31, no. 11, pp. 477–482, 2010.

[16] V. A. Postma, J. A. Wegdam, and I. M. Janssen, "Laparoscopic extirpation of a giant ovarian cyst," *Surgical Endoscopy*, vol. 16, no. 2, p. 361, 2002.

[17] K. A. P. Schultz, S. F. Sencer, Y. Messinger, J. P. Neglia, and M. E. Steiner, "Pediatric ovarian tumors: a review of 67 cases," *Pediatric Blood and Cancer*, vol. 44, no. 2, pp. 167–173, 2005.

[18] D. Alver, C. Gül, A. C. Celayir, and D. Sahin, "A case of ovarian torsion with a serous cyst and coexisting serous cystadenoma in the contralateral ovary," *Journal of Pediatric Surgical Specialties*, vol. 3, pp. 50–52, 2009.

[19] Y. T. Kim, J. W. Kim, and B. H. Choe, "A case of huge ovarian cyst of 21-year-old young woman," *Journal of Obstetrics and Gynaecology Research*, vol. 25, no. 4, pp. 275–279, 1999.

[20] B. Lefebvre, P. Philippart, B. Brandetet, P. M. Da Costa, and X. Vandemergel, "Giant ovarian cystadenoma in adolescent: case report and review of the literature," *Revue Medicale de Bruxelles*, vol. 21, no. 3, pp. 157–159, 2000.

55

A Case of Hemolytic Disease of the Newborn due to Di^a Antibody

Ashif Jethava, Esperanza Olivares, and Sherry Shariatmadar

Department of Pathology, University of Miami, Jackson Health System, Miami, FL, USA

Correspondence should be addressed to Sherry Shariatmadar; sshariat@med.miami.edu

Academic Editor: Mohammad M. A. Faridi

Anti-Di^a is a clinically significant red cell antibody known to cause hemolytic disease of the newborn. Here, we report on a case of mild hemolytic disease of the newborn caused by Di^a antibody. The mother had three prior pregnancies with no history of blood transfusion. She delivered a preterm 35-week-old female newborn by cesarean section. The neonate developed anemia and mild icterus on postnatal day five with hemoglobin of 9500 mg/dL and total bilirubin of 10 mg/dL. The direct antiglobulin test on the neonate's red blood cells was positive. The maternal serum and an eluate from the infant RBCs were negative in routine antibody detection tests but were positive using commercially prepared Di(a+) red cells. The neonate was discharged home in stable condition following treatment with erythropoietin and phototherapy. When a newborn has a positive DAT in the absence of major blood group incompatibility or commonly detected RBC antibodies, an antibody to a low frequency antigen such as Di^a must be considered. Further immunohematology tests are required to determine presence of the antibody and the clinician must be alerted to closely monitor the infant for signs of anemia and hemolysis.

1. Introduction

The first antigen assigned to the Diego blood group system, Di^a, was described by Layrisse et al. in 1955 [1]. They reported an antibody to a low frequency antigen in the serum of a Venezuelan woman (Mrs. Diego) which caused fatal hemolytic disease of the newborn (HDN). The existence of the antibody had been noted briefly in another report one year earlier [2]. The prevalence of the Di^a antigen is known to be different among races, which has made the Diego blood group attractive to anthropologists [3]. It is very rare among Caucasians and Blacks (0.01%) but relatively common among the South American Indians (36%) and Asians of Mongoloid origin (5–15%) which includes the Japanese, Chinese, and Koreans [4–8]. Anti-Di^a has been reported to cause moderate to severe HDN [9–14] and rarely a hemolytic transfusion reaction [15]. Here we report a case of HDN caused by Di^a antibody. The newborn developed anemia and moderate hyperbilirubinemia which required erythropoietin injection and phototherapy.

2. Case Presentation

A 30-year-old South American woman, G4P3L3, with a history of preterm labor, placenta previa, and cesarean section × 3 and no prior history of transfusions gave birth to a preterm 35-week-old female newborn by cesarean section. Records of her antenatal care were not available to us as she presented to our hospital for the first time following arrival from Peru. The newborn infant had a birth weight of 2,900 grams with an Apgar score of 8. Soon after birth, the neonate was noted to have an episode of respiratory distress and drop in oxygen saturation to 82% requiring frequent suctioning and continuous oxygen support. She was admitted to the neonatal intensive care unit for further evaluation and monitoring. Initial chest X-ray demonstrated bilateral perihilar and lower lobe interstitial infiltrates for which she was started on broad spectrum intravenous ampicillin and gentamycin antibiotics. Blood culture, urinalysis, and urine for microscopic examination were ordered and reported as negative. On the fifth day, the neonate was noted to be pale and icteric with clinical signs of anemia. Laboratory findings were as follows: RBC 2.71×10^6 cells/mcl; white blood cell count 11.7×10^9/L; hemoglobin 9.5 mg/dL; hematocrit 26.5%; reticulocyte count 6.5%; platelet count 435×10^9/L; and liver function test showed a total bilirubin of 10 mg/dL with predominance of unconjugated hyperbilirubinemia. Extensive investigation was performed to determine the cause of anemia and hemolysis which included tests for cord blood glucose-6-phosphate dehydrogenase (G6PD) and parvovirus B19, both of which were negative.

Immunohematology workup revealed that both the mother and the infant were blood group O, RhD positive. Direct antiglobulin test (DAT) was ordered on the neonate's and mother's red blood cells. It was weakly positive (1+) with monospecific anti-human globulin (AHG) IgG on the neonate's RBCs and negative on the mother's RBCs. The maternal serum and an eluate prepared from neonate's red blood cells showed negative reactions in routine antibody detection tests, but after testing with cells of rare phenotypes, they demonstrated an alloantibody reacting with the Di(a+) red cells by indirect antiglobulin test (IAT) in the AHG phase.

The neonate was successfully treated with subcutaneous erythropoietin injection three times for a week, followed by intensive phototherapy. The bilirubin level dropped to 6.7 mg/dL within few days of treatment. The infant was discharged home in good clinical condition with the following laboratory findings: RBC 3.18×10^6 cell/μL; hemoglobin 11.2 mg/dL; hematocrit 32.3%; and a reticulocyte count of 2.5%.

3. Methods

Postnatal screening for unexpected RBC antibodies was performed using tube methodology including Low Ionic Strength Solution (LISS) (Clinical Diagnostics, Raritan, NJ) and polyethylene glycol (PeG) techniques (Immucor Inc., Norcross, GA, USA) with commercially prepared screening cells (Medion Grifols Diagnostics AG, Switzerland) at 37°C and indirect antiglobulin test (IAT) according to the manufacturer's instructions. The DAT was performed using the tube methodology with poly- and monospecific IgG anti-human globulin (Bio-Rad Medical Diagnostics, Dreieich, Germany). An antibody elution was performed on the neonate's DAT positive RBCs obtained by acid elution with use of commercial reagents (Gamma ELU-KIT, Immucor, Rodemark, Germany).

The neonate's eluate was tested against two screen cells (Medion Grifols Diagnostics AG, Switzerland) and a panel of six reagent RBCs (three Di(a+) RBCs were included). Maternal serum was tested against three selected cells positive for Di^a antigen at room temperature, 37°C, and IAT phase (Panocell-20, Immucor, Norcross GA, USA).

Determination of RBC antibody specificities in the mother's serum and of the neonate's RBC eluate using commercial RBC panels produced 2+ reactions solely with three Di(a+) test RBCs.

4. Discussion

The Diego blood group system currently consists of 22 antigens, including three pairs of antithetical antigens: Di^a/Di^b, Wr^a/Wr^b, and WU/DISK. The antigens are located on the red blood cell membrane transporter also known as Band 3, encoded by a SLC4A1 gene on chromosome 17q12-q21 [16]. Band 3 acts as an anion exchanger between chloride and bicarbonate ions which helps transport carbon dioxide from the tissues to the lung. It also helps to maintain the structural integrity of the red blood cell membrane by stabilizing membrane lipids [16–18]. The Di^a antigen is fully developed on the red cells of the newborn infants as it is on the red cells of adults. Di^a antibodies are polyclonal IgGs of subclasses IgG1 and IgG3. These antibodies occasionally bind complement and lyses untreated red blood cells [16–18].

Based on genetic studies, there is great variation in the distribution of the Di^a antigen in different races. It is relatively common among the South American Indians and Asian of Mongolian origin and rare in Caucasian and Blacks [5–8]. Because of the different prevalence of the Di^a antigen, it has been of great interest to the field of anthropology and transfusion medicine. Anti-Di^a is known to be dangerous to the fetus and newborn and has been associated with moderate to severe HDN, at least one of which was fatal [9–14].

Monestier et al. described a woman who gave birth to an infant with hyperbilirubinemia and a strongly positive DAT. During the pregnancy and after delivery, the mother had negative RBC antibody screening tests using standard red blood cell panels, but the indirect antiglobulin test between the mother's serum and the father's red blood cells was strongly positive. The antibody was eluted from the newborn infant's red blood cells and was identified as anti-Di^a [14]. Hundric-Haspl reported anemia in a 3-week-old infant who had been discharged home in good condition shortly after birth. The infants DAT was positive shortly after birth while testing of the mother's serum and the eluate of infants RBCs using routine immunohematology tests were negative. Repeat testing following readmission showed similar results on routine tests; however, on testing with extensive panel of red blood cells, anti-Di^a was identified in the mother's serum and the eluate of the infants RBCs [19]. In our case, postpartum antibody screening test of the mother's plasma against common red cell antigens was negative. The newborn initially had no clinical signs of HDN in spite of a positive DAT. Anemia and moderate hyperbilirubinemia were noted five days after birth and successfully treated with phototherapy and erythropoietin injection. The maternal plasma and infant's eluate from red blood cells were negative in routine antibody detection tests but were positive when tested against Di(a+) RBCs.

Development of Di^a antibodies mostly occurs following alloimmunization of a woman who is negative for the Di^a antigen while carrying a fetus who has inherited the antigen from the father [9–14, 19]. The usual immunizing event is delivery and fetomaternal hemorrhage is more commonly encountered with C-section delivery [20]. Immunization can also occur following trauma, amniocentesis, cordocentesis, abortion, or other procedures. In majority of the cases, the presence of Di^a antibodies in the plasma of an immunized pregnant woman cannot be determined by routine screening test, as most antibody screening cells lack the Di^a antigen. Therefore, there may be no serologic evidence that HDN is present and even with standard prenatal care, the diagnosis may not be apparent until after delivery, when the newborn is found to have a positive DAT and clinical signs of HDN. Because of the low frequency of the antigen in our population, finding compatible blood is not difficult if the neonate needs a blood transfusion.

5. Conclusion

Whenever a newborn has a positive DAT result in the absence of major blood group incompatibility or reactivity with common red cell antigens, it is important to consider that the positive DAT may be due to alloimmunization to a low frequency RBC antigen such as Di^a that cannot be detected in routine antibody detection tests. Further testing with rare RBC antigens should be performed to determine the presence of the antibody and the infant should be closely monitored and treated for clinical signs of anemia and hemolysis.

Conflict of Interests

The authors certify that they do not have any affiliation with or financial involvement in any organization or entity with a direct financial interest in the subject matter or materials discussed in the paper (e.g., employment, consultancies, stock ownership, honoraria, and expert testimony). They do not have any commercial or proprietary interest in any drug, device, or equipment mentioned in the paper. They declare that they do not have any conflict of interests. No financial support was used for this work. No previously published figures or tables were used in this paper.

Authors' Contribution

They certify sufficient participation of each author in the conception, design, analysis, interpretation, writing, revising, and approval of the paper.

References

[1] M. Layrisse, T. Arends, and S. R. Dominguez, "Nuevo grupo sanguineo encontrado en descendientes de Indios," *Acta Médica Venezolana*, vol. 3, pp. 132–138, 1955.

[2] P. Levine, E. A. Koch, R. T. McGee, and G. H. Hill, "Rare human isoagglutinins and their identification," *American Journal of Clinical Pathology*, vol. 24, no. 3, pp. 292–304, 1954.

[3] M. Layrisse, "Anthropological considerations of the Diego (Di^a) antigen. Possible application in the studies of Mongoloid and hybrid populations," *American Journal of Physical Anthropology*, vol. 16, no. 2, pp. 173–186, 1958.

[4] R. T. Simmons, J. A. Albrey, J. A. G. Morgan, and e tal, "The Diego blood group: anti—Di^a and Di (a+) blood group antigen found in Caucasians," *Medical Journal of Australia*, vol. 1, no. 10, pp. 406–407, 1968.

[5] M. Layrisse and T. Arends, "The Diego blood factor in Negroid populations," *Nature*, vol. 179, no. 4557, pp. 478–479, 1957.

[6] P. C. Junqueira, P. J. Wishart, F. Ottensooser, R. Pasqualin, P. L. Fernandez, and H. Kalmus, "The Diego blood factor in Brazilian Indians," *Nature*, vol. 177, article 41, 1956.

[7] P. C. Junqueira, P. J. Wishart, F. Ottensooser, R. Pasqualin, P. L. Fernandez, and H. Kalmus, "The *Diego* blood factor in Brazilian Indians," *Nature*, vol. 177, no. 4497, pp. 40–41, 1956.

[8] M. Layrisse and T. Arends, "The *Diego* blood factor in Chinese and Japanese," *Nature*, vol. 177, no. 4519, pp. 1083–1084, 1956.

[9] P. Levine, E. A. Robinson, M. Layrisse, T. Arends, and R. D. Sisco, "The Diego blood factor," *Nature*, vol. 177, no. 4497, pp. 40–41, 1956.

[10] L. M. Alves De Lima, M. E. Berthier, and W. E. Sad, "Characterization of an anti-Dia antibody causing hemolytic disease in a newborn infant," *Transfusion*, vol. 22, no. 3, pp. 246–247, 1982.

[11] G. Kusnierz-Alejska and S. Bochenek, "Hemolytic disease of the newborn due to anti-Di^a and the incidence of Di^a antigen in Poland," *Vox Sanguinis*, vol. 62, pp. 124–126, 1992.

[12] M. A. Chung, E. H. Park, C. H. Lee et al., "A case of hemolytic disease of the newborn due to anti Di^a antibody," *Journal of the Korean Society of Neonatology*, vol. 8, pp. 141–144, 2002.

[13] J. Y. Ting, E. S. Ma, and K. Y. Wong, "A case of severe haemolytic disease of the newborn due to anti-Di(a) antibody," *Hong Kong Medical Journal*, vol. 10, pp. 347–349, 2004.

[14] M. Monestier, D. Rigal, F. Meyer et al., "HDN caused by anti Di^a antibodies," *Archives Françaises de Pédiatrie*, vol. 41, pp. 641–643, 1984.

[15] M. E. Hinckley and D. W. Huestis, "An immediate hemolytic transfusion reaction apparently caused by anti-Di^a," *Revue Française de Transfusion et Immuno-Hématologie*, vol. 22, no. 5, pp. 581–585, 1979.

[16] D. Figueroa, "The Diego blood group system: a review," *Immunohematology*, vol. 29, no. 2, pp. 73–81, 2013.

[17] P. D. Issitt and D. J. Anstee, *Applied Blood Group Serology*, Montgomery Scientific Publications, 4th edition, 1998.

[18] M. K. Fung, C. D. Hillyer, B. J. Grossman, and C. M. Westhoff, *Technical Manual*, AABB, 18th edition, 2014.

[19] Z. Hundric-Haspl, S. Balen-Marunic, E. Tomasic-Susanj, M. Tomicic, and K. Vujaklija-Stipanovic, "Anti-Diego^a red blood cell alloantibody as a possible cause of anemia in a 3-week-old infant," *Archives of Medical Research*, vol. 34, no. 2, pp. 149–151, 2003.

[20] E. S. Sebring and H. F. Polesky, "Fetomaternal hemorrhage: incidence, risk factors, time of occurrence, and clinical effects," *Transfusion*, vol. 30, no. 4, pp. 344–357, 1990.

56

Clinical Phenotype of DiGeorge Syndrome with Negative Genetic Tests: A Case of DiGeorge-Like Syndrome?

Gianluigi Laccetta,[1] **Benedetta Toschi,**[2] **Antonella Fogli,**[3] **Veronica Bertini,**[3] **Angelo Valetto,**[3] **and Rita Consolini**[1]

[1]*Pediatric Department, Faculty of Medicine, Rheumatology and Clinical Immunology Unit, Pisa University, 56126 Pisa, Italy*
[2]*Medical Genetics Unit, Children Department, Pisa University, 56126 Pisa, Italy*
[3]*Cytogenetics and Molecular Genetics Unit, Children Department, Pisa University, 56126 Pisa, Italy*

Correspondence should be addressed to Gianluigi Laccetta; gianluigilaccetta@libero.it

Academic Editor: Jonathan Muraskas

We report a case of DiGeorge-like syndrome in which immunodeficiency coexisting with juvenile idiopathic arthritis, congenital heart disease, delay in emergence of language and in motor milestones, feeding and growing problems, enamel hypoplasia, mild skeletal anomalies, and facial dysmorphisms are associated with no abnormalities found on genetic tests.

1. Introduction

DiGeorge syndrome (DGS) is usually caused by 22q11.2 deletion; the most common deletion includes loss of *TBX1* gene which is an important transcription factor for the development of the heart, thymus, parathyroid glands, palate, and teeth: thus, haploinsufficiency of *TBX1* is thought to be the greatest cause of the disorder [1, 2]. Rarely, most of DGS phenotypes are well explained by *TBX1* gene mutations [3].

We describe a patient with clinical findings of DGS and negative molecular genetic tests.

2. Case Report

The patient was a 5-year-old male who suffered from pain on his right knee since one year prior to presentation. His right knee was swollen and flexed, his right lower limb was hypotrophic, and his left leg was 1 centimeter shorter in length than his right one. The child had valgus heels and turned his feet inward during the walk; he also had difficulties in walking and climbing stairs. ANA (anti-nuclear antibodies), ACA (anti-centromere antibodies), RF (rheumatoid factor), and ASO (antistreptolysin O) titers were negative and CRP (C-reactive protein) was 1.86 mg/dL (normal value: less than

0.50 mg/dL). X-rays of the knee were normal; ultrasonography and magnetic resonance imaging exhibited a distended anterior joint recess filled with fluid. Juvenile idiopathic arthritis was diagnosed (Juvenile Arthritis Damage Index, JADI = 3) and the patient required oral ibuprofen treatment (30 mg/kg per day divided into 2 doses), intra-articular steroids (20 mg of triamcinolone hexacetonide in 0.5 mL of lidocaine 1%), and serial arthrocentesis. There were neither ocular manifestations of iridocyclitis nor uveitis; the child only had hyperopia requiring prescription lenses.

The prenatal course of the child was characterized by the diagnosis of mild hypoplastic left heart, hypoplastic aortic arch, and persistent left superior vena cava draining into the coronary sinus. When the child was 13 days old he successfully underwent nonemergency repair of his hypoplastic aortic arch using autologous pericardium and surgical obliteration of patent ductus arteriosus with extracorporeal circulation. The patient was also diagnosed with bicuspid aortic valve, dysplastic mitral valve, left-ventricular false tendon, and tricuspid insufficiency; he also had a perimembranous ventricular septal defect which spontaneously closed. The child was diagnosed with progressive aortic recoarctation of periductal type when he was 5 months old and underwent cardiac catheterization and balloon angioplasty using properly sized balloons (CB-Balt 4×20 mm, 6×25 mm, and 8×20 mm); balloon angioplasty reduced peak-to-peak gradient from 47 to 0 mmHg. The patient was treated with captopril (0.3 mg/kg, 3 times a day) up to when he was 5 years old and his parents were told to give the child antibiotic prophylaxis for bacterial endocarditis in case of need. On physical examination performed at our institution, a 2/6 holosystolic murmur was heard over heart; cardiac frequency (108 bpm), blood pressure (100/65 mmHg), oxygen saturation (SaO_2 98%), and respiratory rate (21 times/min) were normal. Electrocardiogram showed sinus rhythm, incomplete right bundle branch block, and abnormal ventricular repolarization.

The early course of the child was also characterized by feeding and growing difficulties as he was below the third percentile in weight during his first three years of life; thus, the child was diagnosed with ankyloglossia and underwent surgical treatment twice when he was 3 years old. Rhinoscopy and oropharyngoscopy performed at our institution were normal and physical examination showed that the patient was between the third and the fifteenth percentile both in height (103 cm) and in weight (15.8 kg) according to 2007 WHO growth charts; thus, feeding and growing difficulties were probably caused by ankyloglossia.

The patient also had delay in emergence of language: he was able to speak at 3 years 2 months and needed speech therapy. The child reported neither sensorineural nor conductive hearing loss as otoscopy, tympanogram, and audiometric evaluation were normal. The patient also had delay in motor milestones as he could sit at 12 months and was able to walk at 2 years; when first evaluated by neuropsychiatrists, the child was aged 4 and exhibited shyness, difficulty with social interactions, and deficits in fine motor coordination. Neuropsychiatrists noted difficulties in the area of verbal communication, reading decoding, grammatical skills, and spelling; cognitive assessments were performed using the Wechsler Preschool and Primary Scale of Intelligence-Third Edition (WPPSI-III): full scale IQ was moderately below average (score: 78), performance IQ was just below average (score: 88), and verbal IQ was significantly below average (score: 69). Results of cognitive tests made us suspect that delays in emergence of language and in motor milestones were associated; delay in emergence of language was partially due to ankyloglossia.

With regard to the immune function, serial lymphocyte counts showed that the patient had impaired T-cell production not improving over time; the restricted repertoire of T cells caused dysregulation in B cell compartment; in fact total B cells were reduced. Immunologic evaluation at our institution at 5 years of age revealed a low number of white blood cells; percentage of lymphocytes and that of absolute lymphocyte count were below the normal range. Percentage and number of CD3+, CD4+, and CD8+ cells were decreased for age but CD4+ to CD8+ ratio was normal; CD19+ cells were also reduced. Immunologic screening showed a high level of CD16+/56+ cells, just like patients with DGS [4]. Laboratory findings also demonstrate an accelerated conversion of naïve T cells to memory T cells, as typical of patients with DGS [5]. The patient had a low percentage of

TABLE 1: Immunologic profile of the patient.

Panel	Result	Normal range
CD3+ cells (cells/μL)	950	1092–1216
CD3+ cells (%)	53.9	62.0–69.0
CD4+ cells (cells/μL)	467	529–705
CD4+ cells (%)	26.5	30.0–40.0
CD8+ cells (cells/μL)	351	440–564
CD8+ cells (%)	19.9	25.0–32.0
CD16+/56+ cells (cells/μL)	490	141–264
CD16+/56+ cells (%)	27.8	8.0–15.0
CD19+ cells (cells/μL)	315	370–493
CD19+ cells (%)	17.9	21.0–28.0
CD4+ to CD8+ ratio	1.33	1.30–1.50
Naïve (CD45RA+CD62L+) T CD4+ cells (%)	19.4	24.3–81.0
Naïve (CD45RA+CD62L+) T CD8+ cells (%)	18.3	19.9–66.4
Memory (CD45RA−CD62L+) T CD4+ cells (%)	37.4	3.5–36.2
Memory (CD45RA−CD62L+) T CD8+ cells (%)	59.3	1.9–34.2
IgA (mg/dL)	35	109 ± 35
IgM (mg/dL)	48	85 ± 26
IgG (mg/dL)	586	975 ± 248

γ-globulin in serum protein electrophoresis but total serum proteins were in the normal range; IgA, IgM, and IgG levels were decreased for age. Results of immunologic laboratory tests were the ones in Table 1.

The child suffered from recurrent sinusitis, otitis media, and lower respiratory infections in his early years of life because of impaired lymphocytes production, hypogammaglobulinemia, and feeding difficulty.

The child had enamel hypoplasia and caries experience on his course but calcium-phosphorus metabolism was normal.

The child also had clinodactyly of the bilateral little fingers and protuberant ears; no abnormalities were detected by abdominal ultrasonography performed at our institution. Laboratory tests showed normal hepatic and renal functions.

With regard to congenital heart disease, immunodeficiency coexisting with juvenile idiopathic arthritis, delay in emergence of language and in motor milestones, mild skeletal anomalies (bilateral clinodactyly of the fifth fingers), facial dysmorphism (protuberant ears), and enamel hypoplasia, DGS was considered. Ankyloglossia has not been reported in DGS but it should be considered a kind of oral median dysplasia, just like cleft palate; bicuspid aortic valve has been described in a small percentage of patients with DGS [1]. Therefore, FISH (Fluorescent In Situ Hybridization) analysis with Vysis N25 (22q11.2)/ARSA probe was performed but no microdeletions were identified; automatic sequencing of the TBX1 gene coding sequence made by PCR and 3130xl Genetic Analyzer identified no mutations and computer molecular dynamics simulations showed neither reduced nor modified function of the corresponding T-box transcription factor *Tbx1*. Finally, Array-comparative genomic hybridization (Array-CGH) analysis, performed by standard procedures using both 8X60K and 4X180K oligo platforms (Agilent Technologies, Santa Clara, CA, USA), showed neither microdeletions nor microduplications.

3. Discussion

This infant's presentation is consistent with DGS but genetic tests do not confirm this diagnosis; thus, our patient should be considered a case of DiGeorge-like syndrome. Five disorders (Smith-Lemli-Opitz syndrome, Alagille syndrome, VATER association, Goldenhar syndrome, and CHARGE syndrome) have overlapping features with DGS but our patient has been diagnosed with none of them [1]. At present, the child is followed up by healthcare providers from many specialties.

Conflict of Interests

The authors declare that there is no conflict of interests regarding the publication of this paper.

References

[1] D. M. McDonald-McGinn, B. S. Emanuel, and E. H. Zackai, "EH. 22q11.2 deletion syndrome," in *Gene Reviews—NCBI Bookshelf*, 2013, http://www.ncbi.nlm.nih.gov/books/NBK1523/.

[2] S. Gao, X. Li, and B. A. Amendt, "Understanding the role of *Tbx1* as a candidate gene for 22q11.2 deletion syndrome," *Current Allergy and Asthma Reports*, vol. 13, no. 6, pp. 613–621, 2013.

[3] T. Ogata, T. Niihori, N. Tanaka et al., "TBX1 mutation identified by exome sequencing in a Japanese family with 22q11.2 deletion syndrome-like craniofacial features and hypocalcemia," *PLoS ONE*, vol. 9, no. 3, Article ID e91598, 2014.

[4] Y. Kanaya, S. Ohga, K. Ikeda et al., "Maturational alterations of peripheral T cell subsets and cytokine gene expression in 22q11.2 deletion syndrome," *Clinical and Experimental Immunology*, vol. 144, no. 1, pp. 85–93, 2006.

[5] R. Zemble, E. Luning Prak, K. McDonald, D. McDonald-McGinn, E. Zackai, and K. Sullivan, "Secondary immunologic consequences in chromosome 22q11.2 deletion syndrome (DiGeorge syndrome/velocardiofacial syndrome)," *Clinical Immunology*, vol. 136, no. 3, pp. 409–418, 2010.

57

Neonatal Hyperglycemia due to Transient Neonatal Diabetes Mellitus in Puerto Rico

N. Fargas-Berríos, L. García-Fragoso, I. García-García, and M. Valcárcel

Neonatology Section, Department of Pediatrics, University Pediatrics Hospital, School of Medicine,
Medical Sciences Campus, University of Puerto Rico, San Juan, PR 00936-5067, USA

Correspondence should be addressed to N. Fargas-Berríos; neichma.fargas@upr.edu

Academic Editor: Josef Sykora

Neonatal hyperglycemia is a metabolic disorder found in the neonatal intensive care units. Neonatal diabetes mellitus (NDM) is a very uncommon cause of hyperglycemia in the newborn, occurring in 1 in every 400,000 births. There are two subtypes of neonatal diabetes mellitus: permanent neonatal diabetes mellitus (PNDM) and transient neonatal diabetes mellitus (TNDM). We describe a term, small for gestational age, female neonate with transient neonatal diabetes mellitus who presented with poor feeding tolerance and vomiting associated with hyperglycemia (385 mg/dL), glycosuria, and metabolic acidosis within the first 12 hours of life. The neonate was treated with intravenous insulin, obtaining a slight control of hyperglycemia. An adequate glycemia was achieved at 5 weeks of life. The molecular studies showed complete loss of maternal methylation at the TND differentially methylated region on chromosome 6q24. The etiology of this neonate's hyperglycemia was a hypomethylation of the maternal TND locus. A rare cause of neonatal diabetes mellitus must be considered if a neonate presents refractory hyperglycemia. To our knowledge, this is the first case reported in Puerto Rico of transient neonatal mellitus due to the uncommon mechanism of maternal hypomethylation of the TND locus. Its prevalence in Puerto Rico is unknown.

1. Introduction

Neonatal hyperglycemia is a metabolic disorder found in the neonatal intensive care units [1]. There are several and different etiologies for neonatal hyperglycemia with different clinical pictures and treatments [2].

Neonatal diabetes mellitus (NDM) is a very uncommon cause of hyperglycemia in the newborn, occurring in 1 in every 300,000 to 400,000 live births [1, 3, 4]. NDM presents as insulin requiring persistent hyperglycemia occurring in the first 6 postnatal months, associated with insufficient production of endogenous insulin [1, 3]. NDM is not an autoimmune disorder as insulin-dependent diabetes mellitus in childhood [1, 3]. The insulinopenia of NDM results from abnormal pancreatic islet development, decreased B-cell mass, or B-cell dysfunction [3].

The neonates with NDM are small for gestational age or intrauterine growth retarded and can present with signs of dehydration, weight loss, and glucosuria with or without ketoacidosis or ketonuria. Additionally, they may present with failure to thrive, macroglossia, umbilical hernia, malformations of the brain, heart, or kidneys, hypotonia, deafness, and neurodevelopmental delay [1, 3, 4].

The prevalence of neonatal diabetes mellitus in Puerto Rico is unknown and few cases have been reported [5]. We describe a term, small for gestational age, female neonate with transient neonatal diabetes mellitus in Puerto Rico who presented with poor feeding tolerance and vomiting associated with hyperglycemia, glycosuria, and metabolic acidosis within the first 12 hours of life.

2. Case Presentation

A term, small for gestational age, female neonate was born via spontaneous vaginal delivery at 39 weeks of gestational age to a 23-year-old G2P1A0 woman. The mother received adequate prenatal care and prenatal test results indicated that the mother was hepatitis B surface antigen, VDRL, and HIV negative. The mother had no past medical history for systemic illness and she had several urinary tract infections during the

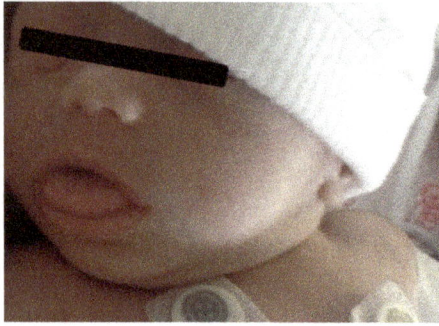

FIGURE 1: TSGA neonate with macroglossia.

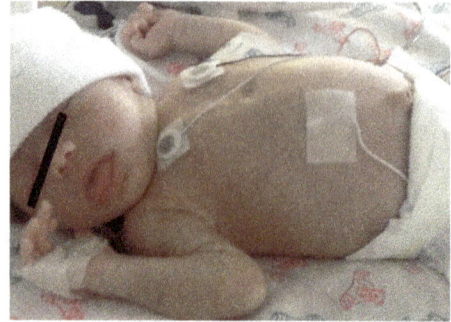

FIGURE 2: TSGA neonate shows an umbilical hernia.

pregnancy. The maternal family history was unremarkable for any systemic illness. The paternal family history was significant for hypertension and type 2 diabetes mellitus. There was no history of consanguinity.

The neonate, who weighed 2,041 g (less than 3rd percentile for gestational age), was vigorous and had a spontaneous cry during birth. The initial blood glucose level was 65 mg/dL. The neonate presented with poor feeding tolerance associated with vomiting and was diagnosed with clinical sepsis. Intravenous antibiotics were administered. The blood glucose levels increased to 206–385 mg/dL with the ingestion of milk formula. The neonate was started on continuous intravenous regular insulin infusion at 13 hours of life. Arterial blood gases analysis revealed pH of 7.266, pCO$_2$ of 25.6 mm Hg, HCO$_3$ 11.8 mmol/L, and base excess −12.7 mmol/L. The insulin infusion was discontinued after adequate glycemic control (104 mg/dL). The neonate was transferred to the Neonatal Intensive Care Unit (NICU) of the University Pediatrics Hospital for evaluation.

On admission to the NICU of the University Pediatrics Hospital, physical examination of the infant revealed normal vital signs (temperature of 36.5°C, heart rate of 145 beats/min, respiratory rate of 33 breaths/min, and mean blood pressure of 53 mm Hg), comfortable breathing at room air, macroglossia, and umbilical hernia (Figures 1 and 2). The neonate presented with blood glucose level of 63 mg/dL on admission. The infant was NPO with TPN CHO 5% and Intralipids 20% to maintain adequate hydration and nutritional requirements. Arterial blood gases analysis was normal with pH of 7.412, pCO$_2$ of 35.6 mm Hg, HCO$_3$ 22.3 mmol/L, and base excess −1.8 mmol/L. The blood glucose levels increased to 320–415 mg/dL and continuous intravenous regular insulin infusion (0.1 units/kg/hr) was started. The carbohydrate infusion was decreased to 3.5 mg/kg/min. Arterial blood gases analysis was performed during the hyperglycemia revealing pH of 7.393, pCO$_2$ of 23.9 mm Hg, HCO$_3$ 14.2 mmol/L, and base excess −8.5 mmol/L.

The laboratory workup revealed glucosuria (more than 1,000 mg/dL) and ketonuria (trace), normal C-reactive protein, ammonia, lactate, insulin level (1 μU/mL), and thyroid stimulating hormone level. The blood glucose levels ranged from 44 to 314 mg/dL. The insulin infusion was discontinued due to hypoglycemia and the carbohydrate infusion was increased. The endocrinologist recommended insulin lispro

injection of 0.5 units if the blood glucose was greater than 200 mg/dL. The blood glucose levels ranged from 46 to 286 mg/dL during the next 3 days.

The abdominal ultrasound was normal, which ruled out any structural disease of the pancreas. The molecular analysis revealed complete loss of maternal methylation at the TND differentially methylated region on chromosome 6q24.

The neonate obtained an adequate glycemia (87 to 118 mg/dL) at 5 weeks of life. The neonate was discharged on enteral feedings with high protein content and without any insulin or hypoglycemic treatment.

3. Discussion

The cause of neonatal hyperglycemia must be thoroughly investigated due to its diverse etiologies, clinical pictures, and treatments. The symptomatology is nonspecific and involves diverse neonatal diagnoses, as sepsis. An uncommon etiology as neonatal diabetes mellitus must be considered if a neonate presents refractory hyperglycemia within the first 6 postnatal months and low birth weight [3].

There are two subtypes of neonatal diabetes mellitus: permanent neonatal diabetes mellitus (PNDM) and transient neonatal diabetes mellitus (TNDM) [1, 3]. Transient neonatal diabetes mellitus (TNDM) accounts for 50–60% of NDM cases and is associated with mutations of sulfonylurea receptors at chromosome 6q24 [1, 3, 6]. This subtype presents soon after birth with a spontaneous remission during infancy. The hyperglycemia may begin in the first 6 postnatal weeks in a term infant and usually improves by 24 months [1]. A number of patients may have a relapse to a permanent form of diabetes mellitus in childhood or adolescence [1, 3, 4]. Permanent neonatal diabetes mellitus (PNDM) is less common and is also characterized by early hyperglycemia. This subtype has no period of remission and must be treated lifelong [3].

Three mechanisms are known to cause TNDM in 90% of cases. All mechanisms involve the altered expression of genes in chromosome 6 due to inappropriate overexpression of the chromosome region 6q24. The three mechanisms are (1) paternal uniparental disomy of chromosome 6 (UPD6pat), (2) unbalanced duplication of 6q24 on the paternal allele, and (3) 6q24 maternal hypomethylation defect [1, 3, 4].

TNDM is effectively treated with insulin and oral sulfonylurea medications and has a spontaneous remission within

1 year, but a small number of patients have relapses in adolescence and adulthood [1, 3, 4]. 50% of patients with 6q24-related TNDM develop permanent diabetes mellitus later in life [1]. PNDM is less common than TNDM but requires lifelong treatment [3]. The prompt diagnosis and treatment of neonatal diabetes mellitus are very important because the adequate control of hyperglycemia promotes a satisfactory weight gain and growth.

Blood samples from the neonate and her parents were sent to the Wessex Regional Genetics Laboratory of the University of Southampton in the United Kingdom. The blood samples were tested for methylation-specific polymerase chain reaction (PCR) of deoxyribonucleic acid (DNA). The DNA-PCR test showed complete loss of maternal methylation at the TND differentially methylated region on chromosome 6q24. Further molecular analyses of the polymorphic loci were performed to determine whether the loss of maternal methylation was caused by paternal uniparental disomy of chromosome 6. The inheritance pattern was not consistent with paternal uniparental disomy. The etiology of this neonate's hyperglycemia was a hypomethylation of the maternal TND locus. The neonate was diagnosed with transient neonatal diabetes mellitus (TNDM) due to 6q24 methylation defect.

The prevalence of neonatal diabetes mellitus in Puerto Rico is unknown and few cases have been reported. Two Puerto Rican infants were identified with NDM due to a KCNJ11 activating mutation [5]. To our knowledge this is the first case reported in Puerto Rico with transient neonatal mellitus due to the uncommon mechanism of maternal hypomethylation of the TDN locus.

Conflict of Interests

The authors declare that there is no conflict of interests regarding the publication of this paper.

References

[1] P. Pun, R. Clark, K.-W. Wan, R. Peverini, and T. A. Merritt, "Neonatal diabetes mellitus: the impact of molecular diagnosis," *NeoReviews*, vol. 11, no. 6, pp. e306–e310, 2010.

[2] P. J. Rozance and W. W. Hay Jr., "Neonatal hyperglycemia," *NeoReviews*, vol. 11, no. 11, pp. e632–e638, 2010.

[3] A. Kataria, R. Palliyil Gopi, P. Mally, and B. Shah, "Neonatal diabetes mellitus: current perspective," *Research and Reports in Neonatology*, vol. 4, pp. 55–64, 2014.

[4] L. E. Docherty, S. Kabwama, A. Lehmann et al., "Clinical presentation of 6q24 transient neonatal diabetes mellitus (6q24 TNDM) and genotype-phenotype correlation in an international cohort of patients," *Diabetologia*, vol. 56, no. 4, pp. 758–762, 2013.

[5] F. Nieves-Rivera and L. González-Pijem, "Neonatal diabetes mellitus: description of two Puerto Rican children with KCNJ11 activating gene mutation," *Puerto Rico Health Sciences Journal*, vol. 30, no. 2, pp. 87–89, 2011.

[6] I. K. Temple, "Diabetes mellitus, 6q24-related transient neonatal," in *GeneReviews at GeneTests Medical Genetics Information Resource*, pp. 1997–2013, University of Washington, Seattle, Wash, USA, 2012, http://www.genetests.org/.

58

Inguinal Hernia Containing Uterus, Fallopian Tube, and Ovary in a Premature Newborn

Kıvılcım Karadeniz Cerit,[1] **Rabia Ergelen,**[2] **Emel Colak,**[1] **and Tolga E. Dagli**[1]

[1]*Department of Pediatric Surgery, School of Medicine, Marmara University, 34899 Istanbul, Turkey*
[2]*Department of Radiology, School of Medicine, Marmara University, 34899 Istanbul, Turkey*

Correspondence should be addressed to Kıvılcım Karadeniz Cerit; kcerit@yahoo.com

Academic Editor: Bernhard Resch

A female infant weighing 2,200 g was delivered at 34 weeks of gestation by vaginal delivery. She presented with an irreducible mass in the left inguinal region at 32 days of age. An ultrasonography (US) was performed and an incarcerated hernia containing uterus, fallopian tube, and ovary was diagnosed preoperatively. Surgery was performed through an inguinal approach; the uterus, fallopian tube, and ovary were found in the hernia sac. High ligation and an additional repair of the internal inguinal ring were performed. Patent processus vaginalis was found during contralateral exploration and also closed. The postoperative course was uneventful. After one year of follow-up, there have been no signs of recurrence.

1. Introduction

Indirect inguinal hernia is the most common congenital anomaly of infancy and childhood with an incidence ranging from 0.8% to 4% [1]. It is seen more often in the first year of life. In premature infants, the incidence increases to 30%. In female infants, sliding inguinal hernias mostly contain the ovary with or without fallopian tube. The presence of the uterus within the hernia sac (hernia uterus inguinale) and incarceration of the adnexa of the uterus are an extremely rare condition in infants [2]. Since only a few cases are described in literature, we herein report a premature female infant who had an inguinal hernia containing uterus, fallopian tube, and ovary.

2. Case Report

A female premature infant was delivered at 34 weeks of gestation (birth weight 2,200 g, height 44 cm, and Apgar score 7/9) by vaginal delivery. No inguinal masses were noted and her external genitalia appeared normal during her first examination. She was referred to the pediatric surgery unit at 32 days of age (weight 3150 g, height 48 cm), with an irreducible mass in the left inguinal region, noticed by her pediatrician a few hours ago. There was no history of irritability, pain, erythema, or vomiting. On physical examination, the patient had an irreducible, soft mass in the left inguinal region. An ultrasonography (US) was performed because an incarcerated ovarian hernia was suspected. A solid mass in left inguinal channel with a clearly visible endometrial lining was seen and an incarcerated hernia containing uterus, fallopian tube, and ovary was diagnosed preoperatively (Figure 1). Surgery was performed through an inguinal approach; the uterus, fallopian tube, and ovary were found in the hernia sac (Figure 2). The organs were freed from the hernia sac. Gentle and careful dissection was required due to strong adhesions between the organs and the hernia sac, which was very thin. The organs were edematous but perfusion appeared normal. The reduction of the hernia contents into the abdomen through the inguinal canal was slightly difficult. A high ligation and an additional repair of the internal inguinal ring were performed to prevent recurrence. During contralateral exploration, a patent processus vaginalis was found and repaired. The postoperative course was uneventful. At one-year follow-up, the patient had neither clinical nor radiological evidence of a recurrence. Pelvic organs appeared normal and in the correct location.

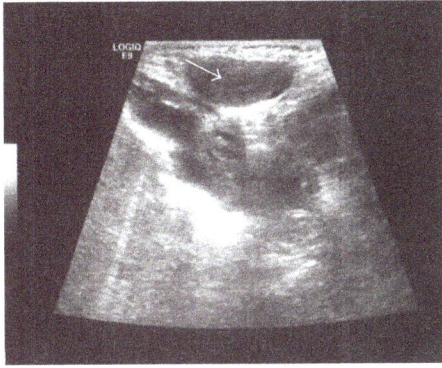

FIGURE 1: Ultrasonography image: a solid mass in right inguinal channel with a clearly visible endometrial lining.

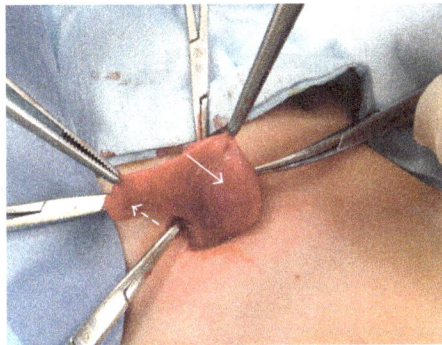

FIGURE 2: Intraoperative findings. Hernia sac containing uterus, fallopian tube, and ovary.

3. Discussion

The current case is a 32-day-old female premature infant that presented with an irreducible indirect inguinal mass. The uterus, fallopian tube, and ovary were identified within an inguinal hernia sac. The hernia contents were reduced into the abdomen through the inguinal canal and a high ligation plus additional repair of the internal inguinal ring were performed.

Processus vaginalis develops at around the sixth month of fetal growth as an evagination of parietal peritoneum. Depending on gender, it is accompanied by the testis or round ligament of the uterus and passes through the inguinal canal up to the scrotum or labium major. Processus vaginalis is relatively small in female infants and obliterates around eight months of gestation. If patency persists, it is termed the canal of Nuck [2].

Inguinal hernia containing an ovary with or without a fallopian tube is not uncommon in female infants. However, an inguinal hernia containing the uterus is extremely rare. The etiology of this pathology is controversial. An anatomic abnormality with primary weakness of the uterine and ovarian suspensory ligaments is suspected. Thomson offered the hypothesis that if there is failure of fusion of the Mullerian ducts leading to excessive mobility of the ovaries plus nonfusion of the uterine cornua, the chance of

herniation of the entire uterus, ovary, and fallopian tube into the inguinal canal is increased [3]. On the other hand, Fowler theorized that elongated ovarian suspensory ligaments were the primary cause or the secondary effect of a hernia [4]. The finding of an anatomic abnormality may compromise fertility; therefore, careful gynecologic follow-up is required until the childbearing age.

The presence of the uterus in an inguinal hernia in boys is attributed to the persistence of Mullerian duct derivatives. Male pseudohermaphroditism is characterized by the presence of Mullerian duct derivatives (uterus, cervix, fallopian tubes, and upper third of the vagina) in phenotypic male patients [5]. Because of the normal female phenotype, analysis of the chromosomes was not performed in the present case.

Due to the rarity of these cases where an indirect hernia sac contains the uterus, fallopian tube, and ovary, different aspects of surgical treatment must be kept in mind. Some authors perform a classic herniorrhaphy with a high ligation through an inguinal approach, while some authors advocate additional closure of the internal ring, as performed in our patient [2]. Suzuki et al. reported one pediatric case with recurrence after reduction of the hernia contents into the abdomen and ligation of the internal ring under laparotomy, in which a high ligation and repair of the inguinal canal under an inguinal approach were performed [6]. Okada et al. recommended simple herniorrhaphy for indirect inguinal hernia containing the uterus, bilateral ovaries, and fallopian tubes [7]. The surgical procedure for inguinal hernia containing uterus is quite different from the cases containing only the ovary as these organs are strongly attached to the hernia sac and it is difficult to free them from the wall of the hernia sac. After freeing these attachments without damaging the organs, we recommend high ligation and additional repair of the internal inguinal ring to prevent recurrence. Furthermore, we also recommend contralateral exploration to prevent the infant from another operation.

Because of the risk of damaging herniated structures during the surgical procedure, a careful preoperative investigation is necessary. US should be routinely performed in female infants with an irreducible palpable inguinal mass [7, 8]. US is an accurate and easily available choice for diagnosis. Preoperative US using a high-frequency transducer is therefore very helpful in reaching a diagnosis with an efficacy considered to be almost 100% [9]. Early recognition by a pediatric surgeon or a neonatologist assures prompt surgical intervention and prevents the injury to the herniated organs in incarcerated inguinal hernias containing uterus, fallopian tube, and ovary.

4. Conclusion

When an atypical inguinal hernia is diagnosed in a premature female infant, we advise prompt ultrasonography in all cases. Early surgical intervention is necessary to prevent the damage of herniated organs, because unexpected reproductive structures may be involved in the hernia sac.

Conflict of Interests

The authors declare that there is no conflict of interests regarding the publication of this paper.

References

[1] E. K. George, A. M. Oudesluys-Murphy, G. C. Madern, P. Cleyndert, and J. G. A. M. Blomjous, "Inguinal hernias containing the uterus, fallopian tube, and ovary in premature female infants," *The Journal of Pediatrics*, vol. 136, no. 5, pp. 696–698, 2000.

[2] V. Cascini, G. Lisi, D. Di Renzo, N. Pappalepore, and P. Lelli Chiesa, "Irreducible indirect inguinal hernia containing uterus and bilateral adnexa in a premature female infant: report of an exceptional case and review of the literature," *Journal of Pediatric Surgery*, vol. 48, no. 1, pp. E17–E19, 2013.

[3] G. R. Thomson, "Complete congenital absence of the vagina associated with bilateral herniæ of uterus, tubes, and ovaries," *British Journal of Surgery*, vol. 36, no. 141, pp. 99–100, 1948.

[4] C. L. Fowler, "Sliding indirect hernia containing both ovaries," *Journal of Pediatric Surgery*, vol. 40, no. 9, pp. E13–E14, 2005.

[5] I. Akıllıoğlu, A. Kaymakcı, I. Akkoyun, Ş. Güven, S. Yücesan, and A. Hiçsönmez, "Inguinal hernias containing the uterus: a case series of 7 female children," *Journal of Pediatric Surgery*, vol. 48, no. 10, pp. 2157–2159, 2013.

[6] N. Suzuki, A. Takahashi, M. Kuroiwa et al., "Diagnosis and treatment of sliding inguinal hernias in infants and children," *Journal of Pediatric Surgery*, vol. 31, pp. 597–601, 1999.

[7] T. Okada, S. Sasaki, S. Honda, H. Miyagi, M. Minato, and S. Todo, "Irreducible indirect inguinal hernia containing uterus, ovaries, and fallopian tubes," *Hernia*, vol. 16, no. 4, pp. 471–473, 2012.

[8] Y.-C. Ming, C.-C. Luo, H.-C. Chao, and S.-M. Chu, "Inguinal hernia containing uterus and uterine adnexa in female infants: report of two cases," *Pediatrics and Neonatology*, vol. 52, no. 2, pp. 103–105, 2011.

[9] G. Jedrzejewski, A. Stankiewicz, and A. P. Wieczorek, "Uterus and ovary hernia of the canal of Nuck," *Pediatric Radiology*, vol. 38, no. 11, pp. 1257–1258, 2008.

59

Separation of the Proximal Humeral Epiphysis in the Newborn: Rapid Diagnosis with Ultrasonography

Rachelle Goldfisher and John Amodio

Department of Radiology, SUNY Downstate Medical Center, 450 Clarkson Avenue, Brooklyn, NY 11203, USA

Correspondence should be addressed to John Amodio; john.amodio@downstate.edu

Academic Editor: Seyed Mohsen Dehghani

Separation of the proximal humeral epiphysis (SPHE) is a well-known occurrence and may occur secondary to trauma, infection, and nonaccidental trauma. Since most newborns do not have the proximal humeral epiphysis ossified at birth, the diagnosis may be difficult to make on routine radiographs. Ultrasonography of the shoulder in the newborn is rapid, noninvasive, and nonionizing imaging techniques which can diagnose SPHE. In this report, we describe and emphasize the diagnostic utility of state-of-the-art ultrasonography for the diagnosis of SPHE.

1. Introduction

Separation of the proximal humeral epiphysis (SPHE) is a well-known occurrence, and may occur secondary to trauma, infection, and nonaccidental trauma. SPHE is known to exist in the newborn after a traumatic delivery.

Since most newborns do not have the proximal humeral epiphysis ossified at birth, the diagnosis may be difficult to make on routine radiographs. Widening of the glenohumeral distance may be a clue on plain film, but it is not always accurate [1].

Ultrasonography of the shoulder in the newborn is rapid, noninvasive, and nonionizing imaging techniques which can diagnose SPHE. Additionally, it can be performed at the bedside. To the best of our knowledge, there have been few reports in the literature demonstrating SPHE in the newborn period with sonography [2–4]. In this report, we describe and emphasize the diagnostic utility of state-of-the-art ultrasonography for the diagnosis of SPHE.

2. Case Report

The patient is an ex 37-week gestational infant who presented with shoulder dystocia. The APGARS at birth were 3, 4, and 7. The infant required positive pressure ventilation and intubation for respiratory distress. Examination in the neonatal ice revealed reduced left arm motion, with swelling, ecchymoses, and tenderness to palpation. Left elbow reflexes were spontaneous and there was a positive left grasp. The infant was not moving the right upper extremity and was diagnosed as having a right Erb's palsy.

X-ray examination of the chest demonstrated a mild air space disease pattern, ossification of the right humeral epiphysis, but the ossification center of the left humeral epiphysis was not clearly visualized (Figure 1). Additionally, the left glenohumeral distance on the left was increased compared to the right. A sonogram of both humeri was obtained which demonstrated a normal ephyseal–humeral relationship on the right (Figure 2(a)); the right femoral epiphysis was located within the normal glenoid labrum (Figure 2(b)). The left humeral epiphysis was displaced from the metaphysis, compatible with epiphyseal separation (Figure 3(a)). The left epiphysis was normally located within the glenohumeral joint (Figure 3(b)). The left shoulder was placed in a sling; subsequent X-ray examination demonstrated healing of the epiphyseal separation (Figure 4).

3. Discussion

The physeal plate is less resistant to trauma in infants and children than are the joint capsule, bone, and ligaments [1].

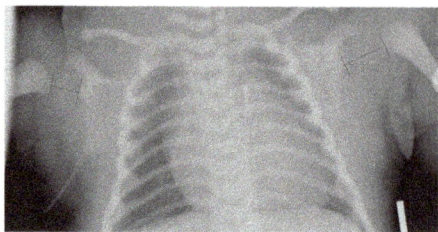

FIGURE 1: AP view of the chest demonstrates the ossification center of the right humerus is within the glenohumeral joint. The ossification center of the left humerus is not visualized. Additionally, the left glenohumeral distance on the left is increased compared to the right.

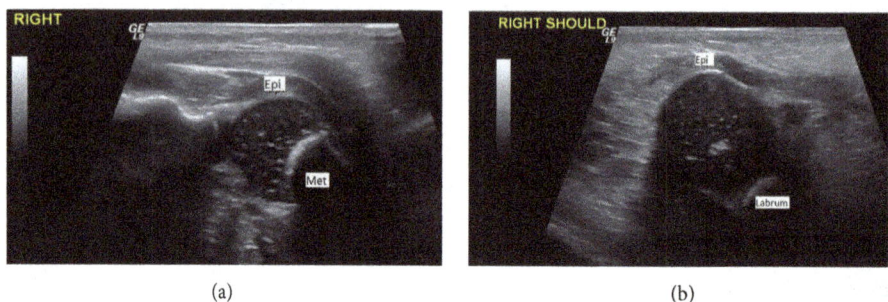

(a)   (b)

FIGURE 2: (a) Longitudinal sonogram of the right shoulder demonstrates the normal relationship of the epiphysis (epi) on the metaphysic (met). (b) Transverse sonogram of the right shoulder demonstrated the right humeral epiphysis within the right glenoid labrum.

Therefore, the path of least resistance of forces applied to the extremities is through the cartilaginous physis. When there is a difficulty delivery, or shoulder dystocia, as in the case presented here, the force applied may be through the proximal humeral physis, resulting in epiphyseal separation from the metaphysis.

Ekengren et al. [4] described 21 infants with 21 epiphyseal separations at birth. Nine of the separations were of the proximal humerus and five of the distal humerus; one of the proximal portion of the femur; five of the distal portion of the femur; and one of the distal portions of the tibia and fibula. Interestingly, according to Lemperg and Liliequist [5] epiphyseal separation of the proximal humerus is rarely accompanied by an injury of the brachial plexus.

Clinically, the infant with an epiphyseal separation of the proximal humerus will move the affected arm little and there is pain and tenderness on physical examination. There may be swelling of the affected region as well as possible hematoma [2].

Broker and Burbach [2] state that the proximal humerus epiphysis ossifies in 15–20% of infants by 39 weeks of gestational age and in 40% at 41 gestational ages. However, the most recent version of Dr. Caffey's textbook [6] states that the proximal humeral ossification center ossifies shortly after birth with 5% and 95% confidence intervals of 37 weeks' gestation and 16 weeks' postnatally, respectively. Nevertheless, the proximal humerus ossification center is not ossified in the majority of full term infants, making plain film evaluation of the injured shoulder quite difficult, if at all possible. A factor which may complicate the diagnosis further is that if the arm is in internal rotation at the time of radiographic examination, the ossification center, if visible, may appear

in a more central position in relationship to the humeral shaft, thus giving the false impression of a normal relationship between the epiphysis and the humerus. An asymmetric position of the humeral shaft with the glenohumeral joint, when compared to the unaffected side, may offer a clue to the diagnosis of epiphyseal separation, when the ossification center is not yet ossified. In such cases, the metaphysis may appear more caudad in relation to the scapula.

Ultrasound is a noninvasive, nonionizing radiation examination which can be rapidly performed at the bedside. The major advantage of sonography is that this technique can image the ossification center, even if it is purely cartilaginous. Thus, the relationship of the epiphysis and metaphysic can readily be identified. In addition, the relationship of the ossification center with the glenohumeral joint can also be easily depicted, Figure 2(a).

MRI can also demonstrate the diagnosis of epiphyseal separation, as well as evaluate the brachial plexus and other soft tissue abnormalities [7]. However, MRI requires transporting the patient to the scanner; special coils are needed to maximize imaging of the affected part and may require that the infant be sedated to minimized motion artifact.

Treatment of epiphyseal separation is usually conservative, with immobilization for several weeks. In general, the prognosis for adequate healing and no residual deformity is excellent, as the plan of cleavage is extra-articular, which insures little or no vascular compromise of the epiphysis [2]. Occasionally, closed reduction may fail. El-adl et al. [7] reported eight cases of SPHE which failed closed reduction; subsequent reduction was performed using k-wires, with subsequent excellent healing and no avascular necrosis of the epiphysis or limb-length deformity.

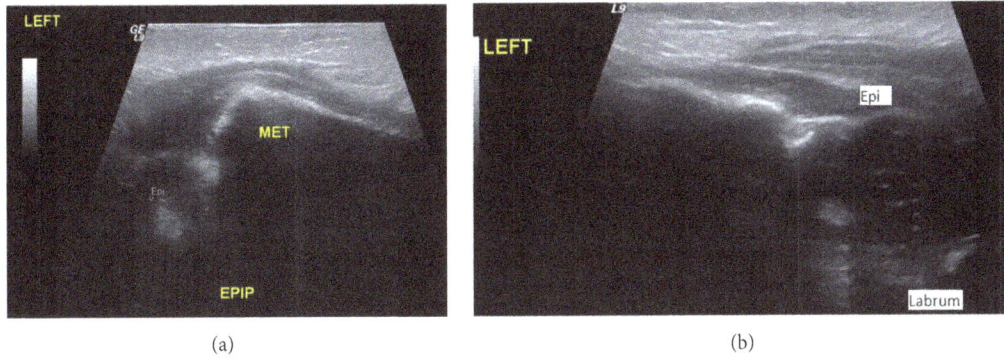

(a)

(b)

FIGURE 3: (a) Longitudinal sonogram of the left shoulder demonstrates separation of the left humeral epiphysis (epi) from the metaphysis (met). (b) Transverse sonogram of the left shoulder shows left humeral epiphysis within the confines of the labrum.

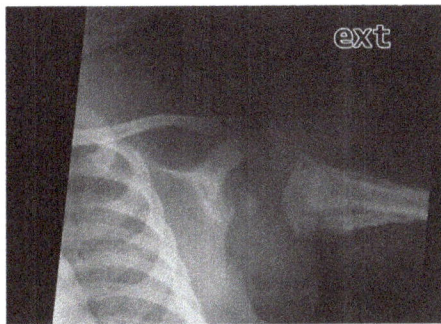

FIGURE 4: AP view of the left shoulder demonstrates abundant new bone along the left humeral shaft compatible with healing and ossification of the epiphysis within the glenoid labrum.

In summary, SPHE should be considered in the differential diagnosis of the neonate with birth trauma who has limitation of motion and tenderness of the arm. The diagnosis may be difficult to make on the basis of plain radiography. Ultrasonography is a rapid bedside examination which can accurately make the diagnosis.

Conflict of Interests

The authors declare that there is no conflict of interests regarding the publication of this paper.

References

[1] S. Carson, D. P. Woolridge, J. Colletti, and K. Kilgore, "Pediatric upper extremity injuries," *Pediatric Clinics of North America*, vol. 53, no. 1, pp. 41–67, 2006.

[2] F. H. L. Broker and T. Burbach, "Ultrasonic diagnosis of separation of the proximal humeral epiphysis in the newborn," *Journal of Bone and Joint Surgery A*, vol. 72, no. 2, pp. 187–191, 1990.

[3] M. Zieger, U. Dorr, and R. D. Schulz, "Sonography of slipped humeral epiphysis due to birth injury," *Pediatric Radiology*, vol. 17, no. 5, pp. 425–426, 1987.

[4] K. Ekengren, S. Bergdahl, and G. Ekstrom, "Birth injuries to the epiphyseal cartilage," *Acta Radiologica*, vol. 19, no. 1B, pp. 197–204, 1978.

[5] R. Lemperg and B. Liliequist, "Dislocation of the proximal epiphysis of the humerus in newborns: report of two cases and discussion of diagnostic criteria," *Acta Paediatrica Scandinavica*, vol. 59, no. 4, pp. 377–380, 1970.

[6] J. Caffey, *Pediatric Diagnostic Imaging*, vol. 2, Mosby, Philadelphia, Pa, USA, 11th edition, 2008.

[7] W. A. El-adl, H. S. A. Elgohary, and M. M. Elshennawy, "Epiphyseal separation of the proximal humerus after birth trauma," *European Journal of Orthopaedic Surgery and Traumatology*, vol. 24, no. 6, pp. 863–867, 2013.

60

Costello Syndrome with Severe Nodulocystic Acne: Unexpected Significant Improvement of Acanthosis Nigricans after Oral Isotretinoin Treatment

Leelawadee Sriboonnark,[1] **Harleen Arora,**[2] **Leyre Falto-Aizpurua,**[2]
Sonal Choudhary,[2] **and Elizabeth Alvarez Connelly**[2]

[1]*Division of Dermatology, Department of Pediatrics, Faculty of Medicine, Khon Kaen University, Khon Kaen 40002, Thailand*
[2]*Miller School of Medicine, Department of Pediatric Dermatology, University of Miami, 1600 NW 10th Avenue,*
 Rosenstiel Medical Science Building, Room 2023, Miami, FL 33136, USA

Correspondence should be addressed to Leelawadee Sriboonnark; drleelawadee@gmail.com

Academic Editor: Ozgur Cogulu

We report the case of 17-year-old female diagnosed with Costello syndrome. Genetic testing provided a proof with G12S mutation in the HRAS gene since 3 years of age with a presentation of severe nodulocystic acne on her face. After 2 months of oral isotretinoin treatment, improvement in her acne was observed. Interestingly, an unexpected significant improvement of acanthosis nigricans on her neck and dorsum of her hands was found as well. We present this case as a successful treatment option by using oral isotretinoin for the treatment of acanthosis nigricans in Costello syndrome patients.

1. Introduction

Costello syndrome is an autosomal dominant inherited disorder with frequent de novo mutation in the HRAS gene [1]. This syndrome has no formal diagnostic criteria. However, it has characteristic craniofacial appearances, hand and wrist posture abnormalities, musculoskeletal and cardiac abnormalities, neurologic problems, psychomotor developmental delay, intellectual disability, and failure to thrive. Cutaneous manifestations in Costello syndrome are common and were described in many literatures [2–4] which included papillomatosis, palmoplantar keratoderma, follicular hyperkeratosis, and acanthosis nigricans [3]. According to up-to-date knowledge, there was no favorable treatment option for these cutaneous findings.

2. Case Presentation

A 17-year-old female was first seen in January 2013 for her complaining of multiple nodulocystic acne on the face persisting for several months. Diagnosis with Costello syndrome was proved since the age of 3 by genetic testing which revealed a mutation (G12S) in the HRAS gene. She also has typical features of this syndrome which included coarse facies (Figure 1), sparse hair, full lips, redundant skin, ulnar deviation of the wrists and fingers, developmental delay, and hydrocephalus which has been operated and drained for several occasions by pediatric neurologist. Hyperkeratotic hyperpigmented plaques on dorsal aspect of her hands and acanthosis nigricans around her neck were also seen and described as typical skin findings commonly found in Costello syndrome as well.

According to her severe nodulocystic acne manifestation, literatures were reviewed and, to date, there was no association between this syndrome and severe nodulocystic acne. However, a prominent history of severe acne with current residual scarring in both her parents was the evidence supporting that severe acne manifestation runs in her family. We then decided to treat her acne initially with oral tetracycline and short course prednisolone 0.5 mg/kg/day without improvement. During that time blood tests were performed including (1) complete hormone panels to exclude adrenal source of hormones since the patient has never menstruated and (2) preisotretinoin laboratory evaluations included

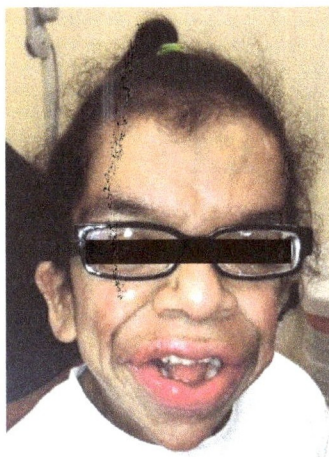

FIGURE 1: Facial manifestation in Costello syndrome.

the pregnancy testing. All results were within normal limits and she was then approved to register in the iPledge system. After discussing risks and benefits, isotretinoin was started at 20 mg orally once a day with significant improvement of her acne after 2 months of the drug administration (Figure 2). Without anticipation, the hyperkeratotic hyperpigmented plaques on dorsal aspect of her hands and the acanthosis nigricans around her neck also had significant improvement from the same isotretinoin treatment as well (Figure 3).

3. Discussion

Costello syndrome is an autosomal dominant inherited disorder with frequent de novo mutation, initially described by Costello [5] in 1971 and 1977. In 2006, Kerr et al. [6] found a heterozygous missense mutation in the protooncogene HRAS where, to date, it has been well accepted that Costello syndrome is caused by HRAS mutations only. Diagnosis of Costello syndrome can be made by typical characteristic of the craniofacial appearances and musculoskeletal, cardiovascular, and neurologic abnormalities as well as psychomotor developmental delayed as described as follows.

List of Abnormalities Found in Costello Syndrome [1]

Craniofacial Appearance

(i) Coarse facial features; full cheeks, full lips, large mouth, and full nasal tip,

(ii) curly, sparse, fine hair,

(iii) wide nasal bridge.

Musculoskeletal System

(i) Diffuse hypotonia and joint laxity,

(ii) ulnar deviation of wrists and fingers and splayed fingers,

(iii) spatulate finger pads and abnormal finger nails,

(iv) positional foot deformity.

Cardiovascular System

(i) Cardiac hypertrophy,

(ii) congenital heart defects,

(iii) aortic dilatation.

Neurologic Abnormalities

(i) Hydrocephalus,

(ii) tethered cord,

(iii) Chiari I malformation.

Psychomotor Development

(i) Developmental delay,

(ii) intellectual disability.

Cutaneous manifestations in Costello syndrome are common and were described in many literatures. Nguyen et al. [3] collected the reported cutaneous signs of Costello syndrome which included (1) loose/redundant/lax skin, (2) deep palmar and/or plantar creases, (3) sparse or thin, curly hair, (4) hyperkeratosis, hyperpigmentation (generalized, localized, or acanthosis nigricans), (5) dysplastic/thin/brittle or deep-set nails, and (6) papillomas.

In our case, the patient showed the nucleotide substitution c.34G > A, resulting in p.Gly12Ser amino acid change representing a mutation (G12S) in the HRAS gene. The patient is also presented with the typical facial manifestations, hand and wrist posture abnormalities, hydrocephalus, and marked cutaneous findings of hyperkeratosis and acanthosis nigricans. Another cutaneous finding found in our patient was the manifestation of severe nodulocystic acne where, to date, literatures reviewed have no association between this finding and Costello syndrome. However, a prominent history of severe acne with current residual scarring in both her parents was the evidence supporting that severe acne manifestation runs in her family.

To date, acanthosis nigricans is apparently a reaction to many stimuli. Many disorders associated with this skin finding included obesity, endocrinologic disorders, and malignancy. Treatment of the underlying disorders which triggered this skin manifestation is the treatment of choice. However, it is possible that acanthosis nigricans which presented in our patient may serve as a direct correlation with HRAS mutation associated with Costello syndrome. Moreover, we have explored other possible related disorders. There were no significant abnormal lipid profiles found from her blood test. Her body weight was normal. The endocrinologic disorders were screened according to the delay of her menstrual period and the results were all normal.

In general, the treatment of hyperkeratosis and acanthosis nigricans in Costello syndrome is mainly for cosmetic purpose; therefore, there was no previous treatment for the cutaneous findings in this patient. Other treatments that have been used in the treatment of acanthosis nigricans are topical keratolytic agents such as urea, salicylic acid, topical tretinoin

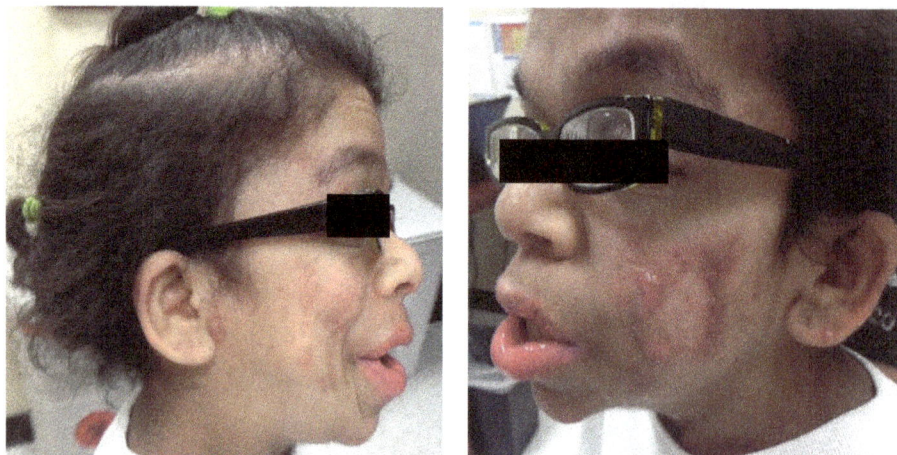

FIGURE 2: Improvement of nodulocystic acne on the face after 2 months of oral isotretinoin treatment.

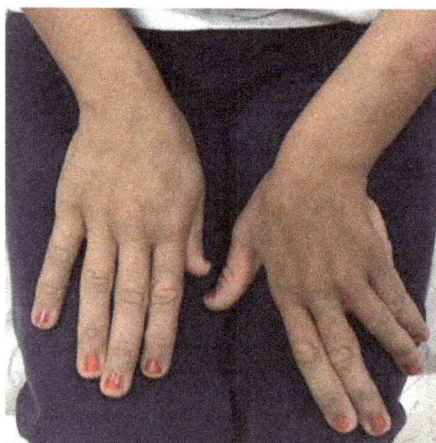

FIGURE 3: Significant improvement of acanthosis nigricans and hyperkeratotic hyperpigmented plaques on the hands after 2 months of oral isotretinoin.

[7], hydroquinone, and ammonium lactate with variable results. Systemic agents which showed benefits in some case reports are etretinate [8], isotretinoin, and metformin [9]. Resolving of acanthosis nigricans around her neck and decreasing of hyperkeratotic hyperpigmented plaques on dorsum of her hands in our patient were interestingly found after 2-month course of oral isotretinoin for the treatment of her acne. We report this finding as a successful treatment option for acanthosis nigricans and hyperpigmented skin found in Costello syndrome.

Conflict of Interests

The authors declare that there is no conflict of interests regarding the publication of this paper.

Acknowledgment

The authors would like to thank Paul Benke, MD, from Joe DiMaggio Children's Hospital, Hollywood, FL, USA, for the genetic testing result.

References

[1] K. W. Gripp and A. E. Lin, "Costello syndrome," in *GeneReviews [Internet]*, R. A. Pagon, M. P. Adam, T. D. Bird, C. R. Dolan, C.-T. Fong, and K. Stephens, Eds., University of Washington, Seattle, Wash, USA, 1993, http://www.ncbi.nlm.nih.gov/books/NBK1507/.

[2] F. Morice-Picard, K. Ezzedine, M.-A. Delrue et al., "Cutaneous manifestations in costello and cardiofaciocutaneous syndrome: rport of 18 cases and literature review," *Pediatric Dermatology*, vol. 30, no. 6, pp. 665–673, 2013.

[3] V. Nguyen, R. L. Buka, B. J. Roberts, and L. F. Eichenfield, "Cutaneous manifestations of Costello syndrome," *International Journal of Dermatology*, vol. 46, no. 1, pp. 72–76, 2007.

[4] D. H. Siegel, J. A. Mann, A. L. Krol, and K. A. Rauen, "Dermatological phenotype in Costello syndrome: consequences of Ras dysregulation in development," *British Journal of Dermatology*, vol. 166, no. 3, pp. 601–607, 2012.

[5] J. M. Costello, "A new syndrome: mental subnormality and nasal papillomata," *Australian Paediatric Journal*, vol. 13, no. 2, pp. 114–118, 1977.

[6] B. Kerr, M.-A. Delrue, S. Sigaudy et al., "Genotype-phenotype correlation in Costello syndrome: HRAS mutation analysis in

43 cases," *Journal of Medical Genetics*, vol. 43, no. 5, pp. 401–405, 2006.

[7] G. L. Darmstadt, B. K. Yokel, and T. D. Horn, "Treatment of acanthosis nigricans with tretinoin," *Archives of Dermatology*, vol. 127, no. 8, pp. 1139–1140, 1991.

[8] N. J. Mork, G. Rajka, and J. Halse, "Treatment of acanthosis nigricans with etretinate (Tigason) in a patient with Lawrence-Seip syndrome (generalized lipodystrophy)," *Acta Dermato-Venereologica*, vol. 66, no. 2, pp. 173–174, 1986.

[9] H. W. Walling, M. Messingham, L. M. Myers, C. L. Mason, and J. S. Strauss, "Improvement of acanthosis nigricans on isotretinoin and metformin," *Journal of Drugs in Dermatology*, vol. 2, no. 6, pp. 677–681, 2003.

61

Acute Lymphocytic Leukemia with Bilateral Renal Masses Masquerading as Nephroblastomatosis

Poonam Thakore, Salim Aljabari, Curtis Turner, and Tetyana L. Vasylyeva

Department of Pediatrics, Texas Tech University Health Sciences Center School of Medicine, Amarillo, TX 79106, USA

Correspondence should be addressed to Tetyana L. Vasylyeva; tetyana.vasylyeva@ttuhsc.edu

Academic Editor: Denis A. Cozzi

Acute lymphoblastic leukemia (ALL) is the most common malignancy in the pediatric patient population. However, renal involvement as the primary manifestation of ALL is rare. We report a case of a 4-year-old boy with bilateral renal lesions resembling nephroblastic rests as the first finding of early stage ALL preceding hematological changes and subsequent classic clinical findings by two weeks. These renal hypodensities completely resolved after one week of induction chemotherapy. This case demonstrates that renal involvement can be the only initial presenting finding of leukemia. Children with lesions resembling nephroblastic rests need appropriate surveillance due to the risk of malignant disease.

1. Introduction

Acute lymphoblastic leukemia (ALL) is the most common malignancy in children between ages of 2 and 5 years [1]. The initial clinical presentation of ALL is nonspecific and may include fatigue, fever, infection, bone pain, organomegaly, and anemia secondary to infiltration of blast cells in bone marrow, peripheral blood, and extramedullary organs. As the disease progresses, other organs, such as the kidneys, may be affected. However, renal involvement in the early stages of ALL is rarely seen [2]. This report details the case of a child with bilateral renal lesions resembling nephroblastic rests as the first finding of ALL preceding the development of the classic features of ALL.

2. Case Report

A four-year-old boy with unremarkable past medical history was seen in the emergency department (ED) with low-grade fever and abdominal pain of a few days duration. A complete blood count (CBC) and abdominal computed tomography (CT) study were performed for evaluation for possible appendicitis. The CBC showed a white blood cell (WBC) count of 8.1×10^9/L with a differential of 22% neutrophils, 68.9% lymphocytes, and an absolute neutrophil count of 1.8×10^9/L,

hemoglobin of 13.3 g/dL, and platelets of 170×10^9/L. Chemistry studies showed blood urea nitrogen of 2.5 mmol/L and creatinine of 33.5 μmol/L. Urinalysis was normal. Although the patient was ultimately diagnosed with viral gastritis and sent home with supportive treatment, CT imaging revealed bilateral renal enlargement with multiple small subcortical and cortical medullary lesions that were hypoenhancing and were determined to be consistent with nephrogenic rests per reading by a pediatric radiologist (Figure 1). In the absence of other significant clinical findings, the renal abnormalities were interpreted as nephroblastomatosis, and the patient was referred to a pediatric nephrology clinic for further follow-up and surveillance for Wilms' tumor transformation. At follow-up, repeat urinalysis was again within normal limits and urine culture was negative. Because of the concern for malignancy such as lymphoma, which can present with similar radiological findings, the need for renal biopsy was discussed with the pediatric oncologist and the pediatric surgeon. However, given the risk versus benefit assessment, close radiologic follow-up was chosen as the management plan instead of biopsy.

Fourteen days after initial presentation, the patient again complained of abdominal pain accompanied by a low-grade fever. Repeat CBC showed WBC of 3.5×10^9/L with a differential of 6% neutrophils, 85% lymphocytes, and

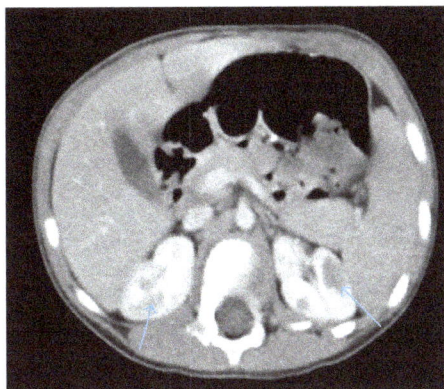

FIGURE 1: CT abdomen with contrast on initial presentation. Arrows showing bilateral hypodense lesions represent leukemic deposits.

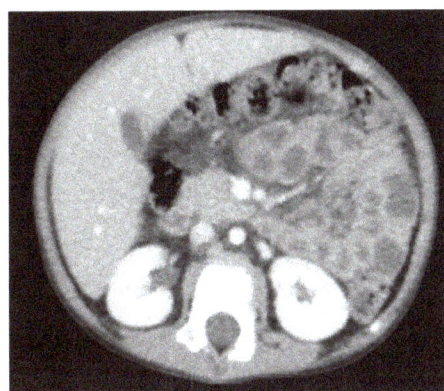

FIGURE 2: CT abdomen with contrast after induction therapy for ALL. Interval resolution of small hypodense subcortical lesions within both kidneys, consistent with favorable response to therapy of leukemic deposits in the kidney.

an absolute neutrophil count of 351×10^9/L, hemoglobin of 11.1 g/dL, and platelet count of 21×10^9/L. The erythrocyte sedimentation rate was 71 mm/hr. The pediatric oncology service was consulted for evaluation for malignancy. Peripheral blood smear was remarkable for the presence of abundant immature lymphoid cells representing 90% of the total white cells. Bone marrow aspirate and biopsy flow cytometry and cytogenetic studies were conclusive for early B cell leukemia.

Treatment was initiated following the guidelines of COG AALL0932. After one week of induction chemotherapy, repeat CT study showed complete interval resolution of all renal hypodensities (Figure 2).

3. Discussion

Renal enlargement in childhood is associated with a broad differential diagnosis including congenital anomalies, hydronephrosis, infection, and malignancy [3]. Leukemic infiltration in the kidney is common in the later stages of ALL in children [4]. However, isolated renal involvement is rare as an initial finding of ALL [3–5]. This patient had significant kidney lesions despite a completely normal initial work-up at

the time of the initial presentation. Thus the initial differential diagnosis by the ED physician did not include malignancy. Moreover, the patient had nonspecific abdominal signs and symptoms with normal urinalysis and negative urine culture making urinary tract infection unlikely. A more complete list of differential diagnoses for similar lesions may include lymphoma, nephroblastomatosis, simple cysts, angiomyolipoma, and metastases in addition to renal leukemic involvement [6]. In the absence of classical signs and symptoms of leukemia, and with the only renal abnormalities on CT imaging, a diagnosis for this patient was elusive.

ALL infiltrates may vary on CT imaging. They may present as enlargement of the kidneys, either unilateral or bilateral, or as low-attenuation focal parenchymal lesions, either unilateral or bilateral and either solitary or multiple [6]. These focal lesions can be difficult to distinguish from nephroblastomatosis, which has a similar radiological picture [6, 7]. In this case, CT imaging showed bilateral renal enlargement with multiple small subcortical and cortical medullary lesions that were hypoenhancing and overall more consistent with nephrogenic rests. Nephroblastomatosis is multifocal or diffuse nephrogenic rests which are defined as persistent foci of embryonic cells beyond 36 weeks' gestation and have the potential to transform into Wilms' tumor [7]. Therefore, this patient was closely followed in the nephrology clinic with repeat imaging studies every 3 months for monitoring for transformation.

In most cases, features of classic leukemia at initial presentation differentiate renal involvement in leukemia from nephroblastomatosis. However, in this case, these classic findings were absent leading the team to conclude that the CT findings were most suggestive of nephroblastomatosis. Although no cytology or histology studies from the lesion were performed, their complete resolution shortly after initiation of ALL specific chemotherapy demonstrates that the lesions were in fact leukemic infiltrates after all.

In conclusion, this case demonstrates that renal involvement may be the initial finding of early stage of ALL. With this in mind, children with lesions resembling nephroblastic rests need to be followed up closely in the pediatric nephrology clinic.

Conflict of Interests

The authors declare that there is no conflict of interests regarding the publication of this paper.

References

[1] K. Kebaili, A. M. Manel, C. Chapelon, P. Taylor, N. Philippe, and Y. Bertrand, "Renal enlargement as presentation of isolated renal relapse in childhood leukemia," *Journal of Pediatric Hematology/Oncology*, vol. 22, no. 5, pp. 454–456, 2000.

[2] N. A. Kalbani, S. Weitzman, M. Abdelhaleem, M. Carcao, and O. Abla, "Acute lymphoblastic leukemia presenting with gross hematuria," *Paediatrics and Child Health*, vol. 12, no. 7, pp. 573–574, 2007.

[3] S. H. G. Ali, F. M. Yacoub, and E. Al-Matar, "Acute lymphoblastic leukemia presenting as bilateral renal enlargement in a child," *Medical Principles and Practice*, vol. 17, no. 6, pp. 504–506, 2008.

[4] R. Pradeep, D. S. Madhumathi, V. Lakshmidevi et al., "Bilateral nephromegaly simulating wilms tumor: a rare initial manifestation of acute lymphoblastic leukemia," *Journal of Pediatric Hematology/Oncology*, vol. 30, no. 6, pp. 471–473, 2008.

[5] E. Erdem, P. Kaylran, G. Ozcelik, A. Ozel, and Z. Yildiz Yildirmak, "Rare presentation of pediatric acute lymphoblastic leukemia: nephromegaly at time of diagnosis," *Indian Journal of Hematology and Blood Transfusion*, vol. 27, no. 1, pp. 43–45, 2011.

[6] M. A. Hilmes, J. R. Dillman, R. J. Mody, and P. J. Strouse, "Pediatric renal leukemia: spectrum of CT imaging findings," *Pediatric Radiology*, vol. 38, no. 4, pp. 424–430, 2008.

[7] R. Anand, M. K. Narula, I. Gupta, V. Chaudhary, S. R. Choudhury, and M. Jain, "Imaging spectrum of primary malignant renal neoplasms in children," *Indian Journal of Medical and Paediatric Oncology*, vol. 33, no. 4, pp. 242–249, 2012.

62

Rahnella aquatilis Sepsis in a Premature Newborn

Canan Kuzdan,[1] **Ahmet Soysal,**[2] **Hülya Özdemir,**[3] **Şenay Coşkun,**[3] **İpek Akman,**[3] **Hülya Bilgen,**[3] **Eren Özek,**[3] **and Mustafa Bakır**[2]

[1]*Istanbul Mehmet Akif Ersoy Thoracic and Cardiovascular Surgery Training and Research Hospital, İstanbul, Turkey*
[2]*Marmara University School of Medicine, Department of Pediatric Infectious Diseases, İstanbul, Turkey*
[3]*Marmara University School of Medicine, Department of Neonatology, İstanbul, Turkey*

Correspondence should be addressed to Canan Kuzdan; drcanankuzdan@gmail.com

Academic Editor: Giovanni Montini

Rahnella aquatilis is an infrequently isolated Gram-negative rod within the Enterobacteriaceae family. The organism's natural habitat is water. The organism is rarely isolated from clinical specimens and it seldom causes infection in immunocompetent individuals. Here we present a one-month-old boy who was born prematurely at 27th week of gestation by cesarean section with a birth weight of 730 g. He developed sepsis caused by *Rahnella aquatilis* during the treatment for ventilator associated pneumonia due to *Stenotrophomonas maltophilia* with ciprofloxacin. He was successfully treated with a combination of amikacin plus meropenem. Although *R. aquatilis* is one of the *saprophyticus* organisms, it may cause life-threatening infection in newborn.

1. Introduction

Rahnella aquatilis is an infrequently isolated Gram-negative rod within the Enterobacteriaceae family. The organism's natural habitat is water [1]. The organism is rarely isolated from clinical specimens and it seldom causes infection in immunocompetent individuals. The infections ascribed to this organism are bacteremia, sepsis, respiratory infection, urinary tract infection, wound infections in immunocompromised patients, and infective endocarditis in patients with congenital heart disease. Here we present a one-month-old boy who was born prematurely at 27th week of gestation by cesarean section with a birth weight of 730 g. He developed sepsis caused by *R. aquatilis* despite ciprofloxacin according to ventilator associated pneumonia caused by *Stenotrophomonas maltophilia*. The mother who underwent bone marrow transplantation 3 years before pregnancy for essential thrombocytosis had reportedly preeclampsia during the last trimester.

2. Case

He was born prematurely at 27th week of gestation by cesarean section with a birth weight of 730 g, APGAR score 8 at 1 minute and 7 at 5 minutes. He was supported by mechanical ventilator for respiratory distress syndrome and was given parenteral nutrition by an umbilical venous catheter. Because of CRP of 10 mg/L and platelets count of 170,000/μL, ampicillin and gentamicin were initiated for suspected septicemia on the first day of his life. There were not any positive cultures (Table 1). On the second postnatal day, after the increase in both oxygen demand and pressure requirement as well as laboratory findings including leukocytes count of 30,000/μL, platelets count of 80,000/μL, and CRP of 42.4 mg/L, the antibiotic regimen was replaced by vancomycin and cefepime (Table 1). Meanwhile on echocardiography, patent ductus arteriosus was determined; then ibuprofen was added. However ibuprofen was discontinued because of side effects such as increased creatinine and thrombocytopenia.

On the 4th postnatal day, fluconazole prophylaxis was given to prevent invasive fungal infection. On the 8th postnatal day, he was extubated but he needed reintubation on the same day. Despite therapy, we observed deep thrombocytopenia (5,000/μL), leukocytes count of 1,000/μL, CRP of 120 mg/L, and clinical deterioration including abdominal distension and hypotension and, thus, cefepime was replaced by meropenem and liposomal amphotericin B as

TABLE 1: All the patient's significant laboratory/microbiological findings and the corresponding therapeutical changes.

Postnatal day	Clinical picture	Leukocytes count (/μL)	Platelets count (/μL)	CRP (mg/L)	Culture	Treatment
1st day	Suspected septicemia	40,000	170,000	10	Negative	Ampicillin and gentamicin
2nd day	Increasing in both oxygen demand and pressure requirement	30,000	80,000	42.4	Negative	Vancomycin and cefepime
8th day	Need for reintubation, abdominal distension, and hypotension	1,000	5,000	120	Negative	Meropenem and liposomal amphotericin B as well as intravenous immunoglobulin as adjuvant therapy
14th day	Pneumonia and atelectasis?	23,000	150,000	36	Negative	Linezolid was added
21st day	Pneumonia, oxygen desaturation, increasing ventilation demand, and suctioning requirement	28,000	110,000	89	S. maltophilia was isolated from endotracheal aspirate culture	Ciprofloxacin was added to liposomal amphotericin B
25th day	Pneumonia, oxygen desaturation, increasing ventilation demand, and suctioning requirement	21,000	33,000	110		Vancomycin and ceftazidime were added to ciprofloxacin; liposomal amphotericin B was discontinued
26th day					The blood cultures taken on 22nd and 23rd day were resulted in on 26th day. R. aquatilis was isolated from blood cultures	Meropenem and amikacin for 21 days

well as intravenous immunoglobulin. An adjuvant therapy was added to antimicrobial regimen (Table 1). At the same time no pathologic finding was found. Any additional finding with respect to necrotizing enterocolitis was not also found. Then, his clinical picture improved.

However, on the 14th postnatal day, his clinical picture deteriorated again. The umbilical venous catheter was removed. Because he developed suspected pneumonia, the antimicrobial treatment was replaced by linezolid, meropenem, and liposomal amphotericin B. Moreover findings were considered as atelectasis, so the appropriate therapy was given (Table 1). On the 19th postnatal day his clinical picture was noted to improve; therefore he was extubated and any microorganism was not isolated from all cultures, so linezolid was stopped. Meropenem and liposomal amphotericin B were continued.

On the 21st postnatal day apnea and bradycardia occurred. He was supported by mechanical ventilator. Ciprofloxacin was added to liposomal amphotericin B, because Stenotrophomonas maltophilia was isolated from endotracheal aspirate culture at the time of clinical deterioration. On the 25th postnatal day, since leukocytes count was 21000/μL, it was determined that platelets count was

33,000/μL and CRP 110 mg/L. Vancomycin was added to antimicrobial regimen, including ciprofloxacin. Liposomal amphotericin B was discontinued. Ceftazidime was added to antimicrobial treatment according to antibiogram susceptibility, because Stenotrophomonas maltophilia was isolated in endotracheal aspirate culture again. At the same time echocardiography did not show any pathologic findings suggesting endocarditis and patent ductus arteriosus was closed. Meanwhile Rahnella aquatilis resistant to piperacillin and cephalosporins, and susceptible to carbapenems and aminoglycosides, was isolated from both blood cultures taken on 2nd day and 3rd day of ciprofloxacin; the antimicrobial regimen was changed to meropenem and amikacin (Table 1). The patient was successfully treated with a combination of amikacin plus meropenem for 21 days. His clinical picture and laboratory findings returned normal. Upon starting full enteral feeding, he was discharged from the hospital.

3. Discussion

Rahnella aquatilis is environmental bacteria commonly isolated from water [1]. To our knowledge, there are 18 reports in the literature about human infection caused by *R. aquatilis*. The majority of these suggested that the infection had been accompanied by diabetes mellitus, alcoholism, cancer, AIDS, and immunosuppression secondary to medications, suggesting that the microorganism may have been an opportunistic pathogen. However, 5 reported cases were in nonimmunocompromised patients [1–5]. The organisms were isolated from blood [1–4, 6–12], wounds [5, 8], urine [8, 13–15], the respiratory tract [8, 16], and stool cultures [8]. In our patient, considering the patient's clinical deterioration, *R. aquatilis* was accepted as active agent because it reproduced in the separate blood cultures. The origin of the *R. aquatilis* strain isolated from our patient is unclear. There were no other reported *R. aquatilis* infections in the hospital during his time there. We did not think of an outbreak due to *R. aquatilis,* so newborn intensive care unit water was not tested for *R. aquatilis*. Our patient was successfully treated with a combination of amikacin plus meropenem. Although *R. aquatilis* is one of the saprophyticus organisms, it may cause life-threatening infection in newborn, especially early preterm and very low birthweight babies.

Conflict of Interests

The authors declare no conflict of interests.

References

[1] N. Caroff, C. Chamoux, F. le Gallou et al., "Two epidemiologically related cases of *Rahnella aquatilis* bacteremia," *European Journal of Clinical Microbiology and Infectious Diseases*, vol. 17, no. 5, pp. 349–352, 1998.

[2] C. L. Chang, J. Jeong, J. H. Shin, E. Y. Lee, and H. C. Son, "Rahnella aquatilis sepsis in an immunocompetent adult," *Journal of Clinical Microbiology*, vol. 37, no. 12, pp. 4161–4162, 1999.

[3] H. Sakata and S. Maruyama, "Study on bacteremia due to community-acquired infection in infants and children without underlying diseases," *Kansenshogaku Zasshi*, vol. 72, no. 11, pp. 1197–1201, 1998.

[4] H. Matsukura, K. Katayania, N. Kitano et al., "Infective endocarditis caused by an unusual gram-negative rod, *Rahnella aquatilis*," *Pediatric Cardiology*, vol. 17, no. 2, pp. 108–111, 1996.

[5] S. Maraki, G. Samonis, E. Marnelakis, and Y. Tselentis, "Surgical wound infection caused by *Rahnella aquatilis*," *Journal of Clinical Microbiology*, vol. 32, no. 11, pp. 2706–2708, 1994.

[6] M. C. Liberto, G. Matera, R. Puccio, T. Lo Russo, E. Colosimo, and E. Focà, "Six cases of sepsis caused by *Pantoea agglomerans* in a teaching hospital," *New Microbiologica*, vol. 32, no. 1, pp. 119–123, 2009.

[7] J. E. Carinder, J. D. Chua, R. B. Corales, A. J. Taege, and G. W. Procop, "Rahnella aquatilis bacteremia in a patient with relapsed acute lymphoblastic leukemia," *Scandinavian Journal of Infectious Diseases*, vol. 33, no. 6, pp. 471–473, 2001.

[8] J. Reina and A. Lopez, "Clinical and microbiological characteristics of *Rahnella aquatilis* strains isolated from children," *Journal of Infection*, vol. 33, no. 2, pp. 135–137, 1996.

[9] G. Funke and H. Rosner, "Rahnella aquatilis bacteremia in an HIV-infected intravenous drug abuser," *Diagnostic Microbiology and Infectious Disease*, vol. 22, no. 3, pp. 293–296, 1995.

[10] H. M. L. Oh and L. Tay, "Bacteraemia caused by *Rahnella aquatilis*: report of two cases and review," *Scandinavian Journal of Infectious Diseases*, vol. 27, no. 1, pp. 79–80, 1995.

[11] J. E. Hoppe, M. Herter, S. Aleksic, T. Klingebiel, and D. Niethammer, "Catheter-related *Rahnella aquatilis* bacteremia in a pediatric bone marrow transplant recipient," *Journal of Clinical Microbiology*, vol. 31, no. 7, pp. 1911–1912, 1993.

[12] P. Goubau, F. van Aelst, J. Verhaegen, and M. Boogaerts, "Septicaemia caused by *Rahnella aquatilis* in an immunocompromised patient," *European Journal of Clinical Microbiology & Infectious Diseases*, vol. 7, no. 5, pp. 697–699, 1988.

[13] E. Domann, G. Hong, C. Imirzalioglu et al., "Culture-independent identification of pathogenic bacteria and polymicrobial infections in the genitourinary tract of renal transplant recipients," *Journal of Clinical Microbiology*, vol. 41, no. 12, pp. 5500–5510, 2003.

[14] P. C. Y. Woo, E. Y. L. Cheung, K.-W. Leung, and K.-Y. Yuen, "Identification by 16S ribosomal RNA gene sequencing of an Enterobacteriaceae species with ambiguous biochemical profile from a renal transplant recipient," *Diagnostic Microbiology & Infectious Disease*, vol. 39, no. 2, pp. 85–93, 2001.

[15] S. R. Alballaa, S. M. H. Qadri, O. Al-Furayh, and K. Al-Qatary, "Urinary tract infection due to *Rahnella aquatilis* in a renal transplant patient," *Journal of Clinical Microbiology*, vol. 30, no. 11, pp. 2948–2950, 1992.

[16] M. Fajardo and M. J. Bueno, "Isolation of *Rahnella aquatilis* in the tracheostomy exudate from a patient with laryngeal cancer," *Enfermedades Infecciosas y Microbiología Clínica*, vol. 18, no. 5, p. 251, 2000 (Spanish).

63

Netherton Syndrome in a Neonate with Possible Growth Hormone Deficiency and Transient Hyperaldosteronism

Chatziioannidis Ilias,[1] **Babatseva Evgenia,**[1] **Patsatsi Aikaterini,**[2] **Galli-Tsinopoulou Asimina,**[3] **Sarri Constantina,**[4] **Lithoxopoulou Maria,**[1] **Mitsiakos George,**[1] **Karagianni Paraskevi,**[1] **Tsakalidis Christos,**[1] **Mamuris Zissis,**[4] **and Nikolaidis Nikolaos**[1]

[1] *2nd Neonatal Intensive Care Unit, G.P.N. Papageorgiou Hospital, Aristotle University Faculty of Medicine,*
 Agias Triados 3B Street, Pefka, 57010 Thessaloniki, Greece
[2] *2nd Dermatology Department, G.P.N. Papageorgiou Hospital, Aristotle University Faculty of Medicine, Thessaloniki, Greece*
[3] *4th Department of Pediatrics, G.P.N. Papageorgiou Hospital, Aristotle University Faculty of Medicine, Thessaloniki, Greece*
[4] *Laboratory of Genetics, Evolutionary & Comparative Biology, Biochemistry & Biotechnology Department,*
 University of Thessaly, Larissa, Greece

Correspondence should be addressed to Chatziioannidis Ilias; drilias@windowslive.com

Academic Editor: Pietro Strisciuglio

Netherton syndrome, a rare autosomal recessive genetic disorder, is classified as an ichthyosiform syndrome. In this report we present the case of a neonate with erythroderma shortly after birth, accompanied by severe hypernatremia, recurrent infections, transient hyperaldosteronism, and signs of growth hormone (GH) deficiency. DNA molecular analysis in the *SPINK5* gene revealed heterozygosity in our index patient for 238insG and 2468delA frameshift mutations in exons 4 and 26, respectively, in the maternal allele and 1431-12G>A splice-site mutation in intron 15 in the paternal allele as well as the missense variation E420K in homozygous state. Combination of the identified mutations along with transient hyperaldosteronism and possible GH deficiency have not been described before. Accordingly, the importance of early multidisciplinary approach is highlighted, in order to reach accurate diagnosis, initiate prompt treatment, and ensure survival with fewer disease complications.

1. Introduction

Netherton syndrome (NS) is a rare autosomal recessive genetic disorder, affecting mainly males. Clinical manifestations of NS are ichthyosiform dermatosis with variable erythroderma, hair shaft abnormalities (trichorrhexis invaginata), and atopic features. Generalized exfoliative erythroderma (with erythema and scaling) is usually the first clinical sign, noted in our case from birth [1, 2]. Additionally, hair shaft disorder is particularly difficult to diagnose in affected neonates. NS diagnosis, often challenging, is based mainly on clinical criteria, skin biopsy with evaluation of LEKTI expression, identification of "bamboo hair," and DNA molecular analysis [3]. We present a case of NS in a neonate with unique genetic defects and concurrent comorbidities.

2. Case Report

Preterm male, appropriate for 35 weeks' gestation, of a primigravida 34-year-old mother was admitted to our hospital at 4 hours of age for respiratory distress and erythroderma. He was born vaginally, after an uneventful pregnancy, from phenotypically healthy, nonconsanguineous parents with no perinatal complications.

Examination at admission revealed a generalized exfoliative erythroderma over the face, trunk, and limbs and excessive scalp scaling (Figures 1(a) and 1(b)). No blisters or pustules were observed. Eyelids and glans penis were swollen while mucous membranes were not involved. Nikolsky and Darier's signs were negative.

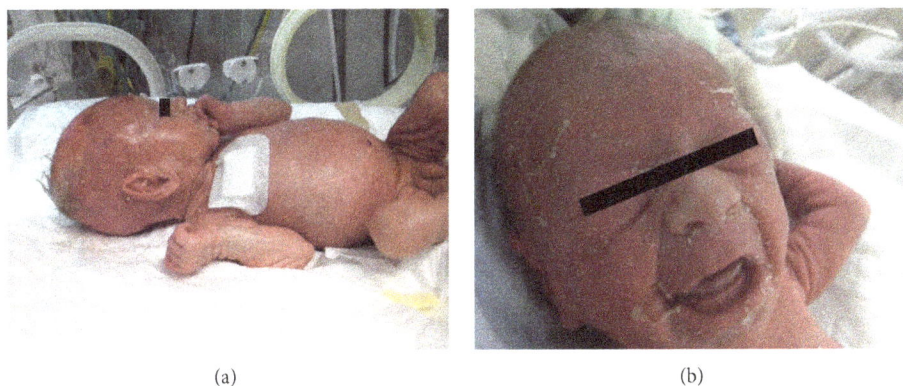

(a)   (b)

FIGURE 1: (a, b) Generalized exfoliation over the face, trunk, and limbs with excessive scalp scaling.

From his 2nd day of life (dol) the neonate presented severe hypernatremia (highest level of sodium at 180 mmol/L (3rd dol) (reference values: 128–150) and weight loss (max at 17% at 4th dol)) due to increased transepidermal water loss. Hypernatremia diagnostic work-up, combined with low potassium levels, normal renin activity value, and mild metabolic alkalosis, was compatible with hyperaldosteronism (aldosterone 392 ng/dL (reference values: 19–141) and renin 4920 ng/dL/hr (reference values: 1100–16700)). During hospitalization recurrent episodes of sepsis occurred due to *Klebsiella pneumoniae, Candida parapsilosis, Staphylococcus haemolyticus* at 9th, 12th, and 27th dol, respectively.

Immunologic studies showed normal IgE 8.6 IU/mL (reference values: <29), immunoglobulin levels, and complement component, excluding immunodeficiencies. TORCH screen and an extensive screening test failed to detect any inherited metabolic diseases.

DNA molecular analysis in the *SPINK5* gene revealed heterozygosity in our index patient for 238insG and 2468delA frameshift mutations in exons 4 and 26, respectively, in the maternal allele and 1431-12G>A splice-site mutation in intron 15 in the paternal allele, as well as the missense variation E420K in homozygous state (Figure 2(a)).

Skin biopsy showed mild acanthosis and hyperkeratosis with loss of the granular layer, findings compatible with nonbullous ichthyosiform erythroderma (Figure 2(b)). Light microscopy of hair pulled from scalp and eyebrows was typical of trichorrhexis invaginata (bamboo hair), with invaginations of the fully keratinized distal hair shaft into the softer, proximal hair shaft (Figure 2(c)).

Failure to thrive and mild developmental delay were also noted. Finally low levels of insulin-like growth factor (IGF-I) 15 ng/mL (reference values: 23–163) with normal IGFBP3 0.79 mg/L (reference values: 0.3–1.4) were indicative of possible growth hormone (GH) deficiency. Thyroid hormone levels, LH, FSH, and ACTH, as well as prolactin levels, were within normal range for his age indicative of intact pituitary gland function. Early morning cortisol levels and 17-OH-progesterone levels were also within normal range excluding classic congenital adrenal hyperplasia.

Emollient applications and topical antibiotics were administered for skin lesions. Transepidermal water loss was reduced by dry wrapping technique and electrolyte imbalance by hydration and finally immunoglobulin (0.4 g/kg/month) was used without significant improvement. Spironolactone was provided for hyperaldosteronism for 57 days, resulting in normal aldosterone levels and subsequent discontinuation.

The infant at 40th dol was discharged suffering from severe failure to thrive. At the age of 10 months erythematous lesions have substantially improved and episodes of sepsis have been reduced. However, severe growth failure, as well as mild developmental delay, still persists.

3. Discussion

Erythroderma of NS in a neonate is one of the most difficult clinical diagnoses. Differential diagnosis includes nonbullous autosomal recessive congenital ichthyoses, bullous ichthyoses, metabolic disorders, immunodeficiency syndromes, infectious diseases, psoriasis, and drug-induced erythroderma [3]. Mutations in serine protease inhibitor Kazal-type 5 (*SPINK5*) gene, located on the chromosome 5q32, coding lymphoepithelial Kazal-type-related inhibitor (LEKTI), lead to LEKTI deficiency and cause the disease [4]. LEKTI acting as a serine protease inhibitor is essential for epidermal cell growth and differentiation, hair morphogenesis, and epidermal permeability barrier. Consequently, unopposed proteolytic activities of epidermal serine proteases induce inflammation and/or loss of antimicrobial protection of mucous epithelium and epidermis [1].

The mutations 2468delA and 238insG alter the open reading frame and introduce a premature termination codon after 26 and 18 codons, respectively. The frameshift mutation 2468delA results in absence of LEKTI 5, as has been shown through immunostaining in the epidermis of a homozygous patient, probably due to nonsense mediated RNA decay [5]. On the other hand, the mutation 1431-12G>A is predicted to perturb splicing and has been shown, through western blot analysis and immunostaining technique, to abolish LEKTI expression [6].

These mutations have been described before in homozygosity as well as in heterozygosity in individuals originating from diverse population groups. For 238insG, especially, it had been previously described in three out of five Greek

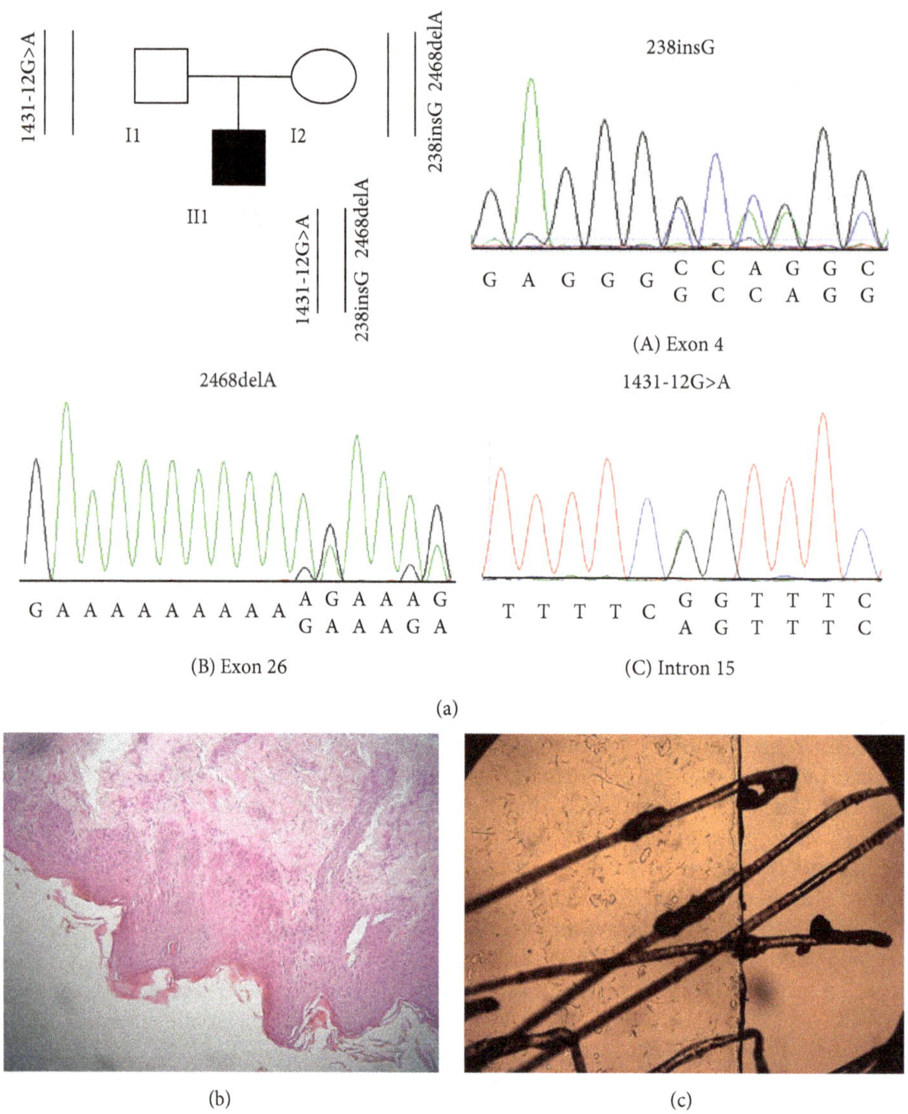

FIGURE 2: A pedigree showing inherited mutations. Filled symbol indicates the affected individual. Chromatograms of the point mutations identified in the affected individual are shown (a). HE, original magnification x200: skin biopsy showing hyperkeratosis, acanthosis, and absence of the granular layer (b). Light microscopy typical of trichorrhexis invaginata (bamboo hair) (c).

patients, making it a common mutation in Greece [7, 8]. Additionally in our case, the variation E420K, although known to be nonpathogenic for NS does alter LEKTI proteolytic activation, has been identified in homozygosity [9].

However, the combination of four different types of mutations (frameshift 2468delA and 238insG, splice-site 1431-12g>A, and missense E420K affecting both alleles) in our index patient is described for the first time in literature and is considered to be pathogenetic.

Absence or impaired function of LEKTI seems to predict clinical severity [4, 8]. Although LEKTI expression was not evaluated on our patient's skin specimen by immunohistochemistry, DNA molecular analysis could be considered indicative. Specifically, 2468delA and 238insG frameshift mutations, already known to cause depletion of LEKTI in homozygous state, in addition to 1431-12G>A splice-site and E420K missense, strongly suggest a significant loss of LEKTI

in our patient considering also clinical course. Finally, the undefined levels of LEKTI along with this first-time reported genotype cannot give firm conclusions for our patient's outcome.

Growth retardation, a common finding in NS patients, is possibly caused either by GH over-processing or circulating bioinactive forms in the pituitary gland due to lack of inhibition of human tissue kallikreins (KLKs) proteases by LEKTI deficiency [10]. In our patient low levels of IGF-I, a mediator of GH, in combination with extreme growth retardation at the age of 10 months were indicative of possible GH deficiency or presence of GH bioinactive forms.

4. Conclusions

In our patient, unique DNA molecular analysis accompanied with transient hyperaldosteronism and possible GH deficiency are described for the first time. Literature supports high mortality and morbidity in infancy with improvement usually occurring during the second year of life. Clinical diagnosis of NS is still challenging; comorbidities variations which can be fatal are described with new combinations of mutations. The present case highlights the importance of an early and accurate diagnosis based on a multidisciplinary approach for the initiation of prompt treatment, in order to ensure survival and avoid severe late complications.

Conflict of Interests

None of the authors have any conflict of interests to declare in relation to this work.

References

[1] J. D. Sun and K. G. Linden, "Netherton syndrome: a case report and review of the literature," *International Journal of Dermatology*, vol. 45, no. 6, pp. 693–697, 2006.

[2] S. Fraitag and C. Bodemer, "Neonatal erythroderma," *Current Opinion in Pediatrics*, vol. 22, no. 4, pp. 438–444, 2010.

[3] S. Chavanas, C. Bodemer, A. Rochat et al., "Mutations in SPINK5, encoding a serine protease inhibitor, cause Netherton syndrome," *Nature Genetics*, vol. 25, no. 2, pp. 141–142, 2000.

[4] N. Komatsu, K. Saijoh, A. Jayakumar et al., "Correlation between SPINK5 gene mutations and clinical manifestations in Netherton syndrome patients," *Journal of Investigative Dermatology*, vol. 128, no. 5, pp. 1148–1159, 2008.

[5] E. Bitoun, S. Chavanas, A. D. Irvine et al., "Netherton syndrome: disease expression and spectrum of SPINK5 mutations in 21 families," *Journal of Investigative Dermatology*, vol. 118, no. 2, pp. 352–361, 2002.

[6] Y. Capri, P. Vanlieferinghen, B. Boeuf, P. Dechelotte, A. Hovnanian, and B. Lecomte, "A lethal variant of Netherton syndrome in a large inbred family," *Archives de Pediatrie*, vol. 18, no. 3, pp. 294–298, 2011.

[7] M. Lacroix, L. Lacaze-Buzy, L. Furio et al., "Clinical expression and new SPINK5 splicing defects in netherton syndrome: unmasking a frequent founder synonymous mutation and unconventional intronic mutations," *Journal of Investigative Dermatology*, vol. 132, no. 3, pp. 575–582, 2012.

[8] E. Sprecher, S. Chavanas, J. J. DiGiovanna et al., "The spectrum of pathogenic mutations in SPINK5 in 19 families with Netherton syndrome: implications for mutation detection and first case of prenatal diagnosis," *Journal of Investigative Dermatology*, vol. 117, no. 2, pp. 179–187, 2001.

[9] P. Fortugno, L. Furio, M. Teson et al., "The 420k LEKTI variant alters LEKTI proteolytic activation and results in protease deregulation: implications for atopic dermatitis," *Human Molecular Genetics*, vol. 21, no. 19, Article ID dds243, pp. 4187–4200, 2012.

[10] B. K. Aydın, F. Baş, Z. Tamay et al., "Netherton syndrome associated with growth hormone deficiency," *Pediatric Dermatology*, vol. 31, no. 1, pp. 90–94, 2014.

64

Niemann-Pick Disease Type C Presenting as a Developmental Coordination Disorder with Bullying by Peers in a School-Age Child

Ryo Suzuki,[1] Atsushi Tanaka,[1] Toshiharu Matsui,[1] Tetsuki Gunji,[1] Jun Tohyama,[2] Aya Nairita,[3] Eiji Nanba,[4] and Kousaku Ohno[5]

[1]Department of Pediatrics, Nagaoka Chuo General Hospital, 2041 Kawasaki-cho, Nagaoka, Niigata 940-8653, Japan

[2]Department of Child Neurology, Nishi-Niigata Chuo National Hospital, 1-14-1 Masago, Nishi-ku, Niigata, Niigata 950-2085, Japan

[3]Division of Child Neurology, Institute of Neurological Sciences, Faculty of Medicine, Tottori University,
36-1 Nishimachi, Yonago, Tottori 683-8504, Japan

[4]Division of Functional Genomics, Research Center for Bioscience and Technology, Tottori University, 86 Nishimachi,
Yonago, Tottori 683-8503, Japan

[5]Sanin Rosai Hospital, 1-8-1 Kaike Shinden, Yonago, Tottori 683-8605, Japan

Correspondence should be addressed to Ryo Suzuki; rsuzuki-tym@umin.ac.jp

Academic Editor: Anibh Martin Das

Niemann-Pick disease type C (NPC) is a rare progressive neurodegenerative disorder, often with onset after normal early childhood development. Juvenile onset NPC patients slowly develop cerebellar symptoms and cognitive impairment and often experience difficulties at school. However, these problems may be overlooked due to the unpublicized nature of NPC, given that it is a rare metabolic disorder. In this report, we present an 11-year-old male NPC patient, who suffered from clumsiness and difficulties in attention and academic and social skills. His symptoms were initially considered to be due to developmental coordination disorder (DCD) coexisting with bullying by peers. DCD is a type of neurodevelopmental disorder defined according to DSM-IV and is characterized by clumsiness that interferes with academic achievement and social integration not due to other general medical conditions. However, a detailed investigation of the patient suggested that the problems could be attributed to the onset of NPC. Clinicians should keep neurodegenerative disorders as differential diagnosis of children with multiple school problems.

1. Introduction

Niemann-Pick disease type C (NPC) is a lysosomal lipid storage disorder with an accumulation of sphingomyelin in reticuloendothelial and parenchymal tissues [1]. The disease is inherited as an autosomal recessive trait and two separate disease gene loci have been identified [2, 3]: the *NPC1* gene on chromosome 18q11-q12 and the *NPC2* gene on chromosome 14q24.3. Clinical features of NPC include a wide spectrum of visceral and neurological signs and symptoms, with age at onset ranging from the perinatal period to late adulthood [1]. For many NPC patients, the onset of the disease is during the juvenile period after normal early development, and they commonly have problems in school, such as poor writing and impaired attention [1]. Here, we report the case of a Japanese male patient who was originally thought to have developmental coordination disorder (DCD), which is characterized by clumsiness that interferes with academic achievement and social integration not due to other general medical conditions [4], coexisting with bullying by peers. However, neurological examination showed typical features of a juvenile onset form of NPC. This case suggests that the early phases of neurodegenerative disorders with multiple school problems can be overlooked or misdiagnosed because of a low index of suspicion among clinicians. Clinicians should consider NPC as a possible cause of degenerative disorders when seeing children with progressive multiple school problems.

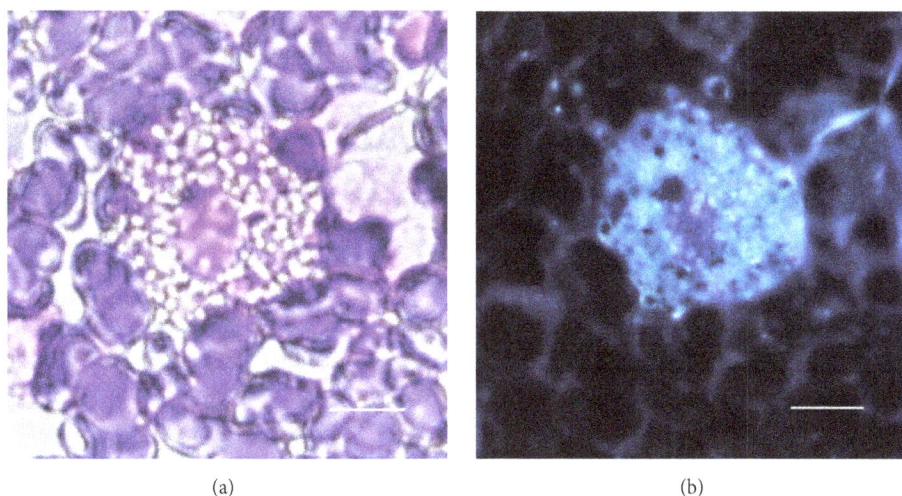

FIGURE 1: (a) High power view of the May-Giemsa-stained bone marrow aspirate. A large macrophage laden with sphingomyelin gives the cytoplasm a foamy appearance. (b) Positive filipin staining of a foam cell is observed on the same field as (a) (scale bar: 10 μm).

2. Case Report

A Japanese boy without a familial history of NPC or consanguineous marriages was born at a weight of 3040 g by vacuum extraction after 40-week gestation. He had been admitted to a newborn nursery for 3 weeks because of meconium aspiration syndrome and prolonged neonatal jaundice. Thereafter, he grew up with normal gross motor milestones: head control attained at 4 months, sitting without support at 7 months, crawling at 8 months, and walking independently at 15 months. After entering elementary school, he had no problem with his schoolwork and initially built successful relationships with his friends, but then he began to be bullied at school when he was around 9 years old. He suffered from pushing, hitting, verbal taunts, and social exclusion by peers. Afterwards, he began to show a depressed appearance and less positive social interaction with classmates and spent more time on his own than with peers. Furthermore, he started to gradually develop difficulties in sustaining close attention to details, declining grades, and clumsiness that interfered with handwriting and activities such as riding a bicycle and playing catch. At 10 years of age, he presented to our pediatric outpatient department complaining of the problems above; however, we misdiagnosed him at this time as having DCD with bullying by peers. Then, we suggested a "wait-and-see" approach after trying supportive care involving the family, school, and other individuals in the child's environment. One and a half years later, at the age of 11 years, he presented to us again because of his progressive clumsiness and notably deteriorated school performance with ongoing bullying episodes. Upon examination, no significant signs were found except for hepatomegaly. On neurological examination, he was alert and oriented, although his speech was slurred with impaired pronunciation. He showed mild facial dyskinesia, slight dysarthria and dysphasia, and exaggeration of deep tendon reflexes in both extremities. Finger-to-nose test was performed correctly, but his movements were slow and slightly awkward. Fine and gross motor clumsiness had

a negative impact on his skills in writing, running, and riding a bike. Although guided and voluntary eye movements were normal, he was unable to perform downward saccadic eye movements in an ophthalmic evaluation, which is a well-known initial sign of NPC [1]. His full-scale IQ was 63 on the Wechsler Intelligence Scale for Children-III. Routine laboratory tests showed normal results, including blood and cerebrospinal fluid, plasma amino acid analysis, and urine organic acid analysis. Cerebral magnetic resonance imaging showed no abnormality. Suspecting NPC from his progressive symptoms, we performed a bone marrow examination as a preliminary test [5]. Cytology of his bone marrow aspirate showed foam cells (Figure 1), supporting the diagnosis of NPC. Furthermore, cytochemical studies on cultured skin fibroblasts showed a significant accumulation of unesterified cholesterol in perinuclear vesicles by cytochemical staining with filipin (Figure 2). In addition, a molecular study of the NPC gene was carried out. Sequencing of all 25 exons of NPC1 and their boundaries was performed on genomic DNA from the patient. We found the compound heterozygous mutations p.P836fsX838 [c.2506 (or 2507) del C] at exon 16 and p.N1156S (c.3467 A>A/G) at exon 22; the former is a newly identified mutation. Following diagnosis, treatment with miglustat was started based on a previously published guideline [5], and we allowed for some additional time to evaluate the effect of the treatment on the patient.

3. Discussion

The patient in this report is a typical case of juvenile onset form of NPC; however, the patient was initially misdiagnosed. Coexistence of his clumsiness and the bullying episode confounded our diagnosis; thus, his symptoms were misinterpreted as those associated with DCD and mediated by bullying. This course to diagnosis will provide instructive information for general pediatricians.

Difficulties in attention, short-term memory, and academic and social skills are more likely to be seen in children

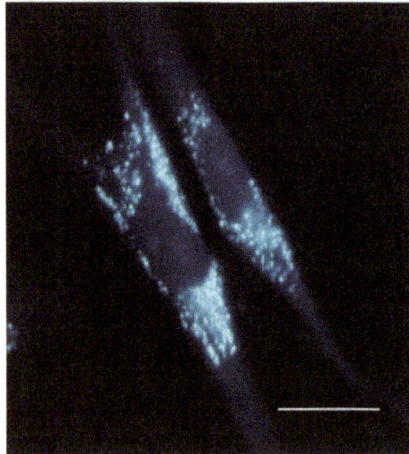

FIGURE 2: Filipin staining is positive in the patient's cultured skin fibroblast cells (scale bar: 20 μm).

with DCD [4, 6]. In addition, being bullied is a common experience and may be related to emotional changes, even for normally developing children [7]. It is important to know that these mimicking conditions may arise as initial signs from large heterogeneous diseases in school-age children, such as adrenoleukodystrophy, subacute sclerosing panencephalitis, and NPC [8]. Psychiatric illnesses and other psychiatric signs, including attention deficit disorder, an Asperger-like presentation, and depressive disorder, have been emphasized as common presentations in adolescence or early adulthood patients [1, 9], but not so far in school-age children with NPC. The majority of NPC patients show characteristic vertical supranuclear gaze palsy, which is often overlooked at the early stage because slow pursuit is often maintained even if saccadic eye movements are already impaired [1]. The NPC Suspicion Index tool is useful for screening NPC based on heterogeneous presentations and family history [10], and it helps physicians unfamiliar with NPC in early identification of patients with suspicion of NPC. The coexistence of bullying may have delayed diagnosis in this case; however, whether or not there is bullying, careful documentation of patient history, physical examinations, and close follow-up are necessary when evaluating patients with multiple school problems.

Bone marrow examination should be considered when NPC is suspected, as the detection of cholesterol accumulating cells in the bone marrow is reported to be helpful for diagnosis before biochemical and histological detection in cultured skin fibroblasts [11]. Cytology of the patient's bone marrow made us strongly suspect NPC as an underlying cause, and the diagnosis was finally confirmed by cytochemical analysis of fibroblasts and genetic analysis.

Genotype-phenotype correlations of NPC are limited because most affected individuals are compound heterozygotes; however, several studies have shown some degree of prediction. No individuals with the I1061T NPC1 mutation, which is a frequent mutant allele in individuals of Western European descent, presented with the severe infantile onset form [12]. Mutations affecting the putative sterol-sensing domain, which is located between amino acid residues 615

and 797, can lead to the absence of stable NPC1 protein and severe neurological phenotype [13]. However, another survey in Japanese subjects did not reveal any clear phenotype-genotype relationships, although the numbers of patients were limited [14]. The patient in this report was found to carry the compound heterozygous mutations p.P836fsX838 [c.2506 (or 2507) del C] at exon 16 and p.N1156S (c.3467 A>A/G) at exon 22 in the NPC1 gene. The former is a newly identified mutation that yields a stop codon downstream of the mutation and the latter missense mutation was previously reported as a pathogenic mutation [2]. Taken together, these mutations could be responsible for the NPC phenotype in this patient.

In the absence of any curative treatment, miglustat has been shown to delay the progression of the neurologic manifestations in a randomized clinical trial [15], and clinical practice settings. As an inhibitor of glycosphingolipids biosynthesis, it reduces lipid storage and cellular pathology in the brain, resulting in its therapeutic effects. It is currently considered as the only approved disease-specific therapy [5], and was approved for treatment of NPC in the EU in 2009 and Japan in 2012.

In summary, we have described a school-age child with juvenile onset form of NPC who developed difficulties in attention, short-term memory, and academic and social skills, and these problems were misinterpreted due to DCD and bullying. General pediatricians need to recognize that these multiple school problems could arise from neurodegenerative disorders and should consider NPC in differential diagnosis of children who present with progressive multiple school difficulties. We hope this report will lead to an improved approach for early diagnosis of children with onset of neurodegenerative disorders and allow better management of NPC patients and their families.

Consent

The patient's guardian gave informed consent for the publication of this case.

Conflict of Interests

The authors declare that there is no conflict of interests regarding the publication of this paper.

Acknowledgments

The authors would like to thank Dr. Takao Komatsubara, Dr. Chisato Hori, and Dr. Kazuo Takeuchi at Nagaoka Chuo General Hospital for their cooperation.

References

[1] M. T. Vanier, "Niemann-Pick disease type C," *Orphanet Journal of Rare Diseases*, vol. 5, article 16, 2010.

[2] E. D. Carstea, J. A. Morris, K. G. Coleman et al., "Niemann-Pick C1 disease gene: homology to mediators of cholesterol homeostasis," *Science*, vol. 277, no. 5323, pp. 228–231, 1997.

[3] S. Naureckiene, D. E. Sleat, H. Lacklan et al., "Identification of HE1 as the second gene of Niemann-Pick C disease," *Science*, vol. 290, no. 5500, pp. 2298–2301, 2000.

[4] R. Blank, B. Smits-Engelsman, H. Polatajko, and P. Wilson, "European Academy for Childhood Disability (EACD): recommendations on the definition, diagnosis and intervention of developmental coordination disorder (long version)," *Developmental Medicine and Child Neurology*, vol. 54, no. 1, pp. 54–93, 2012.

[5] M. C. Patterson, C. J. Hendriksz, M. Walterfang, F. Sedel, M. T. Vanier, and F. Wijburg, "Recommendations for the diagnosis and management of Niemann-Pick disease type C: an update," *Molecular Genetics and Metabolism*, vol. 106, no. 3, pp. 330–344, 2012.

[6] R. Lingam, J. Golding, M. J. Jongmans, L. P. Hunt, M. Ellis, and A. Emond, "The association between developmental coordination disorder and other developmental traits," *Pediatrics*, vol. 126, no. 5, pp. e1109–e1118, 2010.

[7] L. Bond, J. B. Carlin, L. Thomas, K. Rubin, and G. Patton, "Does bullying cause emotional problems? A prospective study of young teenagers," *British Medical Journal*, vol. 323, no. 7311, pp. 480–484, 2001.

[8] J. M. Kwon, "Neurodegenerative disorders of childhood," in *Nelson Textbook of Pediatrics*, R. M. Kliegman, B. F. Stanton, J. W. St Geme III, N. F. Schor, and R. E. Behrman, Eds., pp. 2069–2076, Elsevier Saunders, Philadelphia, Pa, USA, 19th edition, 2011.

[9] M. Sévin, G. Lesca, N. Baumann et al., "The adult form of Niemann-Pick disease type C," *Brain*, vol. 130, no. 1, pp. 120–133, 2007.

[10] F. A. Wijburg, F. Sedel, M. Pineda et al., "Development of a Suspicion Index to aid diagnosis of Niemann-Pick disease type C," *Neurology*, vol. 78, no. 20, pp. 1560–1567, 2012.

[11] J. Tohyama, M. Kato, T. Koeda, and K. Ohno, "Type C Niemann-Pick disease. Detection and quantification of cholesterol-accumulating cells in bone marrow," *Brain and Development*, vol. 15, no. 4, pp. 316–317, 1993.

[12] G. Millat, C. Marçais, M. A. Rafi et al., "Niemann-Pick C1 disease: the I1061T substitution is a frequent mutant allele in patients of Western European descent and correlates with a classic juvenile phenotype," *American Journal of Human Genetics*, vol. 65, no. 5, pp. 1321–1329, 1999.

[13] G. Millat, C. Marçais, C. Tomasetto et al., "Niemann-Pick C1 disease: correlations between NPC1 mutations, levels of NPC1 protein, and phenotypes emphasize the functional significance of the putative sterol-sensing domain and of the cysteine-rich luminal loop," *The American Journal of Human Genetics*, vol. 68, no. 6, pp. 1373–1385, 2001.

[14] T. Yamamoto, E. Nanba, H. Ninomiya et al., "NPC1 gene mutations in Japanese patients with Niemann-Pick disease type C," *Human Genetics*, vol. 105, no. 1-2, pp. 10–16, 1999.

[15] M. C. Patterson, D. Vecchio, H. Prady, L. Abel, and J. E. Wraith, "Miglustat for treatment of Niemann-Pick C disease: a randomised controlled study," *The Lancet Neurology*, vol. 6, no. 9, pp. 765–772, 2007.

65

A Case of Delayed Interval Delivery with a Successful Hospital Move

Toshifumi Yodoshi,[1] Elizabeth Tipton,[2] and Christopher A. Rouse[3]

[1]*Department of Pediatrics, United States Naval Hospital Okinawa, Camp Foster, Futenma, Ginowan, Okinawa, Japan*
[2]*Department of Obstetrics and Gynecology, United States Naval Hospital Okinawa, Camp Foster, Futenma, Ginowan, Okinawa, Japan*
[3]*Department of Neonatology, United States Naval Hospital Okinawa, Camp Foster, Futenma, Ginowan, Okinawa, Japan*

Correspondence should be addressed to Toshifumi Yodoshi; lucky.toshist@gmail.com

Academic Editor: Ursula Kiechl-Kohlendorfer

This report is the first case of delayed interval twin delivery in which the first infant and mother survived without major morbidity following transport to another facility. In addition, this case is only the second report of asynchronous delivery in which both twins survived and neither suffered any major morbidity. A 30-year-old G_5P_{1031} African American female with a diamniotic/dichorionic twin pregnancy presented to U.S. Naval Hospital Okinawa, Japan, at 22 + 5 weeks due to vaginal bleeding. At 23 + 2 weeks, Twin A was born secondary to advanced cervical dilation. Twin A's birth weight was 650 g with APGAR scores of 6 (1 min) and 7 (5 min). Following delivery of Twin A, Placenta A was left in utero with high ligation of the umbilical cord. Due to a scheduled hospital move, the mother and Twin A were transported to the new facility at Camp Foster. Three weeks later, Twin B was delivered at 26 + 4 weeks. Twin B's birth weight was 930 g with APGAR scores of 3 (1 min) and 7 (5 min). Both twins were discharged without IVH, PVL, ROP, or CLD. This case demonstrates the possibility of transporting both the mother and surviving infant A to a higher level of care prior to delivery of subsequent fetuses.

1. Background

The incidence of multiple-fetus pregnancies has dramatically increased over the past two decades due to assisted reproductive technology [1–3]. As a result, second-trimester preterm labor, PPROM, and fetal demise are more commonly encountered by perinatologists [1]. Despite advances in prenatal care, preterm delivery is associated with a high risk of neonatal mortality and morbidity [4]. Gestational age is the most important predictor of neonatal survival in extremely low birth weight babies [5]. In singleton, survival to discharge following delivery at 24, 25, and 26 weeks is 31.2%, 59.1%, and 75.3%, respectively [5]. In multiples, the mortality rate was 32% from 23 to 25 weeks' gestational age, compared to 19.2% from 26 to 27 weeks' gestational age and 11.1% in all gestational age [6]. At these extremely premature gestational ages, even small increases in gestational age have tremendous impact on neonatal survival [5]. Thus, a goal of pregnancy management is to prolong gestation and maximize fetal weight if a mother-fetus dyad is threatened with preterm delivery.

In a multiple-fetus pregnancy, the birth of the first fetus is usually followed by the delivery of the following fetuses. In some cases of multiple pregnancies, however, uterine contractions stop once the first fetus is delivered. The successful delay of the delivery of the second child can be life saving to the subsequent children. In particular, when a first twin is delivered prior to 24 weeks, delayed delivery of the second twin can be associated with reduced perinatal and infant mortality of the second twin [7].

U.S. Naval Hospital Okinawa, Japan, was scheduled to move 3 kilometers from its 55-year-old facility at Camp Lester, Okinawa, Japan, to a new state-of-the-art facility at Camp Foster, Okinawa, Japan, during the time of this case. In the literature, there is one reported case of delayed interval delivery involving transportation to another facility [8]. In this report, the first fetus was delivered at 17 weeks and was nonviable.

We report a case of a patient with a twin pregnancy with the survival of both twins following successful transportation of the mother and Twin A to another facility.

2. Case Presentation

Maternal history is as follows: 30-year-old G_5P_{1031} African American female with history significant for diamniotic/dichorionic twin pregnancy with concordant growth presented to U.S. Naval Hospital Okinawa, Japan, at 22 + 5 weeks with preterm labor and advanced cervical dilation. At 23 + 2 weeks, she experienced PPROM and vaginally delivered Twin A. Following delivery of Twin A, Placenta A was left *in utero* with high ligation of the umbilical cord. Ultrasound demonstrated a reconstituted cervix and a long cervical length. There was no evidence of chorioamnionitis. The mother was administered 7 days of antibiotics to include 3 days of clindamycin and gentamycin and 4 days of oral cephalexin and metronidazole. No tocolytic medications were administered and no cervical cerclage was placed. Due to the scheduled hospital move, she was transported by ground ambulance to the new facility and discharged home after 3 days. She was readmitted at 26 + 3 weeks in active labor. During triage, Twin B demonstrated tachycardia and deep variable decelerations. Twin B was delivered vaginally within one hour of admission with two coordinated pushes. On pathology, Placentas A and B were fused and Placenta B was noted to have a large clot covering 50% of its surface.

Twin A history is as follows: Twin A was delivered at 23 + 2 weeks and was given positive pressure ventilation and surfactant in the delivery room. Her birth weight was 650 g (86th%) with APGAR scores of 6 (1 min) and 7 (5 min). On day of life (DOL) 5, Twin A was transitioned from conventional ventilation to HFOV for worsening respiratory status. On DOL6, dopamine was started for hypotension. The patient was unable to be transported to the new hospital in conjunction with the scheduled NICU move (planned for DOL12) due to worsening clinical status. She stabilized and on DOL16 was transported to the new facility without complications. Her hospital course was significant for no IVH, PVL, ROP, or BPD. She was discharged at 38 + 4 weeks' corrected age with a discharge weight of 2612 g.

Twin B history is as follows: Twin B was delivered at 26 + 4 weeks and was given positive pressure ventilation and surfactant in the delivery room. Her birth weight was 930 g (67th%) with APGAR scores of 3 (1 min) and 7 (5 min). Her hospital course was significant for no IVH, PVL, ROP, or BPD. Twin B was discharged at 35 + 6 weeks' corrected age with a discharge weight of 2666 g.

Hospital move was as follows: The U.S. Naval Hospital Okinawa was scheduled to move 3 kilometers from Camp Lester to Camp Foster. Nine days prior to the scheduled move, Twin A was delivered. Immediately prior to the move, Twin A's condition became more critical. The hospital leadership recognized the high risk of an unstable ELBW transport and chose to keep the Camp Lester NICU open until Twin A was more stable. Concurrently, the new NICU at Camp Foster was opened to provide support to the Labor and Delivery service. For four days the NICU, pharmacy, radiology, laboratory, and respiratory therapy departments provided 24-hour staffing at each location.

3. Discussion

Delayed interval delivery was first reported in the mid-20th century as a means to prolong pregnancy for multifetal gestations after the spontaneous second-trimester delivery of the first fetus. In 1957, Abrams published the first reported case of delayed interval delivery in a patient with normally shaped uterus [9]. Since then, several case reports and case series have been published [10–13]. Although these have clearly demonstrated that delayed interval delivery can be successfully achieved, no standard protocol for management exists because of its very rare occurrence. The use of prolonged bed rest, cervical cerclage, tocolysis, antibiotics, and corticosteroids composes complex, frequently debated issues [14]. In all cases, the umbilical cord of the first-born twin is cut as high as possible inside the cervix [15]. It is remarkable that the remaining placenta and umbilical cord of the expelled fetus do not seem to initiate intrauterine infection [16]. A known risk factor for delayed interval delivery failure is a previous cerclage. Patients with a previous cerclage during pregnancy are less likely to achieve significant latency intervals [17].

Infection is often implicated with preterm labor and preterm birth [18]. All possibilities of infections must be ruled out before attempting delayed interval delivery. In particular, clinical chorioamnionitis must be absent as this can lead to uterine contractions and subsequent delivery. In these cases, broad-spectrum antibiotics are often used to protect against ascending infection [14]. There is controversy about the administration of prophylactic antibiotics. Some authors suggest that antibiotics are not useful in this situation because many low birth weight deliveries occur without placental or amniotic fluid infection [19, 20]. On the other hand, Arias observed that the main reason for failure of delayed interval delivery was intra-amniotic infection [21]. Moreover, as antibiotics often have tocolytic properties, the use of broad-spectrum antibiotics seems justified [21]. In this case, antibiotics were used to mitigate the increased risk of infection associated with PPROM. Because the mother's uterine contractions had quiesced and a long cervical length was noted after the delivery of the first fetus, a tocolytic was not administered and a cervical cerclage was not placed.

Most studies demonstrate that maternal morbidities associated with delayed interval delivery are rare. However, Roman found a 31.6% incidence of serious maternal morbidity related to the delayed interval delivery [22]. All cases were associated with evidence of infection as demonstrated by either clinical signs, positive cultures, or placental pathology. However, most women who had serious morbidity had a negative amniocentesis for subclinical chorioamniotesis prior to undergoing delayed interval delivery [22]. Thus, the risk of a serious, potentially life-threatening maternal complication is difficult to predict and patients must be informed of both fetal and maternal risk during informed consent. In this case, amniocentesis was not performed after the delivery of first fetus.

Delaying the delivery of the second infant has a positive effect on the short-term outcome of that infant [23]. Long-term outcome is comparable to children with the same gestational age [23]. Delayed interval delivery may be attempted when the first baby is born before 24th week of gestational age in order to prolong the second infant's delivery until the 28th to 32nd week. This case is only the second report of delayed interval delivery in which neither twin suffered any major neonatal morbidity (no ROP, IVH, PVL, or BPD). Furthermore, this is the only case reported in which the first infant and mother survived without major morbidity after being transported to another hospital [7].

Interfacility transport of sick and premature infants is a common method to ensure that infants are treated at centers with optimum support. Newborn outcomes are improved if women are transported antenatally, especially for those preterm infants born at less than 30 weeks' gestation [24]. In delayed interval delivery, if infant A is delivered at a location without access to tertiary care, it is possible to transfer the mother to a more appropriate center prior to delivery of subsequent fetuses. While the purpose of this case's transport was to move to a new hospital, it demonstrated the ability to move both infant A and the mother to a center with an increased level of care.

In conclusion, this case demonstrates the possibility of transporting both the mother and surviving infant A without any complications to a higher level of care prior to delivery of subsequent fetuses, using delayed interval delivery.

Conflict of Interests

The authors declare that there is no conflict of interests regarding the publication of this paper.

Acknowledgments

The authors would like to thank Drs. Eric Rabenstein, Antonio Hernandez, and Abel Guerra for assisting with this report.

References

[1] J. Zhang, C. D. Johnson, and M. Hoffman, "Cervical cerclage in delayed interval delivery in a multifetal pregnancy: a review of seven case series," *European Journal of Obstetrics Gynecology and Reproductive Biology*, vol. 108, no. 2, pp. 126–130, 2003.

[2] S. Petousis, A. Goutzioulis, C. Margioula-Siarkou, T. Katsamagkas, I. Kalogiannidis, and T. Agorastos, "Emergency cervical cerclage after miscarriage of the first fetus in dichorionic twin pregnancies: obstetric and neonatal outcomes of delayed delivery interval," *Archives of Gynecology and Obstetrics*, vol. 286, no. 3, pp. 613–617, 2012.

[3] S.-P. Kao, S. Hsu, and D.-C. Ding, "Delayed interval delivery in a triplet pregnancy," *Journal of the Chinese Medical Association*, vol. 69, no. 2, pp. 92–94, 2006.

[4] W. F. Powers and J. L. Kiely, "The risks confronting twins: a national perspective," *American Journal of Obstetrics and Gynecology*, vol. 170, no. 2, pp. 456–461, 1994.

[5] P.-Y. Ancel, F. Goffinet, P. Kuhn et al., "Survival and morbidity of preterm children born at 22 through 34 weeks' gestation in France in 2011: results of the EPIPAGE-2 cohort study," *JAMA Pediatrics*, vol. 169, no. 3, pp. 230–238, 2011.

[6] K. Thai, Q. Y. Lee, K. Lui et al., "Trends in morbidity and mortality of extremely preterm multiple gestation newborns," *Pediatrics*, vol. 136, no. 2, pp. 263–271, 2015.

[7] Y. Oyelese, C. V. Ananth, J. C. Smulian, and A. M. Vintzileos, "Delayed interval delivery in twin pregnancies in the United States: impact on perinatal mortality and morbidity," *The American Journal of Obstetrics and Gynecology*, vol. 192, no. 2, pp. 439–444, 2005.

[8] J. S. Platt and C. Rosa, "Delayed interval delivery military style," *Military Medicine*, vol. 166, no. 3, pp. 278–280, 2001.

[9] R. H. Abrams, "Double pregnancy; report of a case with thirty-five days between deliveries," *Obstetrics & Gynecology*, vol. 9, no. 4, pp. 435–438, 1957.

[10] J. Zhang, B. Hamilton, J. Martin, and A. Trumble, "Delayed interval delivery and infant survival: a population-based study," *The American Journal of Obstetrics and Gynecology*, vol. 191, no. 2, pp. 470–476, 2004.

[11] S. Fayad, A. Bongain, P. Holhfeld et al., "Delayed delivery of second twin: a multicentre study of 35 cases," *European Journal of Obstetrics Gynecology and Reproductive Biology*, vol. 109, no. 1, pp. 16–20, 2003.

[12] S. L. Hamersley, S. K. Coleman, N. K. Bergauer, L. M. Bartholomew, and T. L. Pinckert, "Delayed-interval delivery in twin pregnancies," *Journal of Reproductive Medicine for the Obstetrician and Gynecologist*, vol. 47, no. 2, pp. 125–130, 2002.

[13] B. Arabin and J. van Eyck, "Delayed-interval delivery in twin and triplet pregnancies: 17 years of experience in 1 perinatal center," *American Journal of Obstetrics and Gynecology*, vol. 200, no. 2, pp. 154.e1–154.e8, 2009.

[14] N. Klearhou, A. Mamopoulos, S. Pepes, A. Daniilidis, D. Rousso, and V. Karagiannis, "Delayed interval delivery in twin pregnancy: a case report," *Hippokratia*, vol. 11, no. 1, pp. 44–46, 2007.

[15] F. M. A. Van der Straeten, K. De Ketelaere, and M. Temmerman, "Delayed interval delivery in multiple pregnancies," *European Journal of Obstetrics Gynecology and Reproductive Biology*, vol. 99, no. 1, pp. 85–89, 2001.

[16] A. M. Van Heusden and R. S. G. M. Bots, "Delayed interval delivery in a triplet pregnancy; a case report," *European Journal of Obstetrics and Gynecology and Reproductive Biology*, vol. 38, no. 1, pp. 75–78, 1991.

[17] L. J. Farkouh, E. D. Sabin, K. D. Heyborne, L. G. Lindsay, and R. P. Porreco, "Delayed-interval delivery: extended series from a single maternal-fetal medicine practice," *American Journal of Obstetrics & Gynecology*, vol. 183, no. 6, pp. 1499–1503, 2000.

[18] R. Romero, R. Gómez, T. Chaiworapongsa, G. Conoscenti, J. C. Kim, and Y. M. Kim, "The role of infection in preterm labour and delivery," *Paediatric and Perinatal Epidemiology*, vol. 15, no. 2, pp. 41–56, 2001.

[19] J. Woolfson, T. Fay, and A. Bates, "Twins with 54 days between deliveries. Case report," *BJOG: An International Journal of Obstetrics & Gynaecology*, vol. 90, no. 7, pp. 685–686, 1983.

[20] R. S. Gibbs, R. Romero, S. L. Hillier, D. A. Eschenbach, and R. L. Sweet, "A review of premature birth and subclinical infection," *The American Journal of Obstetrics and Gynecology*, vol. 166, no. 5, pp. 1515–1528, 1992.

[21] F. Arias, "Delayed delivery of multifetal pregnancies with premature rupture of membranes in the second trimester," *American Journal of Obstetrics and Gynecology*, vol. 170, no. 5, pp. 1233–1237, 1994.

[22] A. S. Roman, S. Fishman, N. Fox, C. Klauser, D. Saltzman, and A. Rebarber, "Maternal and neonatal outcomes after delayed-interval delivery of multifetal pregnancies," *The American Journal of Perinatology*, vol. 28, no. 2, pp. 91–96, 2011.

[23] M. Rosbergen, H. P. Vogt, W. Baerts et al., "Long-term and short-term outcome after delayed-interval delivery in multifetal pregnancies," *European Journal of Obstetrics Gynecology and Reproductive Biology*, vol. 122, no. 1, pp. 66–72, 2005.

[24] S. K. Lee, D. D. McMillan, A. Ohlsson, J. Boulton, D. S. C. Lee, and S. Ting, "The benefit of preterm birth at tertiary care centers is related to gestational age," *The American Journal of Obstetrics and Gynecology*, vol. 188, no. 3, pp. 617–622, 2003.

Permissions

All chapters in this book were first published in CRIPE, by Hindawi Publishing Corporation; hereby published with permission under the Creative Commons Attribution License or equivalent. Every chapter published in this book has been scrutinized by our experts. Their significance has been extensively debated. The topics covered herein carry significant findings which will fuel the growth of the discipline. They may even be implemented as practical applications or may be referred to as a beginning point for another development.

The contributors of this book come from diverse backgrounds, making this book a truly international effort. This book will bring forth new frontiers with its revolutionizing research information and detailed analysis of the nascent developments around the world.

We would like to thank all the contributing authors for lending their expertise to make the book truly unique. They have played a crucial role in the development of this book. Without their invaluable contributions this book wouldn't have been possible. They have made vital efforts to compile up to date information on the varied aspects of this subject to make this book a valuable addition to the collection of many professionals and students.

This book was conceptualized with the vision of imparting up-to-date information and advanced data in this field. To ensure the same, a matchless editorial board was set up. Every individual on the board went through rigorous rounds of assessment to prove their worth. After which they invested a large part of their time researching and compiling the most relevant data for our readers.

The editorial board has been involved in producing this book since its inception. They have spent rigorous hours researching and exploring the diverse topics which have resulted in the successful publishing of this book. They have passed on their knowledge of decades through this book. To expedite this challenging task, the publisher supported the team at every step. A small team of assistant editors was also appointed to further simplify the editing procedure and attain best results for the readers.

Apart from the editorial board, the designing team has also invested a significant amount of their time in understanding the subject and creating the most relevant covers. They scrutinized every image to scout for the most suitable representation of the subject and create an appropriate cover for the book.

The publishing team has been an ardent support to the editorial, designing and production team. Their endless efforts to recruit the best for this project, has resulted in the accomplishment of this book. They are a veteran in the field of academics and their pool of knowledge is as vast as their experience in printing. Their expertise and guidance has proved useful at every step. Their uncompromising quality standards have made this book an exceptional effort. Their encouragement from time to time has been an inspiration for everyone.

The publisher and the editorial board hope that this book will prove to be a valuable piece of knowledge for researchers, students, practitioners and scholars across the globe.

List of Contributors

M. S. Yauba
Department of Paediatrics, University of Maiduguri College of Medical Sciences, Maiduguri 752106, Nigeria

H. Ahmed, I. A. Imoudu, M. O. Yusuf and H. U. Makarfi
Department of Paediatrics, Federal Medical Centre, Azare 751101, Nigeria

Zachary Bauman
Henry Ford Macomb Hospital, Clinton Township, MI 48038, USA

Victor Nanagas Jr.
Dayton Children's Hospital, Dayton, OH 45404, USA

Mehjabeen Zaidi, Sonia Qureshi and Fatima Mir
Department of Pediatrics and Child Health, Aga Khan University, Stadium Road, Karachi 74800, Pakistan

Sadia Shakoor
Microbiology, Department of Pathology, Aga Khan University, Stadium Road, Karachi 74800, Pakistan

Saira Fatima
Histopathology, Department of Pathology, Aga Khan University, Stadium Road, Karachi 74800, Pakistan

Pépé Mfutu Ekulu, Orly Kazadi-wa-Kazadi and Michel Ntetani Aloni
Division of Paediatric Haemato-Oncology and Nephrology, Department of Paediatrics, University Hospital of Kinshasa, Faculty of Medicine, University of Kinshasa, Kinshasa, Congo

Paul Kabuyi Lumbala
Division of Cardiology, Department of Paediatrics, University Hospital of Kinshasa, Faculty of Medicine, University of Kinshasa, Kinshasa, Congo

Nanda Ramchandar and Henry A.Wojtczak
Naval Medical Center San Diego, Department of Pediatrics, 34800 Bob Wilson Drive, San Diego, CA 92134, USA

Gema Mira-Perceval Juan, Pedro J. Alcalá Minagorre, Ana M. Huertas Sánchez and Sheila Segura Sánchez
Department of Pediatrics, University General Hospital of Alicante, C/Pintor Baeza 12, 03010 Alicante, Spain

Silvia López Iniesta
Department of Pediatric Hematology and Oncology, University General Hospital of Alicante, C/Pintor Baeza 12, 03010 Alicante, Spain

Francisco J. De León Marrero
Department of Dermatology, University General Hospital of Alicante, C/Pintor Baeza 12, 03010 Alicante, Spain

Estela Costa Navarro and María Niveiro de Jaime
Department of Pathological Anatomy, University General Hospital of Alicante, C/Pintor Baeza 12, 03010 Alicante, Spain

Azhar Farooqui
College of Medicine, Alfaisal University, Riyadh 11533, Saudi Arabia

Susan Gamal Eldin, Muna Dawood Ali, Ali Al Talhi and Ahmad Al Digheari
Department of Pediatrics, Security Forces Hospital, Riyadh 12625, Saudi Arabia

Miriam Michel, Edda Haberlandt, Matthias Baumann and Andreas Entenmann
Department of Pediatrics, Medical University of Innsbruck, Anichstrasse 35, 6020 Innsbruck, Austria

Michaela Wagner
Department of Neuroradiology, Medical University of Innsbruck, Anichstrasse 35, 6020 Innsbruck, Austria

Kevin Rostasy
Medical University of Witten/Herdecke, Department of Neuropediatrics, Dr.-Friedrich-Steiner Strasse 5, 45711 Datteln, Germany

Gonca Keskindemirci, Deniz TuLcu and Gönül Aydoğan
Department of Pediatric Hematology-Oncology, İstanbul Kanuni Sultan Süleyman Educational and Research Hospital, 34303 Istanbul, Turkey

Arzu Akçay
Department of Pediatric Hematology-Oncology, Faculty of Medicine, Acıbadem University, 34742 Istanbul, Turkey

Nuray Aktay Ayaz
Department of Pediatric Rheumatology, İstanbul Kanuni Sultan Süleyman Educational and Research Hospital, 34303 Istanbul, Turkey

Ali Er
Department of Radiology, İstanbul Kanuni Sultan Süleyman Educational and Research Hospital, 34303 Istanbul, Turkey

Ensar Yekeler
Department of Radiology, İstanbul Faculty of Medicine, İstanbul University, 34093 Istanbul, Turkey

Bilge Bilgiç
Department of Pathology, İstanbul Faculty of Medicine, İstanbul University, 34093 Istanbul, Turkey

Luciana Carnevalli Pereira, Ana Paula de Souza Netto, Fernanda Cordeiro da Silva and Cristiane Aparecida Moran
University Nove de Julho (UNINOVE), São Paulo, Brazil

Silvana Alves Pereira
Ana Bezerra University Hospital (HUAB/EBSERH) and Federal University of Rio Grande do Norte (UFRN/FACISA), RN, Brazil

Elie Alam, Marc Mourad and Usamah Hadi
Department of Otolaryngology Head and Neck Surgery, American University of Beirut, P.O. Box 11-0236, Riad El Solh, Beirut 1107-2020, Lebanon

Samir Akel
Division of General Surgery, American University of Beirut, P.O. Box 11-0236, Riad El Solh, Beirut 1107-2020, Lebanon

Sarra Benmiloud, Sana Chaouki, Samir Atmani and Moustapha Hida
Unit of Pediatric Hematology-Oncology, Department of Pediatrics, University Hospital Hassan II, Faculty of Medicine and Pharmacy, University Sidi Mohamed Ben Abdellah of Fez, Morocco

Gulsum Iclal Bayhan
Department of Pediatric Infectious Disease, Yuzuncu Yil University, 65000 Van, Turkey

Ozge Metin and Gonul Tanir
Department of Pediatric Infectious Disease, Dr. Sami Ulus Maternity and Children's Training and Research Hospital, 06080 Ankara, Turkey

Burak Ardicli and Ayse Karaman
Department of Pediatric Surgery, Dr. Sami Ulus Maternity and Children's Training and Research Hospital, 06080 Ankara, Turkey

Tomoo Kise, Hiroshi Yoshimura, Shigeru Fukuyama and Masatsugu Uehara
Division of Pediatric Nephrology, Okinawa Prefectural Nanbu Medical Center-Children's Medical Center, Arakawa 118-1, Haebaru, Okinawa 901-1193, Japan

Christopher Sawyer, Dimitrios Angelis and Robert Bennett
Division of Neonatology, Department of Pediatrics, Texas Tech University Health Sciences Center, Odessa, TX 79763, USA

Alexander K. C. Leung
The Alberta Children's Hospital, The University of Calgary, Calgary, AB, Canada T2M 0H5

Benjamin Barankin
Toronto Dermatology Centre, Toronto, ON, Canada M3H 5Y8

Susana Corujeira
Pediatric Department, Centro Hospitalar São João, Alameda Professor Hernâni Monteiro, 4200-319 Porto, Portugal

Catarina Ferraz, Teresa Nunes and Luísa Guedes Vaz
Pediatric Pulmonology Unit, Pediatric Department, Centro Hospitalar São João, Alameda Professor Hernâni Monteiro, 4200-319 Porto, Portugal

Elsa Fonseca
Pathology Department, Centro Hospitalar São João, Alameda Professor Hernâni Monteiro, 4200-319 Porto, Porto, Portugal

Heves Kırmızıbekmez and Rahime Gül Yesiltepe Mutlu
Pediatric Endocrinology, Zeynep Kamil Obstetrics and Pediatrics Education and Research Hospital, 34668 Istanbul, Turkey

Serdar Moralıoğlu and Ayşenur Cerrah Celayir
Pediatric Surgery, Zeynep Kamil Obstetrics and Pediatrics Education and Research Hospital, 34668 Istanbul, Turkey

Ahmet Tellioğlu
Department of Pediatrics, Zeynep Kamil Obstetrics and Pediatrics Education and Research Hospital, 34668 Istanbul, Turkey

Emel Altuncu, Hulya Bilgen and Eren Ozek
Division of Neonatology, Department of Pediatrics, Faculty of Medicine, Marmara University, 34890 Istanbul, Turkey

Ahmet Soysal
Division of Pediatric Infectious Disease, Department of Pediatrics, Faculty of Medicine, Marmara University, 34890 Istanbul, Turkey

Murat Gunay and Gokhan Celik
Zeynep Kamil Maternity and Children's Diseases Training and Research Hospital, Department of Ophthalmology, 34668 Istanbul, Turkey

Rahim Con
Sanliurfa Obstetrics and Gynecology Hospital, Department of Ophthalmology, 63050 Sanliurfa, Turkey

Sirin Mneimneh, Ali Tabaja and Mariam Rajab
Pediatric Department, Makassed General Hospital, Lebanon

Tiffany Tamse and Avind Rampersad
Florida Hospital for Children, Orlando, FL 32803, USA
University of Central Florida, Orlando, FL 32827, USA

Alejandro Jordan-Villegas
Florida Hospital for Children, Orlando, FL 32803, USA
Orlando Health, Orlando, FL 32806, USA

Jill Ireland
University of Central Florida, Orlando, FL 32827, USA

Hoi Y. Tong, Nicolás Medrano, Alberto M. Borobia and Elena Ramírez
Department of Clinical Pharmacology, Hospital Universitario La Paz, IdiPaz, School of Medicina, Universidad Autónoma de Madrid, Paseo de la Castellana 261, 28046 Madrid, Spain

Carmen Díaz and Paloma Jara
Pediatric Hepatology Department, Hospital Universitario La Paz, IdiPaz, Paseo de la Castellana 261, 28046 Madrid, Spain

Elena Collantes
Pathological Anatomy Department, Hospital Universitario La Paz, IdiPaz, Paseo de la Castellana 261, 28046 Madrid, Spain

A. Hochart, C. Thumerelle, C. Mordacq and A. Deschildre
Département de Pneumologie Pédiatrique, Hôpital Jeanne de Flandre, CHRU Lille, 59 037 Lille, France

L. Petyt
Département d'Imagerie Médicale, Hôpital Calmette, CHRU Lille, 59 037 Lille, France

Caroline Chua and Yahdira Rodriguez-Prado
Division of Neonatology, Department of Pediatrics, University of Central Florida College of Medicine, Nemours Children's Hospital, Orlando, FL 32827,USA

Shilpa Gurnurkar
Division of Endocrinology, Department of Pediatrics, University of Central Florida College of Medicine, Nemours Children's Hospital, Orlando, FL 32827,USA

Victoria Niklas
Division of Neonatology and Newborn Services, Olive View UCLA Medical Center, Los Angeles, CA 91342, USA

Michela Cappella, Vanna Graziani, Claudia Muratori and Federico Marchetti
Department of Paediatrics, Santa Maria delle Croci Hospital, 48121 Ravenna, Italy

Antonella Pragliola and Alberto Sensi
Department of Clinical Pathology, Medical Genetics Unit, Pievesestina, 47522 Cesena, Italy

Khalid Hussain
London Centre for Pediatric Endocrinology and Metabolism, Great Hormond Street Hospital for Children NHS Trust and the Institute of Child Health, London WC1N 3JH, UK

Rama Krishna Sanjeev
Department of Pediatrics, ACMS, India

Seema Kapoor
Division of Genetics, Lok Nayak & Maulana Azad Medical College, New Delhi, India

Manisha Goyal
Department of Paediatrics, Maulana Azad Medical College, New Delhi, India

Rajiv Kapur
Department of Radiology, ACMS, New Delhi, India

Joseph Gerard Gleeson
Neurogenetics Laboratory, Department of Neurosciences and Paediatrics, USA
Rady Children's Hospital, USA
Howard Hughes Medical Institute, CA, USA

Susan R. Mendley
Department of Pediatrics, University of Maryland School of Medicine, Baltimore, MD 21201, USA
Department of Medicine, University of Maryland School of Medicine, Baltimore, MD 21201, USA

Fotios Spyropoulos
Department of Pediatrics, University of Iowa Children's Hospital, Iowa City, IA 52242, USA

Debra R. Counts
Department of Pediatrics, Sinai Hospital, Baltimore, MD 21215, USA

Tiziana Timpanaro, Stefano Passanisi, Alessandra Sauna, Pierluigi Smilari and Filippo Greco
Unit of Clinical Pediatrics, Department of Medical and Pediatric Sciences, University of Catania, Via Santa Sofia, 95123 Catania, Italy

Claudia Trombatore, Monica Pennisi and Giuseppe Petrillo
Radiodiagnostic and Oncological Radiotherapy Unit, University Hospital "Policlinico-Vittorio Emanuele", Via Santa Sofia, 95123 Catania, Italy

Kambiz Masoumi, Arash Forouzan, Ali Khavanin and Mohammad Bahadoram
Department of Emergency Medicine, Imam Khomeini General Hospital, Ahvaz Jundishapur University of Medical Sciences, Ahvaz 6193673166, Iran

Hossein Saidi
Department of Emergency Medicine, Hazrate Rasoul Akram Hospital, Iran University of Medical Sciences, Tehran 14455364, Iran

Hazhir Javaherizadeh
Department of Pediatrics, Abouzar Children's Hospital, Ahvaz Jundishapur University of Medical Sciences, Ahvaz 6135715794, Iran

Vimal Master Sankar Raj and Roberto Gordillo
Department of Pediatric Nephrology, University of Illinois College of Medicine at Peoria (UICOMP), Peoria, IL 61603, USA

Jessica Garcia
Department of Pediatrics, University of Illinois College of Medicine at Peoria (UICOMP), Peoria, IL 61603, USA

Eran Lavi, David Shoseyov and Rebecca Brooks
Department of Pediatrics Mount Scopus, Hadassah-Hebrew University Medical Center, P.O. Box 24035, 91240 Jerusalem, Israel

Natalia Simanovsky
Department of Medical Imaging, Hadassah-Hebrew University Medical Center, Mount Scopus, P.O. Box 24035, 91240 Jerusalem, Israel

Kranti Kiran Reddy Ealla, Surekha Reddy Velidandla, Sangameshwar Manikya and Prasanna M. Danappanavar
Department of Oral and Maxillofacial Pathology, MNR Dental College and Hospital, Sangareddy, Telangana 502294, India

Vijayabaskar Reddy Basavanapalli
Department of Oral and Maxillofacial Surgery, MNR Dental College and Hospital, Sangareddy, Telangana 502294, India

Rajesh Ragulakollu
Department of Pedodontics and Preventive Dentistry, KLR'S Lenora Institute of Dental Sciences, Rajahmundry, Andhra Pradesh 533294, India

Vijayasree Vennila
Department of General Pathology, Kamineni Institute of Medical Sciences, Narketpally, Telangana 508254, India

Ryuta Yonezawa, Kengo Kawamura and Yasuji Inamo
Department of Pediatrics and Child Health, Nihon University School of Medicine, 30-1 Oyaguchi-kamimachi, Itabashi-ku, Tokyo 173-8610, Japan

Tsukasa Kuwana
Department of Emergency and Critical Care Medicine, Nihon University School of Medicine, 30-1 Oyaguchi-kamimachi, Itabashi-ku, Tokyo 173-8610, Japan

Rachelle Goldfisher, Pritish Bawa and John Amodio
Department of Radiology, SUNY Downstate Medical Center, 450 Clarkson Avenue, Brooklyn, NY 11203, USA

Zachary Ibrahim
Department of Pediatrics, SUNY Downstate Medical Center, 450 Clarkson Avenue, Brooklyn, NY 11203, USA

Erica Everest
Cleveland Clinic, 9500 Euclid Avenue, Cleveland, OH 44195, USA
Case Western Reserve University School of Medicine, 10900 Euclid Avenue, Cleveland, OH 44106, USA
Laurie A. Tsilianidis, Anzar Haider, Douglas G. Rogers, Nouhad Raissouni and Bahareh Schweiger
Cleveland Clinic, 9500 Euclid Avenue, Cleveland, OH 44195, USA

Ayuk Adaeze Chikaodinaka
Department of Pediatrics, University of Nigeria Teaching Hospital, PMB 01129, Enugu, Nigeria

Anikene Chukwuemeka Jude
University of Nigeria Teaching Hospital, PMB 01129, Enugu, Nigeria

Anna Tarocco
Pediatric Section, University Hospital S. Anna, Via Aldo Moro 8, 44124 Ferrara, Italy

Elisa Ballardini, Maria Raffaella Contiero, Giampaolo Garani and Silvia Fanaro
Neonatal Intensive Care Unit and Neonatology, University Hospital S. Anna, Ferrara, Italy

Mohammad Ali Kiani and Hamid Reza Kianifar
Pediatric Gastroenterology Ward, Department of Pediatrics, Mashhad University of Medical Sciences, Mashhad 9177948564, Iran

Arash Forouzan, Kambiz Masoumi and Behnaz Mazdaee
Department of Emergency Medicine, Imam Khomeini General Hospital, Ahvaz Jundishapur University of Medical Sciences, Ahvaz 6193673166, Iran

Mohammad Bahadoram
Medical Student Research Committee and Social Determinant of Health Research Center, Ahvaz Jundishapur University of Medical Sciences, Ahvaz 6193673166, Iran

Hassan Ravari
Vascular and Endovascular Surgery Research Center, Imam Reza Hospital, Faculty of Medicine, Mashhad University of Medical Sciences, Mashhad 9177948564, Iran

Joana Martins, P. Nunes, C. Silvestre, C. Abadesso, H. Loureiro and H. Almeida
Pediatric Intensive Care Unit, Professor Doutor Fernando Fonseca Hospital, Lisbon, Portugal

Kam Lun Hon and Albert M. C. Li
Department of Paediatrics, The Chinese University of Hong Kong, Prince of Wales Hospital, Shatin, Hong Kong

Alexander K. C. Leung
Department of Pediatrics, University of Calgary, Calgary, AB, Canada T2M 0H5

Daniel K. K. Ng
Department of Paediatrics, Kwong Wah Hospital, Kowloon, Hong Kong

Fatma Deniz Aygün, Serdar Nepesov, Haluk Çokuğraş and YJldJz CamcJoğlu
Department of Pediatric Infectious Diseases, Clinical Immunology and Allergy, Istanbul University, Cerrahpasa Medical Faculty, 34098 Istanbul, Turkey

Fatma Dursun and Heves KJrmJzJbekmez
Ümraniye Training and Research Hospital, Pediatric Endocrinology, 34766 Istanbul, Turkey

Feyma Meliha Su Dur
Ümraniye Training and Research Hospital, Radiology, Istanbul, Turkey

Ceyhan Fahin
Ümraniye Training and Research Hospital, Pediatric Surgery, Istanbul, Turkey

Murat Hakan Karabulut
Ümraniye Training and Research Hospital, Pathology, Istanbul, Turkey

AsJmYörük
Göztepe Training and Research Hospital, Pediatric Oncology, Istanbul, Turkey

Nancy Spurkeland
Penn State Hershey College of Medicine, Hershey, PA 17033,USA

Gregory Bennett and Chandran Alexander
Department of Pediatrics, Hershey Medical Center, Hershey, PA 17033, USA

Dennis Chang
Department of Pediatrics, Pediatric Cardiology, Hershey Medical Center, Hershey, PA 17033, USA

Gary Ceneviva
Department of Pediatrics, Pediatric Intensive Care, Hershey Medical Center, Hershey, PA 17033, USA

Elvira Ferrés-Amat
Service of Oral and Maxillofacial Surgery, Fundació Hospital de Nens de Barcelona, Consell de Cent 437, 08009 Barcelona, Spain
Department of Oral and Maxillofacial Surgery, Faculty of Dentistry, Universitat Internacional de Catalunya, Josep Trueta s/n, Sant Cugat del Vallès, 08195 Barcelona, Spain
Service of Pediatric Dentistry, Fundació Hospital de Nens de Barcelona, Consell de Cent 437, 08009 Barcelona, Spain

Jordi Prats-Armengol, Javier Mareque-Bueno and Eduard Ferrés-Padró
Service of Oral and Maxillofacial Surgery, Fundació Hospital de Nens de Barcelona, Consell de Cent 437, 08009 Barcelona, Spain
Department of Oral and Maxillofacial Surgery, Faculty of Dentistry, Universitat Internacional de Catalunya, Josep Trueta s/n, Sant Cugat del Vallès, 08195 Barcelona, Spain

Isabel Maura-Solivellas
Service of Pediatric Dentistry, Fundació Hospital de Nens de Barcelona, Consell de Cent 437, 08009 Barcelona, Spain

Eduard Ferrés-Amat
Service of Oral and Maxillofacial Surgery, Fundació Hospital de Nens de Barcelona, Consell de Cent 437, 08009 Barcelona, Spain

Chengming Fan, Can Huang, Jijia Liu and Jinfu Yang
Department of the Cardiothoracic Surgery, The Second Xiangya Hospital, Central South University, Middle Renmin Road 139, Changsha 410011, China

Ayşe Kartal
Department of Child Neurology, Inonu University Faculty of Medicine, Malatya, Turkey

Ayşegül Neşe ÇJtak Kurt, Tuğba Hirfanoğlu, Kürşad AydJn and Ayşe Serdaroğlu
Department of Child Neurology, Gazi University Faculty of Medicine, 06500 Ankara, Turkey

Khaled Khamassi, Habib Jaafoura, Fahmi Masmoudi, Rim Lahiani, Lobna Bougacha and Mamia Ben Salah
Department of Otorhinolaryngology-Head and Neck Surgery, Charles Nicolle Hospital, Boulevard 9 Avril, 1006 Tunis, Tunisia

Sakshi Bami and Valeriy Chorny
Department of Pediatrics, SUNY Downstate Medical Center, 450 Clarkson Avenue, Brooklyn, NY 11203, USA

Yarelis Vazquez, Rachelle Goldfisher and John Amodio
Department of Radiology, SUNY Downstate Medical Center, 450 Clarkson Avenue, Brooklyn, NY 11203, USA

KimMunk, Won Yong Kim and Niels Holmark Andersen
Department of Cardiology, Aarhus University Hospital, Palle Juul-Jensens Boulevard 99, 8200 Aarhus N, Denmark

Lise Gormsen
Department of Psychiatry, Aarhus University Hospital, Risskov Skovagervej 2, 8240 Risskov, Denmark

Christos Salakos
Department of Pediatric Surgery, ATTIKON University Hospital, 1 Rimini Street, Haidari, 12462 Athens, Greece
Department of Pediatric Surgery, "IASO" Maternity and Children's Hospital, 37-39 Kifisias Street, Marousi, 15123 Athens, Greece

Panayiota Kafritsa
Department of Gastroenterology, "IASO" Maternity and Children's Hospital, 37-39 Kifisias Street, Marousi, 15123 Athens, Greece

Yvelise de Verney
Department of Pediatric Surgery, "IASO" Maternity and Children's Hospital, 37-39 Kifisias Street, Marousi, 15123 Athens, Greece

Ariadni Sageorgi
Neonatal Intensive Care Unit, "IASO" Maternity and Children's Hospital, 37-39 Kifisias Street, Marousi, 15123 Athens, Greece

Nick Zavras
Department of Pediatric Surgery, ATTIKON University Hospital, 1 Rimini Street, Haidari, 12462 Athens, Greece

Erica Everest, Laurie A. Tsilianidis, Nouhad Raissouni, Tracy Ballock, Terra Blatnik, Anzar Haider, Douglas G. Rogers and B.Michelle Schweiger
Cleveland Clinic, 9500 Euclid Avenue, Cleveland, OH 44195, USA
Case Western Reserve University School of Medicine, 10900 Euclid Avenue, Cleveland, OH 44106, USA

Gamze Ozgurhan, Mustafa Ozcetin and Zeynep Karakaya
Department of Pediatrics, Suleymaniye Maternity and Children's Training and Research Hospital, Istanbul, Turkey

Aysel Vehapoglu
Department of Pediatrics, Bezmialem Vakif University Medical School, Istanbul, Turkey

Fatih Aygun
Department of Pediatric Intensive Care, Istanbul University Cerrahpasa Medical School, Istanbul, Turkey

Shaza Ali Mohammed Elhassan, Shabina Khan and Ahmed El-Makki
Hamad Medical Corporation, P.O. BOX 3050, Doha, Qatar

Ashif Jethava, Esperanza Olivares and Sherry Shariatmadar
Department of Pathology, University of Miami, Jackson Health System, Miami, FL, USA

Gianluigi Laccetta and Rita Consolini
Pediatric Department, Faculty of Medicine, Rheumatology and Clinical Immunology Unit, Pisa University, 56126 Pisa, Italy

Benedetta Toschi
Medical Genetics Unit, Children Department, Pisa University, 56126 Pisa, Italy

Antonella Fogli, Veronica Bertini and Angelo Valetto
Cytogenetics and Molecular Genetics Unit, Children Department, Pisa University, 56126 Pisa, Italy

N. Fargas-Berríos, L. García-Fragoso, I. García-García and M. Valcárcel
Neonatology Section, Department of Pediatrics, University Pediatrics Hospital, School of Medicine, Medical Sciences Campus, University of Puerto Rico, San Juan, PR 00936-5067, USA

Kıvılcım Karadeniz Cerit, Emel Colak and Tolga E. Dagli
Department of Pediatric Surgery, School of Medicine, Marmara University, 34899 Istanbul, Turkey

Rabia Ergelen
Department of Radiology, School of Medicine, Marmara University, 34899 Istanbul, Turkey

Leelawadee Sriboonnark
Division of Dermatology, Department of Pediatrics, Faculty of Medicine, Khon Kaen University, Khon Kaen 40002, Thailand

Harleen Arora, Leyre Falto-Aizpurua, Sonal Choudhary and Elizabeth Alvarez Connelly
Miller School of Medicine, Department of Pediatric Dermatology, University of Miami, 1600 NW 10th Avenue, Rosenstiel Medical Science Building, Room 2023, Miami, FL 33136, USA

Poonam Thakore, Salim Aljabari, Curtis Turner and Tetyana L. Vasylyeva
Department of Pediatrics, Texas Tech University Health Sciences Center School of Medicine, Amarillo, TX 79106, USA

Canan Kuzdan
Istanbul Mehmet Akif Ersoy Thoracic and Cardiovascular Surgery Training and Research Hospital, İstanbul, Turkey

Ahmet Soysal and Mustafa BakJr
Marmara University School of Medicine, Department of Pediatric Infectious Diseases, İstanbul, Turkey

Hülya Özdemir, Şenay Coşkun, İpek Akman, Hülya Bilgen and Eren Özek
Marmara University School of Medicine, Department of Neonatology, İstanbul, Turkey

Chatziioannidis Ilias, Babatseva Evgenia, Lithoxopoulou Maria, Mitsiakos George, Karagianni Paraskevi, Tsakalidis Christos and Nikolaidis Nikolaos
2nd Neonatal Intensive Care Unit, G.P.N. Papageorgiou Hospital, Aristotle University Faculty of Medicine, Agias Triados 3B Street, Pefka, 57010 Thessaloniki, Greece

Patsatsi Aikaterini
2nd Dermatology Department, G.P.N. Papageorgiou Hospital, Aristotle University Faculty of Medicine, Thessaloniki, Greece

Galli-Tsinopoulou Asimina
4th Department of Pediatrics, G.P.N. Papageorgiou Hospital, Aristotle University Faculty of Medicine, Thessaloniki, Greece

Sarri Constantina and Mamuris Zissis
Laboratory of Genetics, Evolutionary & Comparative Biology, Biochemistry & Biotechnology Department, University of Thessaly, Larissa, Greece

Ryo Suzuki, Atsushi Tanaka, Toshiharu Matsui and Tetsuki Gunji
Department of Pediatrics, Nagaoka Chuo General Hospital, 2041 Kawasaki-cho, Nagaoka, Niigata 940-8653, Japan

Jun Tohyama
Department of Child Neurology, Nishi-Niigata Chuo National Hospital, 1-14-1 Masago, Nishi-ku, Niigata, Niigata 950-2085, Japan

Aya Nairita
Division of Child Neurology, Institute of Neurological Sciences, Faculty of Medicine, Tottori University, 36-1 Nishimachi, Yonago, Tottori 683-8504, Japan

Eiji Nanba
Division of Functional Genomics, Research Center for Bioscience and Technology, Tottori University, 86 Nishimachi, Yonago, Tottori 683-8503, Japan

Kousaku Ohno
Sanin Rosai Hospital, 1-8-1 Kaike Shinden, Yonago, Tottori 683-8605, Japan

Toshifumi Yodoshi
Department of Pediatrics, United States Naval Hospital Okinawa, Camp Foster, Futenma, Ginowan, Okinawa, Japan

Elizabeth Tipton
Department of Obstetrics and Gynecology, United States Naval Hospital Okinawa, Camp Foster, Futenma, Ginowan, Okinawa, Japan

Christopher A. Rouse
Department of Neonatology, United States Naval Hospital Okinawa, Camp Foster, Futenma, Ginowan, Okinawa, Japan

www.ingramcontent.com/pod-product-compliance
Lightning Source LLC
Chambersburg PA
CBHW080504200326
41458CB00012B/4078

9781632424662